Women's Mental Health Across the Lifespan

Women's Mental Health Across the Lifespan examines women's mental health from a developmental perspective, looking at key stressors and strengths from adolescence to old age. Chapters focus in detail on specific stressors and challenges that can impact women's mental health, such as trauma, addictions, and mood and anxiety disorders. This book also examines racial and ethnic disparities in women's physical and mental health, mental health of sexual minorities and women with disabilities, and women in the military, and includes valuable suggestions for putting knowledge into practice.

Kathleen A. Kendall-Tackett, PhD, IBCLC, FAPA, is a health psychologist, board certified lactation consultant, and fellow of the American Psychological Association in both health and trauma psychology. Dr. Kendall-Tackett focuses on women's health with an emphasis on health effects of violence and abuse, trauma and PTSD, maternal depression, and breastfeeding. She is editor in chief of Praeclarus Press and of two peer-reviewed journals: *Psychological Trauma* and *Clinical Lactation*.

Lesia M. Ruglass, PhD, is a licensed clinical psychologist and assistant professor in the Department of Psychology at the City College of New York, where she also directs the OASAS-certified Credentialed Alcoholism and Substance Abuse Counselor (CASAC) program. Her research and clinical interests focus on integrated treatments for trauma, PTSD, and substance use disorders. Dr. Ruglass also maintains a private practice in New York City.

Clinical Topics in Psychology and Psychiatry
Bret A. Moore, PsyD, Series Editor

For a complete list of all books in this series, please visit the series page at: https://www.routledge.com/Clinical-Topics-in-Psychology-and-Psychiatry/book-series/TFSE00310

Women's Mental Health Across the Lifespan: Challenges, Vulnerabilities, and Strengths
edited by Kathleen A. Kendall-Tackett and Lesia M. Ruglass

Treating Disruptive Disorders: A Guide to Psychological, Pharmacological, and Combined Therapies
edited by George M. Kapalka

Cognitive Behavioral Therapy for Preventing Suicide Attempts: A Guide to Brief Treatments Across Clinical Settings
edited by Craig J. Bryan

Trial-Based Cognitive Therapy: A Handbook for Clinicians
by Irismar Reis de Oliveira

Integrating Psychotherapy and Psychopharmacology: A Handbook for Clinicians
edited by Irismar Reis de Oliveira, Thomas Schwartz, and Stephen M. Stahl

Anxiety Disorders: A Guide for Integrating Psychopharmacology and Psychotherapy
edited by Stephen M. Stahl and Bret A. Moore

Women's Mental Health Across the Lifespan

Challenges, Vulnerabilities, and Strengths

Edited by Kathleen A. Kendall-Tackett
and Lesia M. Ruglass

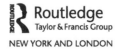

Routledge
Taylor & Francis Group

NEW YORK AND LONDON

First edition published 2017
by Routledge
605 Third Avenue, New York, NY 10017

and by Routledge
2 Park Square, Milton Park, Abingdon, Oxon, OX14 4RN

Routledge is an imprint of the Taylor & Francis Group, an informa business

Library of Congress Cataloging-in-Publication Data
Names: Kendall-Tackett, Kathleen A., editor. | Ruglass, Lesia M., editor.
Title: Women's mental health across the lifespan : challenges,
    vulnerabilities, and strengths / edited by Kathleen A. Kendall-Tackett
    and Lesia M. Ruglass.
Other titles: Clinical topics in psychology and psychiatry.
Description: First edition. | New York, NY : Routledge, 2017. | Series:
    Clinical topics in psychology and psychiatry | Includes bibliographical
    references and index.
Identifiers: LCCN 2016046395| ISBN 9781138182738 (hardcover : alk.
    paper) | ISBN 9781138182745 (pbk. : alk. paper) | ISBN 9781315641928
    (e-book)
Subjects: | MESH: Women's Health | Mental Health | Women—
    psychology | Mental Disorders
Classification: LCC RC451.4.W6 | NLM WA 309.1 | DDC
    362.196890082—dc23
LC record available at https://lccn.loc.gov/2016046395

ISBN: 978-1-138-18273-8(hbk)
ISBN: 978-1-138-18274-5(pbk)

Typeset in Minion Pro
by Swales & Willis Ltd, Exeter, Devon, UK

Contents

Series Editor's Foreword

Women's Mental Health Across the Lifespan: Challenges, Vulnerabilities, and Strengths is the sixth book in one of Routledge's most popular series, Clinical Topics in Psychology and Psychiatry (CTPP). The overarching goal of CTPP is to provide mental health practitioners with practical information that is both comprehensive and relatively easy to integrate into day-to-day clinical practice. It is multidisciplinary in that it covers topics relevant to the fields of psychology and psychiatry and appeals to the student, early career, and senior clinician. Books chosen for the series are authored or edited by national and international experts in their respective areas, and contributors are also highly respected clinicians. The current volume exemplifies the intent, scope, and aims of the CTPP series.

Editors Kathleen A. Kendall-Tackett and Lesia M. Ruglass make a convincing argument for why a comprehensive volume dedicated to women's mental health is needed. Until recently, the emotional well-being of women took a back seat to that of men. Women were often excluded from research protocols. Any conclusions about women's health was based on research results from men, which were often times not applicable. Fortunately, a shift has occurred. Women's issues are integrated more fully into psychological research and outcomes are shaping how we view and treat their psychological conditions. However, until now, there has not been a single authoritative source that adequately covers the psychological challenges women face. This includes information about prevalence rates, biopsychosocial risk factors, and evidence-based interventions.

The reader will find many of this volume's chapters of considerable benefit. Unlike most edited books, editors Kendall-Tackett and Ruglass put together 11 chapters that flow as seamlessly as any authored book. This is in part due to their experiences as writers and editors. It is also a result of the developmental approach they take in helping the reader understand the unique psychological issues women face. After covering the mental health of women from adolescence to older adulthood, the editors provide a deep dive into the various cultural and diversity issues that influence their well-being. They close out the volume with a section that details various clinical issues women deal with that includes mood, anxiety, trauma, and substance use disorders.

In summary, although there is information available on women's mental health, there are few that are as comprehensive, evidence-informed, and practical as the current volume. In addition to being highly respected researchers and writers, Drs. Kendall-Tackett and Ruglass are expert clinicians and educators. Straddling the important sides of practice and science, they have delivered a volume on an important topic that is unparalleled in depth and breadth. As a result of their expertise and high-quality work, this book will undoubtedly collect more users than dust.

Bret A. Moore, PsyD., ABPP
Series Editor
Clinical Topics in Psychology and Psychiatry

About the Editors

Kathleen A. Kendall-Tackett, PhD, IBCLC, FAPA, is a health psychologist and international board-certified lactation consultant, and the owner and editor in chief of Praeclarus Press, a small press specializing in women's health. Dr. Kendall-Tackett is editor in chief of two peer-reviewed journals: *Clinical Lactation* and *Psychological Trauma*. She is fellow of the American Psychological Association (APA) in Health and Trauma Psychology, past president of the APA Division of Trauma Psychology, and a member of the Board for the Advancement of Psychology in the Public Interest. She is clinical professor of nursing at the University of Hawai'i at Manoa and clinical associate professor of pediatrics at Texas Tech University School of Medicine. Dr. Kendall-Tackett specializes in women's-health research, including breastfeeding, depression, trauma, and health psychology, and has won many awards for her work, including the 2016 Outstanding Service to the Field of Trauma Psychology from APA Division 56. Dr. Kendall-Tackett has authored more than 400 articles or chapters, and is currently completing her 35th book, a social history of *The Phantom of the Opera*. Her most recent books include: *Depression in New Mothers*, 3rd edition (2017, Routledge), *Psychology of Trauma 101* (2015, Springer, with Lesia M. Ruglass) and *The Science of Mother–Infant Sleep* (2014, Praeclarus, with Wendy Middlemiss).

Lesia M. Ruglass, PhD, is a licensed clinical psychologist and assistant professor in the Department of Psychology at the City College of New York, where she also directs the Office of Alcoholism and Substance Abuse Services-certified Credentialed Alcoholism and Substance Abuse Counselor (CASAC) program. Dr. Ruglass's research interests include understanding the biopsychosocial mechanisms underlying substance use disorders, assessment and integrated treatment of posttraumatic stress disorder and substance use disorders, and reducing racial/ethnic disparities in mental health and substance use disorder outcomes. She has authored or coauthored 19 peer-reviewed journal articles, is coauthor of the book *Psychology of Trauma 101* (2015, Springer, with Kathleen Kendall-Tackett) and has presented her work at national and international conferences. Dr. Ruglass received her BA in Psychology from New York University, her MA in Psychology from Boston University, and her PhD in clinical psychology from the New School for Social Research in New York City. She is a member of the American Psychological Association and the New York State Psychological Association. Dr. Ruglass also maintains a private practice in New York City.

Preface

I was recently invited to participate in a working group on adverse childhood experiences and obesity by the Office of Women's Health. I was pleased to be involved. As someone who studies trauma, I often think that obesity recommendations fail to recognize the role of trauma in body mass index (BMI). Trauma sensitizes the body and makes it more likely that women (and men) hang on to every calorie, and subsequently have higher BMIs. The more severe the trauma, the greater the increase. This working group brought together both trauma and obesity specialists. The initial recommendation was that women with a BMI >30 should exercise at least five times a week, and should consume no more than 1,200 calories/day.

After a few moments, I raised my hand and suggested that, while I recognized that that was the standard regimen for addressing high BMI, it was not trauma-informed. For one thing, it did not address the role of trauma-related hyperarousal, and until that was addressed, the efforts were likely to fail. Then a physician from the Indian Health Service spoke up and indicated that limiting calories to 1,200/day was likely to be a significant trigger to anyone who had ever been hungry as a child. Another psychologist described her work with lesbian women with high BMIs. Many had significant trauma histories, yet most were part of the body-positive movement in California and refused to acknowledge society's arbitrary designation of >30 BMI as being a problem.

Clearly, the issue of BMI and trauma was much more complicated than the obesity specialists had imagined.

The issues highlighted in that meeting really framed some of the key reasons for why this book is necessary. When we think of women's health, we tend to think in a pretty linear and simplistic way. We don't consider culture or developmental stage. Yet these factors, along with women's mental health, dramatically affect women's physical health. Even something that obesity specialists, and the policy makers influenced by them, thought was straightforward has proven to be anything but.

Women's mental health is textured and varies as much as women themselves. Our goal in this volume is to provide you with an initial glance into the nuances of women's mental health. Only by understanding these can we achieve our ultimate goal: improving the physical and emotional well-being of women.

Kathleen A. Kendall-Tackett

Introduction

Kathleen A. Kendall-Tackett and
Lesia M. Ruglass

Over the past 20 years, we have seen an astonishing increase in knowledge and recognition of women's health as being separate from that of men. Prior to this shift, women were excluded from clinical trials for medications and treatments. The fact that women had monthly cycles, and could become pregnant, was said to "complicate" the findings. Women were treated with regimens developed for men, and researchers never determined whether these treatments were effective for women, let alone safe. To treat women, clinicians need to take into account how women's size and body composition (e.g., smaller stature, higher percentage and different location of body fat) affect treatment. In addition, monthly cycles, pregnancy, postpartum, lactation, and menopause need to be seen as integral to comprehensive care, not merely differences that muck up "perfectly good" research designs.

Part of the push to understand women's physical health came from the U.S. federal government, which insisted that women be included in clinical trials and treatment studies. Another push was consumer driven. Female patients, with conditions such as breast cancer, started to insist that treatments be tailored just for them. They flocked to providers who were female-friendly, and avoided those that were not. Hospitals recognized a potential revenue stream and began opening special women's health clinics.

Women's health has become a particular specialty in health care, even leading to the founding, in the United States, of the Office of Women's Health. All of these changes have been good, but there is still much more to do. Heart disease still kills more women than anything else, yet providers still ignore women's symptoms until it is too late. Many women have births that result in posttraumatic stress disorder (PTSD), and are left to fend for themselves in the postpartum period (in contrast to other cultures where women have support for weeks, or even months).

Even with all of the pieces still missing from a comprehensive approach for women's physical health, we know considerably more about it than we do women's mental health. For example, while there are many books available on women's physical health, there are few that focus on women's mental health. The volumes that are available tend to have a specific focus, such as women's reproductive health. Up until now, there have been no general volumes available that provide a comprehensive overview of women's mental health. The current volume seeks to fill that gap.

Women's mental health has a direct impact on their physical health. For example, depression is a major risk factor for heart disease. That is true for both men and women. If you want to lower heart disease rates, the number-one killer of women, you need to address depression (Kop & Gottdiener, 2005). Childhood abuse increases women's risk for type 2 diabetes by as much as 69%, yet that risk factor is often ignored in diabetes messaging and prevention efforts (Rich-Edwards et al., 2010). Preterm birth is the number-one cause of infant mortality worldwide. Depression and PTSD together during pregnancy increase risk of preterm birth by four times (Yonkers et al., 2014). Women's mental health is not a nice extra. It is critically important to women's physical health.

Women's Mental Health Across the Lifespan covers mental health from a lifespan developmental perspective: from adolescence to old age. Each chapter in Part I examines the challenges and vulnerabilities of each developmental phase, and the particular issues that are more common. The chapter on young adulthood focuses on issues related to childbearing, as that is an experience that the vast majority of women in this age group experience. As our population ages, the needs of women in midlife and old age are also becoming particularly salient.

One noticeable gap in current volumes on women's mental health is the assumption that all women, by virtue of their sex and gender, are the same. We have little written on ethnic-minority women, sexual minorities, or women with disabilities. The studies that do exist highlight specific health disparities in all three groups. And women who identify with more than one identity are at increased risk above and beyond that associated with a single identity. Those seeking to address the mental health of women in these populations often try to do so without first understanding the culture these women belong to. Cultural competence does not refer only to ethnicity. It also refers to these other groups. Part II includes chapters on issues related to race/ethnicity, sexual orientation and gender diversity, and disability. In addition, we have included a chapter on a group that is never described in women's health books: women in the military. As you will see, this population is also unique, and as such, presents unique challenges as well as strengths.

The final part, Part III, covers some common disorders that differentially affect women, including trauma, substance use disorders, depression, and other mood and anxiety disorders. Other texts discuss each of these topics, but rarely as they relate to women specifically. When they do, they rarely address the intersection of these disorders with women's multiple developmental stages and identities. In order to effectively treat these disorders, it's important to understand these differences.

We have truly enjoyed bringing together this talented group of authors. Each brings his or her own voice and most represent the communities they describe. We hope that you find this book to be interesting and helpful in your work.

References

Kop, W. J., & Gottdiener, J. S. (2005). The role of immune system parameters in the relationship between depression and coronary artery disease. *Psychosomatic Medicine, 67*, S37–S41.

Rich-Edwards, J. W., Spiegelman, D., Hibert, E. N. L., Jun, H.-J., Todd, T. J., Kawachi, I., & Wright, R. J. (2010). Abuse in childhood and adolescence as a predictor of type-2 diabetes in adult women. *American Journal of Preventive Medicine, 39*(6), 529–536.

Yonkers, K. A., Smith, M. V., Forray, A., Epperson, C. N., Costello, D., Lin, H., & Belanger, K. (2014). Pregnant women with posttraumatic stress disorder and risk of preterm birth. *JAMA Psychiatry, 71*(8), 897–904.

Author Biographies

Diana Lynn Barnes, PsyD, is in private practice in Los Angeles, California, and has specialized in women's reproductive mental health for over 20 years. She is the past president of Postpartum Support International. Dr. Barnes is the co-author of *The Journey to Parenthood: Myths, Reality and What Really Matters* (Radcliffe, 2007), and the editor of and contributing author to *Women's Reproductive Mental Health Across the Lifespan* (Springer, 2014).

Rebecca P. Cameron, PhD, is a professor of psychology at California State University, Sacramento, and a licensed psychologist in California. She received her doctorate in Clinical Psychology from Kent State University in 1997, and completed a postdoctoral fellowship at Stanford University Department of Psychiatry in 1999. Her research and scholarly interests are in stress, social support, resilience, and health among diverse groups, including people with disabilities and LGBTQ+ individuals.

Aimee N. C. Campbell, PhD, MSW, is an assistant professor of clinical psychiatric social work in the Department of Psychiatry at Columbia University Medical Center and research scientist at New York State Psychiatric Institute in the Division on Substance Abuse. Her research focuses on the development and testing of individual and program-level interventions for substance use disorders and HIV prevention and treatment, including the leveraging of technology-based platforms, with the objective of improving access to and implementation of science-based treatments. Dr. Campbell completed undergraduate training in sociology at the University of Washington and her master's degree and doctorate in social work at Columbia University.

Linda Cedeno, PhD, is a clinical psychologist with a full-time private practice centrally located in Manhattan. Dr. Cedeno works extensively with individuals and couples utilizing approaches including cognitive-behavioral therapy, emotionally focused couples therapy, motivational enhancement, psychodynamic psychotherapy, community reinforcement and family training (CRAFT), compassion-focused therapy, and mindfulness meditation.

Dr. Alette Coble-Temple is a licensed clinical psychologist for the Department of State Hospitals and a professor at John F. Kennedy University in Pleasant Hill, California. As a professional woman with cerebral palsy she believes advocacy, mentorship, and leadership development are essential components to increasing the number of people with disabilities in the employment sector, and ultimately result in healthier living and financial stability.

Zhen Cong, PhD, is currently an associate professor in the Department of Human Development and Family Studies at Texas Tech University. She received her PhD from the School of Gerontology at the University of Southern California. Her research interests include older adults' mental health, intergenerational relationships, and disasters' impact on older adults' well-being.

Colleen Clemency Cordes, PhD, is a clinical associate professor and the director of the Doctor of Behavioral Health program at Arizona State University (ASU). She is a psychologist and completed a postdoctoral fellowship in primary care behavioral health at the Edith Norse Rodgers Veterans Memorial Hospital in 2010. In addition to her work with ASU, she practices as a behavioral health consultant in HonorHealth's federally qualified health center.

helen DeVinney, PsyD, is a member of the core faculty at The George Washington University Professional Psychology program, where she teaches class in psychodynamic psychopathology, gender development, and clinical psychotherapy. Her clinical and research interests are varied, but she is particularly interested in the intersections of psychoanalysis and issues of gender, sexuality, race, and class as vehicles for individual and communal social justice.

Tia R. Dole, PhD, is a licensed clinical psychologist practicing in New York City. Dr. Dole is the site director for Psychological Services and Training at North Central Bronx Hospital. Her clinical interests include the treatment of psychosis, trauma, and working with adolescents struggling with identity issues. In her private practice, Dr. Dole specializes in working with families and individuals and families of color.

Ethan Eisen, PhD, received his doctorate in clinical psychology from The George Washington University in 2016, and completed his clinical internship at the VA Long Beach Healthcare System. His research and scholarly interests include posttraumatic stress disorder and moral injury, as well as the role of diverse identities in Israeli society, where he currently resides.

Maria Espinola, PsyD, is an assistant professor in the Department of Psychiatry at the University of Cincinnati College of Medicine. She earned her doctorate degree in clinical psychology at Nova Southeastern University. Dr. Espinola completed her predoctoral fellowship on multicultural psychology at Boston University School of Medicine and her postdoctoral training on women's psychology at Harvard Medical School.

CPT Jackie Hammelman, PhD, is a clinical psychologist in the U.S. Army. She is a member of the APA Division of Military Psychology.

Denise A. Hien, PhD, ABPP, is a professor in clinical psychology at the Gordon F. Derner Institute for Advanced Psychological Studies at Adelphi University, and adjunct senior research scientist at Columbia University College of Physicians and Surgeons, Division on Substance Abuse. She and her group conduct programmatic research on women's mental health and addictions, with continuous funding from the National Institute on Drug Abuse and National Institute on Alcoholism and Alcohol Abuse for 20 years.

Dr. Teresa López-Castro is a licensed clinical psychologist and assistant professor in Psychology at the City College of New York, specializing in the integrative treatment of trauma-related disorders. She has published and presented internationally on advancing the field of treatment research through novel methodologies and therapeutic targets.

Linda R. Mona, PhD, is a licensed clinical psychologist at the VA Long Beach Healthcare System specializing in providing mental health services to veterans with disabilities and chronic health conditions. She also serves as a healthcare services consultant, providing training to integrated healthcare settings and allied health clinical service providers on disability, diversity, and inclusion strategies.

Yaolin Pei, MS, is currently a PhD student in the Department of Human Development and Family Studies at Texas Tech University. Her research focuses on aging, the well-being of older adults, and intergenerational relationships.

Dr. Jessica Punzo is a licensed clinical psychologist and director of the Anti-Violence Project at the Center on Halsted, which is the Midwest's most comprehensive community center dedicated to advancing community and securing the health and well-being of the LGBTQ people of Chicagoland. Dr. Punzo is also an adjunct faculty member at The Chicago School of Professional Psychology. She is very passionate about psychological trauma and is thus involved in various national traumatic stress organizations through membership and active leadership roles.

Tanya Saraiya is a second-year doctoral student in the Clinical Psychology PhD program at Adelphi University. She is also a research fellow at the TRACC program—Translational Research in Addictions at City College and Columbia University. Tanya is interested in investigating the efficacy and effectiveness of posttraumatic stress disorder andsubstance use disorder treatments through examining health disparities among minority groups and developing new treatments based on neural and behavioral laboratory-based research studies.

Arlene (Lu) Steinberg, PsyD, is a psychologist/psychoanalyst in private practice and treasurer of the Division of Psychoanalysis (39) of the American Pscyhological Association, had been past president of Psychoanalysis for Social Responsibility, section 9 of Division 39, and will be co-editor with Judie Alpert of an upcoming special issue of the journal *Psychoanalytic Psychology* on Sexual Boundary Violations in 2017.

Kimberly D. Thompson, PhD, is a clinical psychologist involved in a variety of professional activities, including clinical practice, teaching at the graduate level, speaking to lay and professional audiences, and writing. Her clinical and research interests focus on perinatal women and children from birth through age five. She lives and works in Lubbock, Texas.

Margaret Wolff is a doctoral candidate at the City University of New York Graduate School of Public Health and Health Policy in New York, NY. Her research focuses on using multidimensional constructs of sexual orientation to understand the structural factors that undergird substance abuse and sexual health disparities among sexual-minority women.

Part I

Women's Mental Health in Lifespan Perspective

Chapter One
Mental Health of Women: A Focus on Adolescent Girls

Tia R. Dole

A common refrain that is often heard when adults refer to adolescence is, "I wouldn't want to be a teenager nowadays!" There is a perception that the issues that young people face, especially young girls, are much more challenging in today's world than in previous generations. Whether this perception is true remains to be seen. However, for adolescent girls in our society, there are a whole host of factors that affect development and mental health. Some of these factors are relatively new (e.g., social media), and some have been a part of modern society for a long time (e.g., depression, body image, or serious mental health conditions). Adolescent girls in the United States face challenges that are both unique to their culture and common across different types of societies. For the purposes of brevity, most of the research presented in this chapter is focused on adolescent girls from a Western perspective. However, it will include the different diasporas that exist within Western society. Nonetheless, many of the themes could be generalized to other cultures.

This chapter will focus on salient topics related to mental health issues for adolescent girls. These topics include self-esteem, depressive symptoms, disordered eating behaviors, and social media. However, in exploring these topics, one will note that the underlying theme linking them is self-esteem. The interrelatedness of self-esteem and mental health in adolescent girls cannot be overstated. In essence, how an adolescent girl perceives herself has an untold impact on how she dates, how she eats, her mood, drug use, sexual behavior, and most importantly, her resilience. Hence, I will start this chapter with a discussion of self-esteem, how it has been examined, and its impact on girls. In the following sections, we will see how this construct plays a significant role in the mental health of adolescent girls overall, and how interventions that are based on improving self-esteem, or a sense of self-efficacy, can have a significant impact on the way that a girl develops into an adult.

Self-Esteem

Self-esteem, or the positive or negative evaluation of oneself (Rosenberg, 1986), is a concept that is often examined with regard to adolescent girls. How a young girl perceives herself can have far-reaching consequences on her behavior and outcomes, including physical health and criminal behavior (Trzesniewski et al., 2006). Self-esteem is typically measured using tools such as the Rosenberg Self-Esteem Scale (Rosenberg, 1986). Initially it was thought to measure a single construct called "self-esteem." However, over time this measure has been found to have two subscales that are related, but separate (Farruggia, Chen, Greenberger, Dmitrieva, & Macek, 2004; Martin, Thompson, & Chan, 2006; Owens, 1994). These constructs are "Self-Worth" (one's evaluation of one-self), and "Self-Deprecation" (the degree to which an individual denigrates one's self-worth, abilities, or usefulness). Recent research has found that, for girls progressing through adolescence, self-esteem is not a static construct; it is dynamic. In fact, Baldwin and Hoffmann (2002) found a curvilinear relationship between self-esteem and time. Starting from age 12, some girls experience a drop in self-esteem that starts to recover around the age of 17, with negative life events having a significant impact on an adolescents' self-esteem. Interestingly, for boys, self-esteem increased through the age of 14, decreased to age 16, and then increased through early adulthood. In essence, girls struggle with maintaining a positive image of themselves throughout adolescence in ways that boys do not seem challenged. Race and culture also impact the complicated trajectory of self-esteem in adolescent girls (Twenge & Crocker, 2002).

Impett, Sorsoli, Schooler, Henson, and Tolman (2008), examining research literature from a feminist developmental perspective, suggest that the differences between boys and girls are derived from differences within the power hierarchy in our society, and girls' focus on relationships. Traditionally, development is seen through the lens of male development, primarily focused on individuation and individualism (Erikson, 1968). This is in contrast to examining development from a feminist perspective, or an alternative perspective, in which relationships between individuals retain their importance over time. Consequently, with the value in our society on individualism, the way that girls grow and change is not as valued, and thus, the innate way that girls make sense of their world is not considered worthwhile. Girls have a strong emphasis on relationships and their esteem is based heavily on the way that they are relating to each other, and how others are relating to them. In fact, we find that how girls negotiate relationships and how they think about themselves have important implications for self-esteem. Consequently, perhaps one of the underlying factors impacting the precipitous drop in self-esteem for girls in mid-adolescence especially is related to the fact that the way girls gain confidence in themselves is undervalued in our society.

Research by Impett et al. (2008) and Impett, Henson, Breines, Schooler, and Tolman (2011) suggests that girls who have higher relationship authenticity, meaning that a young girl's behavior reflects what she thinks and feels, also have higher self-esteem. These findings suggest that teaching young women to be "true to themselves" in their interactions with others will increase their chances of feeling good about who they are as a person. These findings also suggest that girls may be at an inherent disadvantage in terms of acquiring a positive sense of self if they are not taught the value of being authentic in interpersonal relationships. In fact, some recent research has supported this hypothesis. It appears that authenticity in interpersonal relationships can serve as a mediator between childhood maltreatment and negative outcomes, such as depression, poor self-esteem, and trauma symptoms for college-aged women (Theran & Han, 2013). For adolescent girls, lack of authenticity with parents was related to depression (Theran, 2011). Thus, interventions focused on girls feeling more comfortable with who they are may be essential in improving functioning.

Race and ethnicity also play a role in the development and maintenance of self-esteem. Some research has shown that self-esteem manifests differently across cultures. In fact, some research has found that, for African American girls, the trajectory of plummeting self-esteem through adolescence was not found (Gray-Little & Hafdahl, 2000; Twenge & Crocker, 2002). Crocker and Major (1989) speculate that stigmatized groups (like African Americans) may attribute negative feedback from others as based in prejudice, or failures to perform as related to prejudice, even when they are not. Blacks may also be protected from poor self-esteem by in-group comparisons, in which people compare themselves to other similarly "disadvantaged" individuals. Thus, role failure is not perceived of as harshly. Other research has found that Blacks are less likely to base their esteem on the approval of others, and that basing one's self-esteem on the approval of others mediated the relationships between self-esteem and race (Ziegler-Hill, 2007).

Some researchers suggest that, instead of employing methods to improve self-esteem overall (as one would do for White adolescent girls), for Black girls one should use the improvement of self-esteem as a way of decreasing risky sexual behaviors that may lead to increased risk of HIV infection (Adams, 2010). This study also found that for Black girls, in particular, social support led to decreased self-deprecation scores.

There have been several factors that mediate and moderate the development and maintenance of self-esteem in adolescent girls. One significant area of research has been in the role of sports participation and its association with better outcomes for girls, including improved self-esteem, self-worth, and a positive body image (Findlay & Coplan, 2008; Marsh & Jackson, 1986; Richman

& Schaffer, 2000). Some research has found that these robust results are even more complex, with perceived peer acceptance mediating the relationship between sports participation and self-esteem (Daniels & Leaper, 2006). In fact, Adachi and Willoughby (2014) recently conducted a study in which high levels of self-esteem predicted greater involvement in sports, not the inverse. Their conclusions suggested that a young woman's enjoyment of the sport is what impacted self-esteem, rather than simply participating in sports themselves.

Predictors of Higher Self-Esteem

Much of the research on self-esteem tends to be focused on trends which predict negative outcomes. However, research has pointed to factors that are associated with higher self-esteem. A seminal study by Birndorf, Ryan, Auinger, and Aten (2005) using the National Education Longitudinal Study (Kaufman, Bradby, & National Center for Education Statistics, 1992) database found that some predictors of higher self-esteem were being African American or Latina, positive family communications, safety, and religious community.

The importance of this type of research cannot be overstated. Examining why some girls are more resilient is essential to developing effective programs like Girls on the Run (Martin, Waldron, McCabe, & Choi, 2009) that help build self-esteem and a sense of efficacy. Some protective factors are somewhat dependent on self-esteem as well. Cooper (2009) found that for African American adolescent girls, self-esteem served as a mediating factor between father–daughter relationship quality and academic achievement. Girls who reported having a positive relationship with their father also reported higher self-esteem and higher academic performance. Other protective factors include being of Black or Latina descent (Bachman, O'Malley, Freedman-Doan, Trzesniewski, & Donnellan, 2011), a sense of self-efficacy or mastery (Lightsey, Burke, Ervin, Henderson, & Yee, 2006), being emotionally stable, extraverted, or conscientious (Erol & Orth, 2011).

Depression

The effects of depressive disorders for adolescent girls have untold consequences. In their seminal paper, "The Development of Depression in Children and Adolescents," Cicchetti and Toth (1998) described what could be considered to be a condition that occurs with relative frequency, with between 15% and 20% of young people experiencing depression during their adolescence (Harrington, Rutter, & Fombonne, 1996). Cicchetti and Toth (1998) noted that the long-term consequences of depression are fairly far reaching, with a significantly increased risk for major depressive disorder in adulthood, and other comorbid conditions like anxiety disorders, conduct disorders, and substance abuse.

In the United States, the rates of a major depressive episode for adolescent girls between the ages of 12 and 17 are 17.3% (11.4% for all adolescents in that same age range) (Center for Behavioral Health Statistics and Quality, 2015). Thus, nearly 20% of girls meet criteria for a depressive episode. This number is not inclusive of girls who have subthreshold depressive symptoms. These alarming numbers point to an urgent need for intervention in the United States. However, the etiology of depression in adolescent girls is fairly complicated: the intersection of genetics, negative life events, and environment can cause, or increase, vulnerability to depressive symptoms. Thompson, Parker, Hallmayer, Waugh, and Gotlib (2011) found that adolescent girls who experienced what they describe as "early adversity" (e.g., having a mother diagnosed with recurrent major depressive disorder), and who also had specific nucleotide polymorphism related to oxytocin, reported the highest levels of depression and anxiety. Thus, the effects of genetics and home environment can combine to impact a young girl's functioning.

There appears to be a natural connection between self-esteem and depression in adolescents. Consequently, much of the research in these fields explicitly examines the relationships between them. For instance, rates of depression in adolescents are directly related to low self-esteem, with adolescents who experience low self-esteem subsequently experiencing higher rates of depression (Orth, Robins, Widaman, & Conger, 2014). As with self-esteem, depression in adolescence follows an inverted U-shaped curve, beginning in early adolescence and continuing until approximately age 17, when it begins to decrease (Rawana & Morgan, 2014). This same pattern is shown for adolescent boys, though boys have lower initial levels of depression (Rawana & Morgan, 2014).

Pubertal Timing

There are also factors that may influence rates of depression, such as pubertal timing, though some of this research is mixed (Ellis, 2004). The concept of pubertal timing affecting subsequent adolescent psychological well-being was originally called the Stage Termination Hypothesis (Peskin & Livson, 1972; Petersen & Taylor, 1980). This hypothesis posited that behavioral problems in adolescence occurred because early pubertal timing did not allow girls to complete essential developmental milestones in early to middle childhood. Keenan, Culbert, Grimm, Howell, and Stepp (2014) found an inverse relationship between pubertal timing and depression, with early-onset puberty being associated with increased depression. Overall, African American girls have a slightly earlier onset for puberty, and consequently reported higher rates of depression, thus race served as a moderating factor.

Markotte, Fortin, Potvin, and Papillon (2002) conducted a study that indicated that, for adolescents transitioning to high school, self-esteem, negative stressful life events, and body image mediated the relationship between pubertal status and depressive symptoms. In other words, girls with less body appreciation, more negative events, and lower self-esteem evidenced greater depressive symptoms, with a modest effect with regard to pubertal status. Other research has found that it's the *perception* of early puberty that impacts externalizing behaviors for adolescent girls (Carter, Caldwell, Matsuko, Antonucci, & Jackson, 2011). This means that it's not the early pubertal timing that is linked to depression, but girls feeling like it's come too soon.

There have been many factors that are related to the development of depressive symptoms in adolescent girls. For instance, romantic activities (e.g., dating) for adolescent girls have been linked to depressive symptoms, eating-disorder symptoms, anxiety, and externalizing behaviors (Starr et al., 2012). Chan, Kelly, and Toumbourou (2013) found that for adolescent girls, when controlling for variables like school commitment, ethnicity, and peers who consume alcohol, family conflict predicted depressive symptoms, which subsequently led to heavy alcohol use in later adolescence. Furthermore, smoking is associated with higher rates of depression, even when controlling for socioeconomic status (Beal, Negriff, Dorn, Pabst, & Schulenberg, 2013).

As seen above, there are many factors that impact the development of depressive symptoms in adolescent girls. However, the risks of depressive symptoms can also be potentially life threatening.

Depression in girls can lead to problematic behaviors, such as non-suicidal self-injury (NSSI), suicidal ideation, and externalizing behaviors, among others. Behaviors like NSSI are linked with emotional dysregulation and interpersonal difficulties, and NSSI typically begins during adolescence (Adrian, Zeman, Erdley, Lisa, & Sim, 2011; Ross & Heath, 2002). The long-term consequences of using NSSI in an effort to regulate emotions are related to the negative impact on both physical health and psychological functioning. In addition to NSSI, suicide rates have sky-rocketed in the last 15 years. A recent study by the Centers for Disease Control and Prevention (2016) showed that, between 1999 and 2014, the suicide rate for girls between the ages of 10 and 14 increased 200%, from 0.5 per 100,000 to 1.5 per 100,000 (for boys of the same age range the rate is 2.6 per 100,000), with poisoning being the most common method. These statistics are alarming, and early intervention for suicide prevention has increased in recent years to address what is now being called an "epidemic."

Interventions for Depression

Fortunately, there have been several studies which provide support for effective interventions for adolescents coping with depressive symptoms. Cognitive-behavioral therapy, in particular, has been found to be particularly effective for treating depressive symptoms in adolescents (Spirito, Esposito-Smythers,

Wolff, & Uhl, 2011), while combining selective serotonin reuptake inhibitors and cognitive-behavioral therapy has been shown to be the most effective intervention for adolescents with depression (Brent et al., 2008). However, whether girls are willing to engage with treatment is the interesting question. Caporino and Karver (2012) found that, for adolescent girls, receiving psychopharmacology alone was not acceptable. Girls were more likely to be open to psychotherapy (cognitive-behavioral therapy, interpersonal therapy, or family therapy), or psychopharmacology *and* psychotherapy combined, and symptom severity did not change the acceptability of the medication-only possibility. What this means in terms of intervention is that girls don't want just medication; they want the opportunity for talk therapy first. Family therapy, in particular, may have a significant impact on improved functioning for adolescent girls, particularly since familial conflict has been directly related to negative outcomes such as self-injury (Adrian et al., 2011; Chan et al., 2013). Thus, we have the treatment available; it simply needs to be implemented.

Disordered Eating

According to the *Diagnostic and Statistical Manual and Mental Disorders-5* (DSM-5: American Psychiatric Association (APA), 2013), eating disorders are defined by the presence of anorexia nervosa (AN), bulimia nervosa (BN), and binge-eating disorder (BED). AN is defined as the restriction of caloric intake relative to the needs of the body, resulting in low body weight, while BN is defined by binge eating followed by "inappropriate" behaviors, such as self-induced vomiting, to avoid weight gain (APA, 2013). Finally, BED is defined as eating significantly more food than other people would in a short time frame (APA, 2013). All three of these disorders have significant and potentially long-term effects on the body and psychological functioning (Spoor, Stice, Burton, & Bohon, 2007). In fact, AN remains the most dangerous of all mental health conditions, with a mortality rate of up to 10% (Arcelus, Mitchell, Wales, & Nielsen, 2011). Thus, the risks and consequences of developing an eating disorder for young girls are quite significant.

In the United States, the rates of eating disorders are less than depression: 2.7% of 13–18-year-olds have a lifetime prevalence of a "severe" eating disorder, but the number increases to 3.8% for girls in the same age range (Merikangas et al., 2010). More troubling, these numbers do not include subthreshold, or "problem" eating behaviors. Some studies have found that rates of subthreshold pathological eating are much higher than threshold rates. Stice, Marti, Shaw, and Jacobins (2009) found that subthreshold rates of AN, BN, and BED are 6.1%, 4.6%, and 4.6% respectively. These rates are twice the threshold rates, and consequently represent a large portion of young girls affected by the long-term consequences of disordered eating in terms of functional impairment and poor body image.

Andrew, Tiggemann, and Clark (2015) report that perceived body acceptance and body appreciation were associated with healthier eating habits, or "intuitive eating," while self-objectification and social comparison were negatively associated with healthier eating habits. In fact, over time, body appreciation leads to decreased dieting, alcohol use, and cigarette smoking. It is likely that the girls in their study who perceived that their body was accepted by those important to them, possibly through subtle non-judgmental messages about appearance, may have been less likely to experience preoccupation with appearance and instead feel respect and appreciation for their body (Tylka & Wood-Barcalow, 2015, p. 470).

These results have been found in other studies. When controlling for socioeconomic status as well as race/ethnicity, academic achievement, and other factors typically related to positive "youth development," decreases in body objectification also led to an increase in self-esteem and a decrease in depressive symptoms (Impett et al., 2011).

Paxton, Neumark-Sztainer, Hannan, and Eisenberg (2006), in their study examining the impact of body dissatisfaction on adolescent girls, found that body dissatisfaction was a risk factor for both low self-esteem and depressive mood over a long period of time during adolescence (approximately five years) for girls, but not for boys. They purport that these three constructs (body dissatisfaction, self-esteem, and depressive mood) have a "spiral relation." Essentially, low self-esteem is a risk factor for body dissatisfaction, which can in turn result in depressed mood. As with all of the constructs being examined during the course of this chapter, none of these constructs exists separately. For adolescent girls, there are a host of factors that contribute to resilience and dysfunction. These studies have been replicated elsewhere (Ferreiro, Seoane, & Senra, 2012; Rodgers, Paxton, & McLean, 2014).

Cross-culturally, there are differences with body dissatisfaction as well. Bucchianeri et al. (2016) found that Asian adolescents (boys and girls) had the highest levels of body dissatisfaction among all ethnic groups studied (e.g., White, Black, "Other," or Hispanic). However, while higher body dissatisfaction was associated with disordered eating behaviors, the relationship was not moderated by race/ethnicity for girls (it was in boys). Thus, for girls, ethnicity was not a potential protective or risk factor for disordered eating habits.

There are a number of factors which may protect or help girls who are experiencing problematic behaviors related to eating. Interventions that are focused on health, body acceptance, and decreasing weight stigma are key factors in not only improving healthy eating, but also problematic behaviors like alcohol consumption. Based on their research with adolescent girls in the United Kingdom, Cribb and Haase (2015) speculate that girls who experience more social support may counter the negative impact of the internalization of body ideals, and the overall influence of the media. Peer groups have been found to have a significant impact on the development of body image, both positive and negative, depending on the context (Ferguson, Winegard, & Winegard, 2011). Other factors that may serve as protective factors for preventing the development of disordered eating habits include lower body mass index (BMI), healthier eating habits, high self-esteem, and a low to moderate degree of perfectionism (Westerberg-Jacobson, Edlund, & Ghaderi, 2010).

There have been a number of treatments developed to help adolescent girls cope with and overcome threshold and subthreshold eating disorders; however, they remain somewhat hard to treat, particularly in the context of the high mortality rate associated with AN (Arcelus et al., 2011). More recently, intensive family therapies have shown a great deal of promise. Interventions such as intensive family therapy (both single-family and multiple-family) have been found to be effective (Lock, 2015; Marzola et al., 2015) for girls with AN. Overall, treatments for this population (young girls) have not been studied extensively, and there is a dearth of literature addressing effective treatments for BN and BED (Lock, 2015; Lock & Fitpatrick, 2007). One study conducted by a large group of researchers (Pretorius et al., 2009) did find a significant improvement with BN utilizing an online cognitive-behavioral therapy treatment. More creative applications of well-established psychotherapies will likely be forthcoming, particularly in light of the "digital age" that young people experience from birth.

Social Media

Social media has exploded since the advent of Friendster and Facebook, and today there are many "apps," or applications, that adolescents use on their phones or devices to connect with other young people. Parents are often concerned about their child's "exposure" to social media apps due to fears around bullying, access to inappropriate material, and lack of connection to real-life people. However, despite widespread concerns among parents and clinicians alike, some researchers posit that there hasn't been consistent evidence of the negative effects of social media on young people (Ferguson, Muñoz, Garz, & Galindo, 2014).

One major concern regarding social media has been focused on how exposure to social media could affect an adolescent girl with regard to body image. Some research has found no effect of social media on body dissatisfaction, life satisfaction, or eating-disorder symptoms (Ferguson et al., 2014). One relationship that they did find was between social media and peer competition. They concluded that social media usage did not predict negative outcomes (Ferguson et al., 2014). Other researchers have found that social media has a negative impact on body image and an increase in disordered eating behaviors (Latzer, Spivak-Lavi, & Katz, 2015). Furthermore, lower sense of empowerment and low parental involvement (in conjunction with social media exposure) led to increases in disordered eating behaviors. Internalization of thin body ideals can lead to a drive for thinness and greater body dissatisfaction (Bearman, Presnell, Martinez, & Stice, 2006).

With regard to mood, there has been some concern that social media has a negative impact on young people, and that social media use is linked with depression and/or anxiety. In a study conducted by Feinstein, Bhatia, Hershenberg, and Davila (2012), the authors found that depressed mood did not predict an increase of social media, but that depressed young people simply enacted their "existing pathologies" on the social media plane in the same way they would in person. Unfortunately, at this juncture there is not a great deal of research with regard to social media and adolescent girls specifically. However, research conducted on teens, young adults, and women found that Facebook usage and selected technology usage predicted clinical symptoms. For instance, more Facebook friends predicted bipolar mania, histrionic personality disorder, and narcissism (Rosen, Whaling, Rab, Carrier, & Cheever, 2013). Another detrimental effect was a penchant for multitasking.

Overall, the research of the effect of social media on adolescents remains in its infancy. However, one thing that is clear is that social media is slowly (or perhaps rapidly) becoming woven in our society. It is likely that, as stated above, social media usage and interactions reflect real-life interactions. Until more research is conducted, the effect of social media on adolescent girls remains to be seen.

Conclusions

Some conclusions that could be gleaned from the above discussion of mental health issues in adolescent girls are as follows:

- Young women today are bombarded with a whole host of negative feedback, negative life events, and the temptation to cope with negative events in ways that "work" initially, but have long-term negative consequences.
- These consequences include struggling with mental health issues such as depression (young women have a significant increase of depression during adolescence). Other consequences that young women face include low self-esteem, particularly for White adolescent girls, as a result of the internalization of a negative self-concept. And finally, disordered eating habits can emerge, coupled by negative body image, and these are fairly difficult to overcome.
- However, research also shows that girls are remarkably resilient. Most of them bounce back out of adolescence, intact and productive through adulthood.

- For those who struggle to recover from childhood maltreatment, genetic loading, or simply the negative influence of the media, research has shown that early intervention with a focus on psychotherapy for individuals and families is considered acceptable to young girls, and effective overall.
- Medication has also been found to be effective for treating other more serious mental health conditions. Thus, we already have interventions that we know work; it's often simply a matter of implementing the right treatment at the right time.

References

Adachi, P.J.C., & Willoughby, T. (2014). It's not how much you play, but how much you enjoy the game: The longitudinal associations between adolescents' self-esteem and the frequency verses enjoyment of involvement in sports. *Journal of Youth and Adolescence, 43,* 137–145.

Adams, P. (2010). Understanding the different realities, experience and use of self-esteem between black and white adolescent girls. *Journal of Black Psychology, 36*(3), 255–276.

Adrian, M., Zeman, J., Erdley, C., Lisa, L., & Sim, L. (2011). Emotional dysregulation and interpersonal difficulties as risk factors for non-suicidal self-injury in adolescent girls. *Journal of Abnormal Child Psychology, 39*(3), 389–400.

American Psychiatric Association. (2013). *Diagnostic and statistical manual of mental disorders: DSM-5.* Washington, D.C.: American Psychiatric Association.

Andrew, R., Tiggemann, M., & Clark, L. (2015). The protective role of body appreciation against media-induced body dissatisfaction. *Body Image, Sep 15,* 98–104.

Arcelus, J., Mitchell, A.J., Wales, J., & Nielsen, S. (2011). Mortality rates in patients with anorexia nervosa and other eating disorders. A meta-analysis of 36 studies. Archives of Mitchell, *Archives of General Psychiatry, 68,* 724–731.

Bachman, J.G., O'Malley, P.M., Freedman-Doan, P., Trzesniewski, K.H., & Donnellan, M.B. (2011). Adolescent self-esteem: Differences by race/ethnicity, gender, and age. *Self and Identity, 10*(4), 445–473.

Baldwin, S. A., & Hoffmann, J. P. (2002). The dynamics of self-esteem: A growth-curve analysis. *Journal of Youth and Adolescence, 31,* 101–113.

Beal, S.J., Negriff, S., Dorn, L.D., Pabst, S., & Schulenberg, J. (2013). Longitudinal associations between smoking and depressive symptoms among adolescent girls. *Prevention Science, 15,* 506–515.

Bearman, S.K., Presnell, K., Martinez, E., & Stice, E. (2006). The skinny on body dissatisfaction: a longitudinal study of adolescent girls and boys. *Journal of Youth and Adolescence, 35*(2), 229–241.

Birndorf, S., Ryan, S., Auinger, P., & Aten, M. (2005). High self-esteem among adolescents: Longitudinal trends, sex differences and protective factors. *Journal of Adolescent Health, 37*(3), 194–201.

Brent, D., Emslie, G., Clarke, G., Wagner, K.D., Asarnow, J.R., Keller, M., ... Zelazny, J. (2008). Switching to another SSRI or to venlafaxine with or without cognitive behavioral therapy for adolescents with SSRI-resistant depression: The TORDIA randomized controlled trial. *JAMA : The Journal of the American Medical Association, 299*(8), 901–913.

Bucchianeri, M.M., Fernandes, N., Loth, K., Hannan, P.J., Eisenberg, M.E., & Neumark-Sztainer, D. (2016). Body dissatisfaction: Do associations with disordered eating and psychological well-being differ across race/ethnicity in adolescent girls and boys? *Cultural Diversity and Ethnic Minority Psychology, 22*(1), 137–146.

Caporino, N.E., & Karver, M.S. (2012). The acceptability of treatments for depression to a community sample of adolescent girls. *Journal of Adolescence, 35*(5), 1237–1245.

Carter, R., Caldwell, C.H., Matsuko, N., Antonucci, T., & Jackson, J.S. (2011). Ethnicity, perceived pubertal timing, externalizing behaviors, and depressive symptoms among Black adolescent girls. *Journal of Youth and Adolescence, 40*(10), 1394–1406.

Center for Behavioral Health Statistics and Quality. (2015). *Behavioral health trends in the United States: Results from the 2014 National Survey on Drug Use and Health.* HHS Publication No. SMA 15-4927, NSDUH Series H-50. Rockville, MD: Substance Abuse and Mental Health Services Administration.

14 • Tia R. Dole

Centers for Disease Control and Prevention. (2016). *Increase in Suicide in the United States, 1999–2014*. Retrieved from: http://www.cdc.gov/nchs/products/databriefs/db241.htm.

Chan, G.K., Kelly, A.B., & Toumbourou, J.W. (2013). Accounting for the association of family conflict and heavy alcohol use among adolescent girls: The role of depressed mood. *Journal of Studies on Alcohol and Drugs, 74*(3), 396–405.

Cicchetti, D., & Toth, S.L. (1998). The development of depression in children and adolescents. *American Psychologist, 53*(2), 221–241.

Cooper, S.M. (2009). Associations between father–daughter relationship quality and the academic engagement of African American adolescent girls: Self-esteem as a mediator? *Journal of Black Psychology, 35*(4), 495–516.

Cribb, V.L., & Haase, A.M. (2015). Girls feeling good at school: School gender environment, internalization and awareness of socio-cultural attitudes associations with self-esteem in adolescent girls. *Journal of Adolescence, 46,* 107–114.

Crocker, J., & Major, B. (1989). Social stigma and self-esteem: The self-protective properties of stigma. *Psychological Review, 96,* 608–630.

Daniels, E., & Leaper, C. (2006). A longitudinal investigation of sport participation, peer acceptance, and self-esteem among adolescent boys and girls. *Sex Roles, 55,* 875–880.

Ellis, B.J. (2004). Timing of pubertal maturation in girls: An integrated life history approach. *Psychological Bulletin, 130,* 920–958.

Erikson, E. (1968). *Identity, youth, and crisis*. New York: W. W. Norton.

Erol, R.Y., & Orth, U. (2011). Self-esteem development from age 14 to 30 years: A longitudinal study. *Journal of Personality and Social Psychology, 101,* 607–619.

Farruggia, S., Chen, C., Greenberger, E., Dmitrieva, J., & Macek, P. (2004). Adolescent self-esteem in cross-cultural perspective: Testing measurement equivalence and a mediation model. *Journal of Cross-Cultural Psychology, 35,* 719–733.

Feinstein, B.A., Bhatia, V., Hershenberg, R., & Davila, J. (2012). Another venue for problematic interpersonal behavior: The effects of depressive and anxious symptoms on social networking experience. *Journal of Social and Clinical Psychology, 31*(4), 356–382.

Ferguson, C.J., Muñoz, M.E., Garza, A., & Galindo, M. (2014). Concurrent and prospective analyses of peer, television and social media influences on body dissatisfaction, eating disorder symptoms and life satisfaction in adolescent girls. *Journal of Youth and Adolescence, 43*(1), 1–14.

Ferguson, C.J., Winegard, B., & Winegard, B.M. (2011). Who is the fairest one of all? How evolution guides peer and media influences on female body dissatisfaction. *Review of General Psychology, 15*(1), 11–28.

Ferreiro, F., Seoane, G., & Senra, C. (2012). Gender-related risk and protective factors for depressive symptoms and disordered eating in adolescence: A 4-year longitudinal study. *Journal of Youth and Adolescence, 41*(5), 607–622.

Findlay, L.C., & Coplan, R.J. (2008). Come out and play: Shyness in childhood and the benefits of organized sports participation. *Journal of Canadian Behavioral Science, 40,* 153–161.

Gray-Little, B., & Hafdahl, A. (2000). Factors influencing racial comparisons of self-esteem: A quantitative review. *Psychological Bulletin, 126,* 26–54.

Harrington, R., Rutter, M., & Fombonne, E. (1996). Developmental pathways in depression: Multiple meanings, antecedents, and endpoints. *Development and Psychopathology, 8,* 601–616.

Impett, E. A., Sorsoli, L., Schooler, D., Henson, J. M., & Tolman, D. L. (2008). Girls' relationship authenticity and self-esteem across adolescence. *Developmental Psychology, 44,* 722–733.

Impett, E. A., Henson, J. M., Breines, J., Schooler, D., & Tolman, D. L. (2011). Embodiment feels better: Girls' body objectification and well-being across adolescence. *Psychology of Women Quarterly, 35,* 46–58.

Kaufman, P., Bradby, D., & National Center for Education Statistics. (1992). *National education longitudinal study of 1988: Characteristics of at-risk students in NELS:88*. Washington, DC: U.S. Department of Education, Office of Educational Research and Improvement, National Center for Education Statistics. http://doi.org/10.3886/ICPSR09389.v1.

Keenan, K., Culbert, K.M., Grimm, K.J., Howell, A.E., & Stepp, S.D. (2014). Timing and tempo: Exploring the complex association between pubertal development and depression in African American and European American girls. *Journal of Abnormal Psychology, 123*(4), 725–736.

Latzer, Y., Spivak-Lavi, Z., & Katz, R. (2015). Disordered eating and media exposure among adolescent girls: The role of parental involvement and sense of empowerment. Involvement and sense of empowerment. *International Journal of Adolescence and Youth, 20*(3), 375–391.

Lightsey, O.R., Jr., Burke, M., Ervin, A., Henderson, D., & Yee, C. (2006). Generalized self-efficacy, self-esteem, and negative affect. *Canadian Journal of Behavioural Science/Revue canadienne des sciences du comportement, 38*, 72–80.

Lock, J. (2015). An update on evidence-based psychosocial treatments for eating disorders in children and adolescents. *Journal of Clinical Child and Adolescent Psychology, 44*(5), 707–721.

Lock, J., & Fitzpatrick, K.K. (2007). Evidenced-based treatments for children and adolescents with eating disorders: Family therapy and family-facilitated cognitive-behavioral therapy. *Journal of Contemporary Psychotherapy, 37*(3), 145–155.

Marcotte, D., Fortin, L., Potvin, P., & Papillon, M. (2002). Gender differences in depressive symptoms during adolescence: Role of gender-typed characteristics, self-esteem, body image, stressful life events, and pubertal status. *Journal of Emotional and Behavioral Disorders, 10*, 29–42.

Marsh, H.W., & Jackson, S.A. (1986). Multidimensional self-concepts, masculinity, and femininity as a function of women's involvement in athletics. *Sex Roles, 15*, 391–415.

Martin, C.R., Thompson, D.R., & Chan, D.S. (2006). An examination of the psychometric properties of the Rosenberg Self-Esteem Scale (RSES) in Chinese acute coronary syndrome (ACS) patients. *Psychology, Health & Medicine, 11*, 507–521.

Martin, J.J., Waldron, J.J., McCabe, A., & Choi, Y.S. (2009). The impact of 'Girls on the Run' on self-concept and fat attitudes. *Journal of Clinical Sport Psychology, 3*, 127–138.

Marzola, E., Knatz, S., Murray, S.B., Rockwell, R., Boutelle, K., Eisler, I., & Kaye, W.H. (2015). Short-term intensive family therapy for adolescent eating disorders: 30-month outcome. *European Eating Disorders Review, 23*(3), 210–218.

Merikangas, K.R., He, J., Burstein, M., Swanson, S.A., Avenevoli, S., Cui, L., Benjet, C., Georgiades, K., & Swendsen, J. (2010). Lifetime prevalence of mental disorders in U.S. adolescents: Results from the National Comorbidity Study-Adolescent Supplement (NCS-A). *Journal of the American Academy of Child and Adolescent Psychiatry, 49*(10), 980–989.

Orth, U., Robins, R.W., Widaman, K.F., & Conger, R.D. (2014). Is low self-esteem a risk factor for depression? Findings from a longitudinal study of Mexican-origin youth. *Developmental Psychology, 50*, 622–633.

Owens, T.J. (1994). Two dimensions of self-esteem: Reciprocal effects of positive self-worth and self-deprecation on adolescent problems. *American Sociological Review, 59*, 391–407.

Paxton, S.J., Neumark-Sztainer, D., Hannan, P.J., & Eisenberg, M.E. (2006). Body dissatisfaction prospectively predicts depressive mood and low self-esteem in adolescent girls and boys. *Journal of Clinical Child and Adolescent Psychology, 35*(4), 539–549.

Peskin, H., & Livson, N. (1972). Pre-and post-pubertal personality and adult psychological functioning. *Seminars in Psychiatry, 4*, 343–353.

Petersen, A.C., & Taylor, B. (1980). Puberty: biological change and psychological adaptation. In J. Adelson (Ed.), *Handbook of adolescent psychology* (pp. 117–158). New York: Wiley.

Pretorius, N., Arcelus, J., Beecham, J., Dawson, H., Doherty, F., Eisler, I., . . . Schmidt, U. (2009). Cognitive-behavioural therapy for adolescents with bulimic symptomatology: The acceptability and effectiveness of internet-based delivery. *Behaviour Research and Therapy, 47*(9), 729–736.

Rawana, J.S., & Morgan, A.S. (2014). Trajectories of depressive symptoms from adolescence to young adulthood: The role of self-esteem and body-related predictors. *Journal of Youth and Adolescence, 43*(4), 597–611.

Richman, E.L., & Schaffer, D.R. (2000). "If you let me play sports:" How might sport participation influence the self-esteem of adolescent females? *Psychology of Women Quarterly, 24*, 189–199.

Rodgers, R.F., Paxton, S.J., & McLean, S.A. (2014). A biopsychosocial model of body image concerns and disordered eating in early adolescent girls. *Journal of Youth and Adolescence, 43*(5), 814–823.

Rosen, L.D., Whaling, K., Rab, S., Carrier, L.M., & Cheever, N.A. (2013). Is Facebook creating "iDisorders"? The link between clinical symptoms of psychiatric disorders and technology use, attitudes and anxiety. *Computers in Human Behavior, 29*(3), 1243–1254.

Rosenberg, M. (1986). *Conceiving the self.* Malabar, FL: Krieger.

Ross, S., & Heath, N. (2002). A study of the frequency of self- mutilation in a community sample of adolescents. *Journal of Youth and Adolescence, 31*, 67–77.

Spirito, A., Esposito-Smythers, C., Wolff, J., & Uhl, K. (2011). Cognitive-behavioral therapy for adolescent depression and suicidality. *Child and Adolescent Psychiatric Clinics of North America, 20*(2), 191–204.

Spoor, S.T., Stice, E., Burton, D., & Bohon, C. (2007). Relations of bulimic symptom frequency and intensity to psychosocial impairment and health care utilization: Results from a community-recruited sample. *International Journal of Eating Disorders, 40*, 505–514.

Starr, L.R., Davila, J., Stroud, C.B., Clara Li, P.C., Yoneda, A., Hershenberg, R., & Ramsay Miller, M. (2012). Love hurts (in more ways than one): Specificity of psychological symptoms as predictors and consequences of romantic activity among early adolescent girls. *Journal of Clinical Psychology, 68*(4), 403–420.

Stice, E., Marti, C.N., Shaw, H., & Jacobins, M. (2009). An 8-year longitudinal study of the natural history of threshold, subthreshold, and partial eating disorders from a community sample of adolescents. *Journal of Abnormal Psychology, 118*(3), 587–597.

Theran, S.A. (2011). Authenticity in relationships and depressive symptoms: A gender analysis. *Personality and Individual Differences, 51*(4), 423–428.

Theran, S.A., & Han, S.C. (2013). Authenticity as a mediator of the relation between child maltreatment and negative outcomes for college women. *Journal of Aggression, Maltreatment & Trauma, 22*(10), 1096–1116.

Thompson, R.J., Parker, K.J., Hallmayer, J.F., Waugh, C.E., & Gotlib, I.H. (2011). Oxytocin receptor gene polymorphism (rs2254298) interacts with familial risk for psychopathology to predict symptoms of depression and anxiety in adolescent girls. *Psychoneuroendocrinology, 36*(1), 144–147.

Trzesniewski, K.H., Donnellan, M.B., Moffitt, T.E., Robins, R.W., Poulton, R., & Caspi, A. (2006). Low self-esteem during adolescence predicts poor health, criminal behaviour and limited economic prospects during adulthood. *Developmental Psychology, 42*(2), 381–390.

Twenge, J., & Crocker, J. (2002). Race and self-esteem: Meta-analyses comparing Whites, Blacks, Hispanics, Asians, and American Indians and comment on Gray-Little and Hafdahl (2000). *Psychological Bulletin, 128*, 371–408.

Tylka, T.L., & Wood-Barcalow, N.L. (2015). A positive complement (special issue). *Body Image, 14*, 115–117.

Westerberg-Jacobson, J., Edlund, B., & Ghaderi, A. (2010). Risk and protective factors for disturbed eating: A 7-year longitudinal study of eating attitudes and psychological factors in adolescent girls and their parents. *Eating and Weight Disorders, 15*(4), 208–218.

Ziegler-Hill, V. (2007). Contingent self-esteem and race: Implications for the Black self-esteem advantage. *Journal of Black Psychology, 33,* 51–74.

Chapter Two
Women's Mental Health and Reproductive Events During Young Adulthood (Ages 20-39)

Diana Lynn Barnes

Across the female lifespan, women's mental health is governed by the continuous hormonal fluctuations that occur from puberty to menopause (Dossett, 2014). For women of reproductive age, there is a heightened sensitivity to the extraordinary hormonal changes that occur during pregnancy and in the postpartum with increased vulnerability to depression (Bromberger et al., 2009; Soares, 2013; Steiner, Dunn, & Born, 2003; Stewart, Gucciardi, & Grace, 2004). During young adulthood, women are encountering any number of psychosocial stressors as they navigate relationships, create families, and build careers. The degree of stress along with the existence or absence of adequate emotional support mediates the risks for the onset of mood and anxiety disorders during these delicate reproductive years (Beck, 2002b; Puryear, 2007). Although not all women of childbearing age either choose or are able to have children, the focus of this chapter is the psychological experience of women who do become mothers at some point in young adulthood because the reproductive milestone of childbearing is so intricately and frequently intertwined with psychological well-being during this time.

Birth

When considering women's mental health across the lifespan, there is no period of greater psychological and emotional vulnerability than during the reproductive years. Research indicates more psychiatric admissions around childbearing than at any other time in the female life cycle (Gavin et al., 2005; Munk-Olson, Larsen, Pedersen, Mors, & Mortensen, 2006). Studies indicate that, when left untreated, antenatal depression is a highly significant predictor of depression in the postpartum period (Katon, Russo, & Gavin, 2014). Untreated mood disorders during the peripartum period, the period around pregnancy and birth, rob new mothers of the very things they need to deepen the connection with their newborn, even while their baby is still in utero: motivation, enthusiasm, energy, joy, and a strong sense of feeling emotionally present.

Pregnancy

Despite the cultural myths that pregnancy is a period of ultimate fulfillment and emotional completeness, it can also be a time of emotional fragility that embodies much more than just the physical experience of growing a human being. Pregnancy involves a psychological gestation (Barnes, 2014) that brings together the elements of a woman's life story, her relationship with her own mother and her partner, along with her current life circumstances and what she believes society expects from her in this role. As laboring women bring their past with them into the birthing experience, they also bring the stories they have heard about birth, their own previous birth experiences, as well as the birth stories others have shared with them (Simkin, 2006).

Physiology and psychology are delicately interwoven during the nine months of pregnancy; as a woman's physical well-being affects her mind and her moods, so the reverse is true. Although we previously believed that the womb is a protected space that automatically shields the growing infant from a mother's emotional life during the peripartum, this no longer holds true. Undue stress elevates cortisol and studies conclude that those women whose mental health is compromised during pregnancy are at an increased risk of delivering a preterm and/or low-birthweight infant (Field, Diego, & Hernandez-Reif, 2006). In addition, untreated mood disorders during pregnancy disrupt the blossoming maternal–fetal attachment in utero that is so critical for the healthy psychological, social-emotional, and cognitive development of that child, not only in infancy but across the lifespan (Axness & Evans, 2014).

Some studies identify a woman's acceptance of her pregnancy as a fundamental developmental task whose resolution is a critical and integral part of the psychosocial adaptation to pregnancy (Davis-Floyd, 2004; Lederman & Weis, 2009). Whether or not a woman embraces her pregnancy influences her relationship with her baby beginning in utero while also affecting her ability to psychologically prepare for childbirth and motherhood. However, pregnancy and childbirth represent an emotional paradox for the expectant mother. While acceptance of her pregnancy deepens the sense of relationship between a mother and her infant that is so vital for a psychologically stable transition to motherhood, childbirth implies the first of many separations from her infant as well as a woman's own separation from her former sense of herself in the world as she carves out another way of seeing herself in the world.

Labor Day

Although our culture designates childbirth as the dividing line between pregnancy and motherhood—the split between past and present—contemporary understanding recognizes it as a psychologically pivotal transition in a woman's life (Barnes, 2014; Choi, Henshaw, Baker, & Tree, 2005; Smith, 1999). Just as the stage of transition during labor propels the baby from the cushion of the intrauterine environment into an unknown world, so does the experience of childbirth act as connective tissue between two disparate realms—the known one without a child and the unfamiliar universe called motherhood. For any number of women, being thrust into the present without an opportunity to integrate the life that came before baby can be destabilizing and terrifying, leaving them much more prone to depression and anxiety in the postpartum period (Barnes, 2014). Childbirth is a marker for the realization that her life will never be the same. Joy for the baby that has arrived often coexists with a profound sadness and grief as the life that she knew begins to vanish from the foreground.

Labor and delivery are psychologically complex events replete with intense emotions that run the gamut from euphoria to terror, embarrassment, joy, anxiety, impatience, and feelings of helplessness, empowerment, and even ambivalence (Barnes, 2007). For some women, childbirth is the most natural of physiological processes and for others, labor and delivery are mysterious, frightening, and unpredictable events where the unexpected *is* expected. A woman's perception of her pregnancy and of her birth experience sets the tone for the early weeks and months of the postpartum period, and frequently becomes a barometer by which she measures her own self-esteem.

While the intensity of women's feelings about negative aspects of their birth experiences may fade or shift over time, what seems to remain constant is women's impressions of the kind of attentive care they received (Simkin, 1991; Waldenstrom, 2004). When women feel respected, emotionally supported, and cared about during birth, that often has a long-term positive effect on the overall tone of the story a woman shares about her children's birth, even years after her grown children leave home. The sensitivity of birth professionals to a woman's needs during birth speaks to the critical importance of human connection as a fundamental requirement for an empowering birth that goes far beyond the medical logistics of getting a baby through the birth canal.

The conclusions from a number of studies that evaluated women's satisfaction with their birth experiences identified several contributing factors. A woman was more likely to report a satisfying outcome if she felt involved in decision making during childbirth, if she felt freedom from fear, and/or experienced a sense of emotional safety and unconditional acceptance from those professionals and family members who attended the birth (Hodnett, 2002; Lowe, 2002; Simkin, 1991, 1992). When a woman can reflect back on her experience with a sense that her overall vision for her birth was met, and that she had a voice in her own experience, she is more likely to feel empowered, to experience childbirth as transformational, even spiritual, with a sense of awe and pride for what she and her body were able to accomplish together (Hodnett, 2002; Simkin, 1992).

The Process of Birth, Historically Speaking

A look back at the historical progression of childbirth confirms the significance of psychological support as a fundamental prerequisite for the laboring woman (Leavitt, 1986). The birthing experiences of women in colonial America reveal a dramatically different scenario than the medicalized hospital births of the current era. Women gave birth at home, surrounded by other women who could offer emotional support and advice through shared experience.

Although midwives helped navigate the events of labor and delivery, a woman mostly took charge of her own birth experience. Women chose the physical setting for birth; they decided which of their female neighbors, friends, or relatives would attend and what assistance they needed to feel most comforted during labor and childbirth. Many of their female attendants stayed on for days or even weeks following delivery in order to support the new mother during the "lying-in period" as she made the transition to motherhood (Leavitt, 1986). Men only attended births on the rare occasion that other women were not available. Physicians were seldom called, and only in cases where labor failed to progress normally.

During this era, however, prevailing beliefs and messages about pregnancy and birth set the stage for the emergence of "social childbirth" (Wertz & Wertz, 1977). A woman's pregnancy and birthing experience were anything but a cause for celebration; instead pregnancy spelled trepidation and dread. Religious teachings accentuated women's fears. In Genesis, it was said that "I will greatly increase your pangs in childbearing; in pain shall you bring forth children" (Genesis, 3:16). Biblical caution in tandem with poor birth outcomes where maternal and infant mortality was common left women anticipating their own deaths each time they became pregnant. The idea that women could bond over childbirth, offer each other encouragement and relief from the terrors of labor and the anticipated threats to self that were associated with impending childbirth acted as a catalyst for the social nature of birth during this time (Leavitt, 1986).

By the 20th century, however, the traditions that embraced childbirth as a social event began to change as doctors became a routinely integral part of the landscape of childbirth, attending nearly half of the nation's babies (Cassidy, 2006; Leavitt, 1986). Although home births were still considered the norm, the dynamics around the birthing bed shifted as technology and medicine slowly took priority over the emotional experience of childbearing women and the presence of midwives in American births declined significantly. By the 1940s, more than half of all births in the United States happened in hospitals; by 1973, midwives had just about disappeared from the scene (Cassidy, 2006). It was now understood that a hospital birth meant a medicated birth. In comparison, those countries that recognize birth as a natural process, not an illness to be treated, and where midwives attend most of the births have a much lower rate of surgical deliveries (Gaskin, 2011). In the Netherlands, for example, where home births are quite common, and the culture of childbirth embraces normality, there are considerably lower rates of obstetrical interference (Christiaens, Neiuwenhuijze, & deVries, 2013).

Childbirth Without Fear

British obstetrician Grantley Dick-Read believed that education and support were the precursors to a positive, even painless, birth experience, having observed that women suffered during labor because they were anxious and frightened. His observations were rooted in scientific understanding that fear complicates childbirth by signaling the body to shut down normally existing processes in response to the fight-or-flight reflex. He promoted these views in his groundbreaking book *Childbirth Without Fear* (Dick-Read, 1984), which set the tone for the natural childbirth movement, and gained momentum by the middle of the 20th century.

He recognized that a woman's physical alertness and emotional calm during labor and birth facilitated the initial bonding between mother and infant—what he referred to as "mother love" (Dick-Read, 1984). He encouraged breastfeeding, and reintroduced the idea that loving care was critical to a successful birth experience, inviting husbands, those who could quell their own anxieties, into the birthing room to provide the much-needed psychological support. His work was the catalyst for other natural-birth approaches and philosophies like that of Fernand Lamaze, whose 1984 classic, *Painless Childbirth: The Lamaze Method,* set forth the idea that, during pregnancy, women could be conditioned to become desensitized to pain during childbirth. The Lamaze method also led to our more contemporary understanding that birth is a normal human process that doesn't automatically require drugs or medical intervention to proceed.

Along with this renewed awareness of natural birth came the added insight that the language used to describe birth cues women's emotions, which in turn influences their attitudes and that becomes a huge determinant of a woman's birth experience (Simkin, 2012). With the advent of hypnobirthing came a stark change in birth language. The word contraction was replaced by surges and waves; pain was merely pressure; no longer were there birth coaches, only birth companions, and a baby is birthed, not delivered (Cassidy, 2006).

Coming Full Circle

The word midwife finds its origins in the language of Old England. It derives from the word *mit*, meaning "with" and *wif*, which means woman (O'Boyle, 2014). The idea of being with a woman during her birthing experience emphasizes the critical importance of psychological support in fostering her power to birth. Drs. John Kennell and Marshall Klaus happened upon the significance of emotional support during childbirth while doing research on maternal bonding (Cassidy, 2006; Klaus, Kennell, & Klaus, 2012).

In 1975, there was no word for a woman who was not a midwife, but whose role was to provide physical and emotional support to the laboring woman through reassurance and encouragement; consequently, Dana Raphael, in her book, *The Tender Gift* (1955), was the first to borrow from the Greek language and refer to these special caregivers as *doulas*. Klaus and Kennell initiated a groundbreaking study (Klaus, Kennell, & Klaus, 1993) that looked at the potential benefits of a doula-attended birth using two groups of laboring women—those with doulas and those without. The conclusions from their research indicated that, in women who had doulas present at their births, there was a 25% reduction in the length of labor, a 50% reduction in caesarean births, and epidural requests for pain management were significantly reduced by 60% among those women who had doula support (Klaus, Kennell, & Klaus, 1993). Dr. Michel Odent, well known in the international birth community for his influence on birth practices, identifies the doula as an essential part of the transition to motherhood (Odent, 2012). He maintains that the doula as a nurturing and maternal presence that a woman can rely on before, during, and after birth furthers the "rediscovery of authentic midwifery" (Odent, 2012).

When Pregnancy Looks Different

Traditionally, pregnancy concerns have focused on both the physical well-being of the growing infant in utero and the mother's physical well-being as a contributory factor in her baby's healthy development. There was very limited recognition of the connection between a woman's state of mind and the look of her pregnancy. Even less attention was paid to the significance of psychosocial stress as a tipping point for what has been described in some literature as reproductive dysfunction (Amon et al., 2012).

The possibility that a woman could be totally unaware she was pregnant seems to defy all logic and rational thought. Yet, approximately one out of 475 women experience a pervasive denial of their pregnancies (Amon et al., 2012) in which they carry to term without any concrete knowledge that they are carrying a baby. This phenomenon emerges within a psychosocial context in which women feel threatened by the possible repercussions, e.g., abandonment, if they should reveal their pregnancies (Meyer & Oberman, 2001; Miller, 2003). In essence, the mind signals the body to suppress any conscious acknowledgment of a pregnancy, which then results in a woman's misinterpretation of pregnancy-related symptoms that continues through labor and delivery (Miller, 2003; Spinelli, 2003). As example, pregnancy-related weight gain is attributed to overeating; a young woman may have occasional bleeding throughout the pregnancy which seems to confirm her negation of the pregnancy. Pregnancy tests may even be negative. Because there is no awareness of a pregnancy, women consequently receive no prenatal care (Friedman, Heneghan, & Rosenthal, 2007). Even labor is misidentified as severe gastrointestinal distress, or the need to have a bowel movement (Bonnet, 1993). Families often partner in this denial with no suspicions that a baby is coming, even when they are in the room next door as she labors.

Most often, these young women give birth in the bathroom with no understanding of what is really occurring, and sadly, these babies frequently die, and their mothers are charged with murder. Neonaticide is the term used to describe the death of an infant within the first 24 hours of life (Resnick, 1969). In later recalling the events of labor and delivery, women describe dissociative symptoms around their infants' births. Many report depersonalization and derealization in which they feel like observers, rather than participants in what is occurring; in the immediate aftermath of labor and delivery, they often firmly believe their baby is deceased (Spinelli, 2001). In a state of shock, panic, and shame at the sudden realization they have birthed a baby whom they believe is stillborn, women frequently take steps to dispose of the infant, not knowing what else to do.

A review of the psychosocial histories of women who deny their pregnancies in this way reveals a backdrop of personal trauma, along with family chaos and dysfunction, including substance abuse, physical, emotional, and/or sexual trauma, and family violence (Spinelli, 2001, 2003). In any number of cases, women have given birth before, attending to their older children with love and care. Their backgrounds generally show no prior interaction with law enforcement or department of children's services (Twomey, 2009).

Sometimes women acknowledge the reality of a pregnancy but their feelings are blunted instead of the heightened emotional sensitivity one would expect to see (Miller, 2003). In this affective denial, there are very few preparations made for the baby's arrival, there is no talk about the baby, no visualizing of the relationship; instead there is an avoidance of anything that might be a reminder of the impending birth. It can appear that this expecting mother is having difficulty adjusting to the idea of becoming a mother, for the first time or again, but in fact, the baby is a traumatic reminder of the dramatic changes in her life she would hope to avoid.

For women who experience a psychotic denial of their pregnancies, the fact of a baby on the way is so intolerable that these pregnancies are embraced in a delusional way (Friedman et al., 2007; Miller, 2003). A woman might perceive that there is a blood clot causing her symptoms, or a tumor that needs to be excised. An indepth look at her psychiatric history along with current psycho-social stressors often uncovers clues to understanding how a pregnancy took such a turn.

Just as a pregnancy can be denied, it can also be created in the mind of a young woman who longs for a child. Pseudocyesis is a clinical syndrome in which a woman who is not pregnant maintains a delusional belief that she is (Rosch, Sajatovic, & Sivec, 2003). Her conviction is supported by the emergence of somatic signs that give the appearance of a pregnancy. Among the reported symptoms of pseudocyesis are amenorrhea, enlarged breasts and abdomen, changes in the uterus as well as around the nipples and areolae. Some women report sensations of fetal movement in addition to the objective symptoms of pregnancy, including nausea, vomiting, and weight gain (Brockington, 2000). Abdominal ultrasound, however, shows an absence of any developing fetus or placenta. Most women who develop a phantom pregnancy suffer from depression or anxiety. Undue emotional stress caused by psychological conflicts or needs acts as a catalyst for the neuroendocrine changes associated with this disorder (Tarin, Hermenegildo, Garcia-Perez, & Cano, 2013).

Recurrent pregnancy losses, infertility, impending menopause coupled with the intense yearning or even fear of a pregnancy are some of the pathways to the emergence of symptoms (Ibekwe & Achor, 2008). Cultures that place a high value on a woman's ability to produce children have higher rates of this disorder (Savs, Derganc, & Licina, 2012). Pseudocyesis needs to be understood as the interplay between psychological, sociocultural, and endocrine factors that create a powerful connection between the mind and body.

Infertility

There is an unspoken and unconscious agreement that a woman has with her own body. When she is ready to have children, she will conceive quickly, carry to term without interruption, and give birth without incident (Barnes, 2014; Raphael-Leff, 2013). Embedded in this non-negotiable contract is a vision of the relationship with her imagined child, along with the fantasies and dreams of what the future holds. When any of these elements of the reproductive timeline fall short of what a woman firmly anticipates, the stark realization that her body will not be able to do what she believes nature intended it to do has profound repercussions for her feelings about herself, her emotional life, and even her mental health (Ismail, Crome, & O'Brien, 2006; Miles, Keitel, Jackson, Harris, & Licciardi, 2009). One study found that depressive symptoms in women with infertility are similar to those found in women with chronic illnesses, such as cancer, bypass surgery, and HIV-positive status (Domar, Zuttermeister, & Friedman, 1993).

Reproductive Technology

Worldwide, more than 70 million couples are affected by infertility (Ombelet, Cooke, Dyer, Serour, & Devroey, 2008). According to a 2012 Centers for Disease Control report, utilizing key statistics from the National Survey of Family Growth (2006–2010), 6.7 million women in the United States aged 15–44 will experience infertility. The American Society for Reproductive Medicine (ASRM) defines infertility as "no evidence of conception after 1 year of trying in a couple where the female partner is less than age 35, and after 6 months of trying when the female partner is age 35 and older (ASRM, 2008). In primary infertility, a woman has never been pregnant, whereas in secondary infertility a woman has been pregnant in the past (ASRM, 2013).

Assisted reproductive technology instills hope because it offers the promise of fulfilling the vision of motherhood and family, and there are a wide range of options available to women, depending on the causes of her infertility and her age. In an intrauterine insemination sperm from either the intended father or a sperm donor is placed directly into the uterus immediately prior to, or during, ovulation to facilitate conception. In vitro fertilization (IVF) involves the removal of oocytes, either from the intended mother or from an egg donor, that are fertilized with sperm from the husband, partner, or donor. The resulting embryo is transferred to the woman's uterus. Sometimes frozen embryos are also used. When a woman is unable to carry a pregnancy to term, IVF with a gestational surrogacy is another option. In this procedure, the fertilized embryos are transferred into the uterus of the surrogate who then hopefully carries the pregnancy to term.

At the same time that technologically induced conception brings hope that almost anything is possible in order to have a baby, it also acts as a catalyst for a whole range of psychological questions and emotional issues (Notman, 2011). The woman who carries a baby to whom she is not genetically related may have very specific wants about hair and eye color in order to create a sense of genetic connection in her own mind. When a woman receives a baby from the union of a gestational surrogate and her husband's sperm, she becomes the adoptive mother with no genetic or biological ties. There may even be envy that the infant who is born belongs to her husband, and she is not the *real mother*. Women frequently worry about how and when or even whether they will talk to their child about his/her origins. Some women feel shame that they have had to go to such great lengths to birth a child, withholding the information from family and friends, hoping no one will suspect.

Conception

The longing to produce a child permeates a woman's psyche at so many different levels. The inability to conceive can feel as though a death has occurred (Schwerdtfeger & Shreffler, 2009). And in many ways it has. Each unsuccessful attempt at procreation not only means that a woman must deal with the potential loss of a future baby, but it also requires her to cope with the painful loss of the dreams, expectations, and hope that are an integral part of the reproductive story she has been scripting since childhood (Jaffe & Diamond, 2011).

Sometimes, the fractured vision feels even more devastating than the physical and emotional challenges of the infertility itself. With each new menstrual cycle, with each procedure, a woman may feel as though she is caught in a relentless succession of hanging on to optimism and possibility followed by the devastating letdown that occurs when she realizes once again that conception has failed to take place, followed once more by a push for renewed hope that the next try will result in the pregnancy she is working so hard to achieve. The loss of control a woman feels over her situation, her body, and her sense of self as a woman are exacerbated by infertility treatments that leave her feeling even less in control, and often feeling as though her body is being invaded by relentless testing and procedures (Greil, 2002).

The failure to conceive has a pervasive effect that extends beyond a woman's reproductive capabilities. Infertility frequently stirs doubts about her competency in other areas of her life (Raphael-Leff, 2013; Valentine, 1987). This self-doubt also plays a role in the downward spiral into depression.

The Biological Clock

For contemporary women, the pattern of their reproductive lives is dramatically different than in previous generations. This is due in large part because, over the years, women have had increasingly more autonomy over their own bodies, and no longer feel confined to traditional ideals and structures around childbearing. Today, women have choices as to when they get pregnant, how to get pregnant, with whom to get pregnant, and even if they'd like to be pregnant at all (Raphael-Leff, 2013). Delaying motherhood, however, until a woman feels that the pieces of her life are in place, whether professionally, economically, or emotionally, has physical ramifications due to the age-related decline in fertility, commonly referred to as the biological clock (Winkler, 2014). While women in the 1950s were generally bearing children in their 20s, it is not unusual for women of this generation to have their first child between age 27 and 30 (Matthews & Hamilton, 2009). The numbers of women giving birth after 40 has doubled within the last ten years (Raphael-Leff, 2013).

Perinatal Loss

Any discussion about infertility must also include a conversation about perinatal loss and its psychological impact. Perinatal loss refers to a range of reproductive events related to conception, pregnancy, and birth (Callister, 2006). This includes infertility along with miscarriage, stillbirth, preterm birth, birth of a child with anomalies, and neonatal death. Most first-trimester miscarriages result from chromosomal abnormalities that interfere with fetal development. An ectopic pregnancy, in which conception takes place outside the uterus, generally in one of the fallopian tubes, often necessitates a medical termination and is also considered an early-pregnancy loss. Beyond 20 weeks, fetal death is termed a stillbirth and occurs in approximately 1% of pregnancies (MacDorman & Gregory, 2015).

The emotional content of a woman's grief is not limited to sadness. Positive feelings and hopeful expectations are most often replaced by shock, anger, and despair. Studies suggest that the emotional repercussions following pregnancy loss run the gamut from anger and helplessness to anxiety and depression (Geller, Kerns, & Klier, 2004; Lim & Cheng, 2011; Lok & Neugebauer, 2007; Shreffler, Greil, & McQuillan, 2011). There may be feelings of intense despair, frustration, resentment, irritability, powerlessness, and rage. Women often feel ashamed of the surprising bitterness they feel in the company of other women who do have children.

Some women feel a sense of guilt, alienation, and isolation (Adolfsson, Larsson, Wimja, & Bertö, 2004). They may experience feelings of emptiness with worry that the void will remain unfulfilled, and that they will never again be able to experience joy (Arnold & Gemma, 2008). A woman may blame herself for the fetal demise, believing she is responsible, and that she failed to protect her baby in utero.

In some cases, psychological symptoms associated with miscarriage may persist as long as one year following the loss (Lok & Neugebauer, 2007). One Finnish study conducted between 1987 and 1994 that looked at suicide rates of women who had experienced miscarriage in the last year of their lives found significantly higher numbers of suicides than among women who had given birth and among women in the general population of reproductive age (Gissler, Hemminki, & Lonnqvist, 1996). The study by Lok and Neugebauer (2007) that addressed psychological morbidity following miscarriage identified a number of predisposing risk factors that included a pre-existing history of perinatal loss, prior psychiatric illness, childlessness, a lack of social/partner support, as well as a woman's ambivalence toward the fetus.

Attempting to grieve the losses that often recur with infertility while trying to maintain a sense of hopefulness about a positive outcome can feel emotionally complicated. A woman's psychological distress following pregnancy loss is further complicated by the realities of her infertility. Giving herself permission to mourn each successive loss may feel as though she is giving into the realities of her situation. Research suggests that women who face reproductive challenges have significantly poorer mental health overall than those women without reproductive issues (Badenhorst & Hughes, 2007; Schwerdtfeger & Shreffler, 2009).

A study by Schwerdtfeger and Shreffler (2009) assessing women's emotional reactions to their infertility found that, among women who experienced pregnancy loss, their responses included anger at God, feeling cheated by life, feeling as though their infertility was a punishment, feelings of inadequacy, and that their bodies have failed them, undermining their sense of themselves as women. Longitudinal research that looked at psychological morbidity in a sample of 280 miscarrying women found that, immediately after the loss, approximately 25% scored high enough on the Beck Depression Inventory to meet criteria for a depressive episode (Lok, Yip, Lee, Sahota, & Chung, 2010).

Despite the frequent generalization of Kubler-Ross' four stages of grieving in dying individuals to all kinds of grief experiences (1969), there is no timetable to grief. It is neither time-limited, nor is it linear. With perinatal loss, the intensity of one's grief is not determined by the length of the pregnancy (Badenhorst & Hughes, 2007; Lim & Cheng, 2011). Perinatal loss has been described as an ambiguous loss (Lang et al., 2011). While there is an intense psychological experience, there is the physical absence of the fetus or infant.

This ambiguity is compounded by society's minimization of this special kind of loss coupled with a lack of understanding as to why a woman's grief may be prolonged and so intense. Consequently, women often feel disenfranchised in their grief as compared to those women who experience traditionally accepted losses (Cacciatore, 2013; Jaffe & Diamond, 2011). They may find it difficult to validate their own emotional experience when it's not backed by the prevailing cultural beliefs around grieving. Mourning the death of an elder parent, for example, is made easier because there are memories to call upon, a story to tell, and religious or cultural rituals to facilitate the grieving process. This kind of death represents a loss of the past, unlike a perinatal death, which represents the loss of the future (Arnold & Gemma, 1994). The growing body of research understands that for some women perinatal loss is experienced as a traumatic event (Shakhar & Fleisig, 2014; Turton, Hughes, Evans, & Fainman, 2001), with studies documenting clinically recognized posttraumatic symptoms in women whose reproductive challenges include infertility, high-risk pregnancies, and pregnancy loss (Brier, 2004; Carter, Misri, & Tomfohr, 2007; Lok & Neugebauer, 2007).

Understanding the Grief of Perinatal Loss

The seemingly incontrovertible belief that when we're ready for motherhood, our bodies will obey and our babies will just come is shattered by the reality of a pregnancy loss. There is a wonderful naiveté about a first pregnancy that disappears with the pain of loss. Even a full-term pregnancy with a successful outcome can never restore that innocence. A pregnancy will never be experienced in the same way again. It changes the relationship a woman has with her own body.

Furthermore, the pain of pregnancy loss does not automatically resolve in the next pregnancy. A subsequent pregnancy following a miscarriage is not a replacement for the pregnancy that came before. In most cases, women predict another loss, and there is an unwavering stance that "I'll believe it when I see it" and they are actually holding their babies in their arms.

Anxiety takes center stage for women who are pregnant again after perinatal loss. As protection against anticipated loss, women often sequester any positive feelings about the pregnancy by lowering their expectations, pulling back from excitement, or even blocking out the loss as self-protection against any possibility of incurring the emotional devastation caused by previous losses (Cote-Arsenault & Donato, 2010; Van, 2012). In a psychological process termed "emotional cushioning" (Cote-Arsenault & Donato, 2010), women regulate their emotional connection to the fetus in any number of ways. For example, they may delay sharing the news about the pregnancy or put off any of the usual physical preparations that are made before the baby comes home (Côté-Arsenault, Donato, & Earl, 2006; Côté-Arsenault & Marshall, 2000). Depending on where the prior loss occurred along the gestational line often becomes a marker in a subsequent pregnancy for when she feels like she can hopefully stop holding her breath.

Even with a successful birth after pregnancy, the sense of vulnerability often continues with mothers feeling more hypervigilant and overprotective with the next child (Côté-Arsenault & Freije, 2004). And when there is recurrent perinatal loss, the feeling of being betrayed by her own body can result in an unraveling of a woman's self-worth and sense of femininity (Shakhar & Fleisig, 2014).

Because the threat and possibility of repeated loss persist, the heightened anxiety and hypervigilance that are symptoms of posttraumatic stress (American Psychiatric Association, 2013) dominate the emotional landscape. There is a complete loss of trust in her body's ability to sustain a pregnancy, so she may spend much of the pregnancy checking for signs that this unborn child is still alive. It is difficult to feel close and connected to someone you expect to lose. Consequently, the terror that comes with anticipated loss in a subsequent pregnancy often disrupts the developing attachment relationship in utero and leaves some women that much more vulnerable to depressed mood.

Helping Women Cope

Grief is a normal reaction to loss, and bereavement is an integral part of the human experience. Because of the seemingly pervasive cultural discomfort with sadness and mourning, there is a mistaken idea that resolving a perinatal loss requires a woman to put the loss behind her as though it never occurred. Women frequently hear that message, in the well-intentioned, but clearly misguided, comments of friends and family following perinatal loss: "It wasn't meant to be"; "At least you have other children"; "Don't worry, you can always have another child"; "One day, this will all be behind you"; "This was God's plan for you." On the contrary, these kinds of comments are less than reassuring, and actually stifle the grieving process, leaving women more isolated in their pain and despair, and much more vulnerable to psychological repercussions, including prolonged depression. A study by Van (2012) concluded that feeling connected to others helped women cope with their grief reactions.

Grieving is a necessary part of healing, but how a woman processes her grief is determined by a number of factors: her ethnicity and religion, the specific beliefs of her culture around death and loss, as well as her feelings of attachment (Jaffe & Diamond, 2011). Although women are likely to employ protective strategies like emotional cushioning to cope with loss, when women are encouraged to talk about their experiences in a compassionate and supportive environment in which they feel heard, they tend to cope more effectively with their grief than women who did not have the opportunity to connect (Cacciatore, 2007; Swanson, Chen, Graham, Wognar, & Petras, 2009; Van, 2012).

Creating a Bridge between the Past and the Future

An early study by Peppers and Knapp (1980) found that maternal attachment begins long before conception. Even before giving birth, planning the pregnancy, confirmation and acceptance of the pregnancy, experiencing the beginnings of fetal movement and the realization of the fetus as an individual are key events that contribute to the formation of maternal–infant attachment. That attachment between a mother and her child exists across the lifespan and, while fetal demise certainly curtails maternal–infant connection, the existence of that child-to-be and what might have been is never forgotten (Arnold & Gemma, 2008).

Grief is the struggle to maintain relatedness to that which was and to what is now. Validation of one's loss is essential to a healthy grieving process (Robinson, Baker, & Nackerud, 1999). Deliberate rumination and preoccupation with the loss serve a function in allowing a woman (and also her partner) to fully process what has occurred (Black & Wright, 2012). In a subsequent pregnancy, societal tenets about moving beyond her grief, and starting over create an emotional conflict for the grieving woman, who becomes caught between an attachment for the baby that was, and a blossoming connection with the baby that will come to be (O'Leary, 2004).

Attachment bonds are not automatically surrendered because of loss. However, they can be reshaped and transformed in such a way as to enhance emotional access to the development of new attachments (Romanoff & Terenzio, 1998). Creating a psychological space in which a woman can feel the freedom to maintain a connection to the baby who died is highly adaptive. It paves the way for her to feel emotionally available for all other relationships, not just for a future child (Attig; 2001; Cote-Arsenault, 2003; O'Leary, 2004).

Becoming Mom

The culture of motherhood upholds the idea that childbirth is just another day in the life of a woman, marked, of course, by the specialness of having a baby; not to be viewed, however, as much more than a temporary interruption in the responsibilities and obligations of daily life. The peripartum period brings a woman face to face with the inconsistencies between the expectations shaped by societal lore and the real story of pregnancy, birth, and motherhood (Barnes, 2007). Much of the psychology of pregnancy, and the mental health of women in the postpartum, is organized around the myth that babies are born and nothing much changes.

There is the added fiction that motherhood is natural, instinctive, and spontaneous, that a baby is born and everything falls into place. The societal fallacy of the maternal instinct inevitably leads to disappointment, discouragement, and even feelings of failure in new mothers (Barnes, 2014). Maternal archetypes of mothers as all-knowing, forever loving, and relentlessly available dismiss the demands and the nuances of this extraordinary relationship between a new mother and her infant. The psychological stress created by these misguided ideas leaves vulnerable women even that much more vulnerable to mood and anxiety disorders in the peripartum (Beck, 2002a).

Learning to be a Mother

As a baby is born, so a mother is also born as she is delivered into a role she has been preparing for long before her baby is even conceived. Each woman's understanding of motherhood is unique. The story of her life creates a tapestry of sensations, emotions, and mental representations from which her own meanings of motherhood emerge. Although there may be many teachers along the way, the greatest sense of a woman's maternal identity finds its origins in the memories and recollections of her attachment to her own mother (Menken, 2008). It is her earliest experiences with her primary attachment figure that shapes a woman's adult attitudes and beliefs about what it means to become a mom. Ideas about her own mother as mother to her are not only a powerful influence on her behavior as a mother to her infant now, but the single best predictor of the kind of attachment relationship she establishes with her own infant by one year of age (Fonagy, Steele, & Steele, 1991). How was she loved and mothered and nurtured? Did she feel she was a bother or a burden to her own mother? The emotional template created by the earliest attachment experience becomes embedded in a woman's mind and in her visceral responses to motherhood (Barnes, 2014). It has been suggested that postpartum depression is a response to unmet attachment needs (Whiffen & Johnson, 1998).

There is an ongoing and all-consuming internal and external dialogue that exists in the minds of new mothers during gestation that continues into the postpartum period (Stern, 1998). Often, the discourse resides comfortably in the periphery of a woman's awareness but catapults into consciousness after the baby comes, shattering any preconceived ideas she may have about motherhood. The life-altering transition from pregnancy to motherhood requires a dramatic change in self-perception along with a shift in existing priorities, behaviors, values, and relationships with others (Barnes, 2014; Lederman & Weis, 2009).

The expected joy of motherhood is often accompanied by unforeseen terror as a new mother realizes she is responsible for the very survival of another (Stern, 1998), at the same time that she herself is attempting to keep her head above water. She may begin to question her ability to be sufficiently nurturing and emotionally engaged with her infant so as to create a solid psychological foundation for that child's healthy development across his/her life. A mother's capacity to reach out to others for support, whether husband, partner, family members, or friends, can help to buffer the sense of isolation and loneliness so many women experience in the early weeks and months postpartum (Dennis, 2003; Evans, Donelle, & Hume-Loveland, 2012; Surkan, Peterson, Hughes, & Gottlieb, 2006).

Time for Growth

At the same time that the early months of motherhood are filled with upheaval and a frequent sense of feeling lost, it has also been recognized as a pivotal life transition that engenders personal growth (Taubman-Ben-Ari, Shlomo, Sivan, & Dolizki, 2009, Tedeschi & Calhoun, 2004). Experiences that are life altering, like the transition to motherhood, challenge a woman's existing self-concept and her feelings about herself in the world (Calhoun & Tedeschi, 2001). Motherhood affords women the opportunity to rescript a life narrative that may have kept them stuck in old story lines that disempowered them (Bailey, 1999).

For some women, the transition to motherhood opens the door to an increased sense of purpose and meaning in life. Women gain self-esteem, increased confidence, competence, and a growing self-awareness of positive aspects of themselves (Wells, Hobfoll, & Lavin, 1999). For other women, immersion into motherhood brings with it increased patience and a deepening insight about the meaning of love and empathy along with an increasing sensitivity to all children, not just their own (Nelson, 2003). The birth of a child becomes a catalyst for the psychological rebirth of a woman in which past and present merge to create a new sense of oneself in the world (Raphael-Leff, 1991). Giving voice to the nuances and complexities of women's authentic experiences of motherhood empowers them (Barnes, 2006, 2014).

Family and Work Balance: Having it All

Approximately 80% of women who work during pregnancy return to their employment within the first year of their infant's life (US Department of Labor, 2015). At some point during pregnancy or in the postpartum period, almost all working mothers consider whether they will be able to manage the simultaneous responsibilities of a demanding career and the obligations of their families. Society has told women they can have it all, but with very little support as to how to do it all. Cultural messages about good mothers leave many women in the precarious emotional position of feeling wrong about any of the choices they make for themselves and for their families following the births of their children. The phrase "being there" has become synonymous with good mothering.

As a result, the career woman with needs of her own who carves out an identity separate from her children is judged as a bad mother who is indifferent to their needs (Agonito, 2014). And the successful career woman who opts out of the workforce temporarily or permanently to stay home with her children is demeaned for seemingly have abandoned her career. However, societal judgments fail to acknowledge that it might have been a decision filled with ambivalence and distress, and in some cases a choice that was forced upon her (Mason & Ekman, 2007). The postpartum mother who wants to be at home full time is regarded as unfulfilled and uninteresting.

Contemporary women find themselves wedged between their own needs and the misguided expectations imposed by societal myths; cultural ideology becomes embedded in women's consciousness to the extent that they are now their own judge and jury in the individual decisions they make. In the privacy of the therapy room, postpartum women speak with shame and guilt at any wish they might have about decisions and choices. There is the guilt-ridden mom who struggles to reclaim even a piece of the self she knew before motherhood but worries that her daughter will perceive her as unavailable. There is the career woman who is headed back to her position filled with anxiety at the thought of separation and the imagined long-term repercussions for her daughter's development. Although most mothers experience some anxiety at the thought of separating from their infant, heightened maternal separation anxiety has a deleterious effect on maternal mental health, including symptoms of anxiety and depression (Hock & Schirtzinger, 1992; Hsu, 2004). Excessive fearfulness about separation may also interfere with a woman's capacity to balance infant care with other activities, including return to employment (Cooklin, Rowe, & Fisher, 2011).

While some early studies do confirm higher levels of psychological distress among working mothers (Aneshensel, Frerichs, & Clark, 1981; McLanahan & Adams, 1987; Radloff, 1975), other studies conclude that married women with children who are employed outside the home are less depressed and in better emotional health (Ahrens & Ryff, 2006; Barnett & Hyde, 2001; Gove & Geerken, 1977). Their explanation is that multiple roles enhance access to resources; these supports that help women cope more effectively with the added stress of employment actually enhance emotional resilience.

An early study by Symonds (1986) concluded that functioning women who are unable to identify and realize their own needs because they have been socialized to find their identity by nurturing and caring for others have higher levels of depression. Other studies suggest that depression results from the psychological pull some women experience between the benefits of employment and their beliefs in the traditional archetype of mother (Hilbrecht, Shaw, Johnson, & Audrey, 2008; Hock & DeMeis, 1990; Quesenberry, Trauth, & Morgan, 2006). In particular, the study by Hock and DeMeis (1990) examined the effects of women's conflicts between their employment preference and employment status and found that depressive symptoms were highest among those mothers who preferred employment, but stayed at home. Homemakers who wanted a career had the lowest self-esteem of any of the groups that were questioned about their preferences (Hock & DeMeis, 1990).

Another study concluded that employed mothers who work in high-quality jobs reported fewer depressive symptoms than those women working in low-quality jobs (Usdansky, Gordon, Wang, & Gluzman, 2011). The sense of accomplishment and confidence that women in high-quality jobs are more likely to experience has a positive impact on maternal mental health (Usdansky et al., 2011). Another consideration in supporting women's mental health following childbirth is the length of maternity leave. One study found that fewer than 12 weeks' maternity leave was not only associated with higher levels of maternal depression and lowered self-esteem, but mothers were less engaged with their infants and less knowledgeable about their children's development (Feldman, Sussman, & Zigler, 2004).

Women with postpartum depression face additional unique challenges in managing the stress overload that is generally expected when balancing employment and family. Many women return to work within 6 weeks after maternity leave, or sooner, depending on their individual circumstances. As a consequence of their depression, they may feel emotionally unprepared to return to work with its accompanying stress and so there is increased absenteeism (Goodman & Crouter, 2009). Women often have difficulties in extending their medical disability after a normal birth or problems finding suitable childcare, which only exacerbates their depressive symptoms. Because they may feel shame and embarrassment about how they are feeling, they rarely share how they are feeling. However, when they do report symptoms of depression, they are often stigmatized and blamed for their illness by coworkers and/or employers (Selix & Goyal, 2015). They may be perceived as weak and lacking personal strength to cope with an illness that others may believe is "all in your head."

So What Works

Flexible hours, flexible work conditions, and more job autonomy with employers who genuinely understand and support the challenges postpartum women face have been associated with lower work stress and better job performance (Galinsky, Bond, & Friedman, 1996). Shorter work hours, and higher childcare quality, facilitate an easier transition for women returning from maternity leave (Nichols & Roux, 2004). Women who return to employment after giving birth have unique needs that are critical to address. Helping women build communities of social support, accessing resources, and creating strategies for coping with the expected stress are at the foundation of successful adaptation during this transition to motherhood (McCubbin & McCubbin, 1993).

The cultural idealization of motherhood dominates the psychological landscape for women during the years of young adulthood. Even societal mandates that view childbearing as a biological imperative have a significant emotional impact on women whether or not they bring children into their lives. And when there is reproductive loss, it pokes holes in a woman's sense of herself that extends beyond her ability to reproduce. Societal fabrications about the experience of pregnancy and the postpartum period as euphoric and automatic set up in the minds of women unrealistic and unreasonable expectations that are impossible to fulfill. These myths negate the authentic and unique experience of each woman during this tender period. Understanding the developmental requirements of the reproductive years and the influence of the psychosocial milieu on mental health should be a focused concern for all health providers who care for women at this time in their lives.

References

Adolfsson, A., Larsson, P., Wimja, B., & Bertö, C. (2004). Guilt and emptiness: Women's experiences of miscarriage. *Health Care for Women International, 25,* 543–560.

Agonito, R. (2014). *The last taboo: Saying no to motherhood.* New York: Algora Publishing.

Ahrens, C.J.C., & Ryff, C.D. (2006). Multiple roles and well-being: Sociodemographic and psychological moderators. *Sex Roles, 55*(11–12), 801–815.

American Psychiatric Association. (2013). *Diagnostic and statistical manual of mental disorders,* 5th edn. Washington, D.C.: American Psychiatric Publishing.

American Society for Reproductive Medicine. (2008). Definitions of infertility and recurrent pregnancy loss. *Supplement to Fertility and Sterility, 2008 Compendium of Practice Committee Reports,* 90, S60.

American Society for Reproductive Medicine. (2013). Retrieved from https://www.asrm.org/Templates/Results.aspx?q=primary%20and%20secondary%20infertility%20definition

Amon, S., Putkonen, H., Weizmann-Henelius, G., Almiron, M.P., Formann, A.K., Voracek, M., & Klier, C.M. (2012). Potential predictors in neonaticide: The impact of the circumstances of pregnancy. *Archives of Women's Mental Health, 15*(3), 167–174.

Aneshensel, C.S., Frerichs, R.R., & Clark, V.A. (1981). Family roles and sex differences in depression. *Journal of Health and Social Behavior, 22,* 379–393.

Arnold, J.H., & Gemma, P.B. (1994). *A child dies: A portrait of family grief.* Philadelphia: The Charles Press Publishers.

Arnold, J., & Gemma, P.B. (2008). The continuing process of parental grief. *Death Studies, 32,* 658–673.

Attig, T. (2001). Relearning the world: Making and finding meanings. In R.A. Neimeyer (Ed.), *Meaning reconstruction and the experience of loss.* Washington, D.C.: American Psychological Association.

Axness, M., & Evans, J. (2014). Pre and perinatal influences on female mental health. In D.L. Barnes (Ed.), *Women's reproductive mental health across the lifespan* (pp. 3–26). New York: Springer.

Badenhorst, W., & Hughes, P. (2007). Psychological aspects of perinatal loss. *Best Practice and Research Clinical Obstetrics and Gynaecology, 21*(2), 249–259.

Bailey, L. (1999). Refracted selves? A study of changes in self-identity in the transition to motherhood. *Sociology, 33*(2), 335–352.

Barnes, D.L. (2006). Postpartum depression: Its impact on couples and marital satisfaction. *Journal of Systemic Therapies, 25*(3), 25–42.

Barnes, D.L. (2007). *The journey to parenthood: Myths, reality and what really matters.* Oxford: Radcliffe Publishers.

Barnes, D.L. (2014). The psychological gestation of motherhood. In D.L. Barnes (Ed.), *Women's reproductive mental health across the lifespan* (pp. 75–90). New York: Springer.

Barnett, R.C., & Hyde, J.S. (2001). Women, men, work and family—An expansionist theory. *American Psychologist, 56*(10), 781–796.

Beck, C.T. (2002a). Postpartum depression: A metasynthesis. *Qualitative Health Research, 12*(4), 453–472.

Beck, C.T. (2002b). Revision of the postpartum depression predictors inventory. *Journal of Obstetric, Gynecologic & Neonatal Nursing, 31*(4), 394–402.

Black, B.P., & Wright, P. (2012). Posttraumatic growth and transformation as outcomes of perinatal loss. *Illness, Crisis & Loss, 20*(3), 225–237.

Bonnet, C. (1993). Adoption at birth: Prevention against neonaticide. *Child Abuse and Neglect, 17,* 501–513.

Brier, N. (2004). Anxiety after miscarriage: A review of the empirical literature and implications for clinical practice. *Birth, 31,* 138–142.

Brockington, I. (2000). Obstetric and gynecological conditions associated with psychiatric disorder. In M.G. Gelder, J.J. Lopez-Ibor, & N. Andreasen (Eds.), *New Oxford Textbook of Psychiatry, v2* (pp. 1195–1209). Oxford: Oxford University Press..

Bromberger, J.T., Kravvitz, H.M., Matthews, K., Youk, A., Brown, C., & Feng, W. (2009). Predictors of first lifetime episodes of major depression in midlife women. *Psychological Medicine, 39,* 55–64.

Cacciatore, J. (2007). Effects of support groups on posttraumatic stress responses in women experiencing stillbirth. *Omega, 55*(1), 71–90.

Cacciatore, J. (2013). Psychological effects of stillbirth. *Seminars in Fetal and Neonatal Medicine, 18*(2), 76–82.

Calhoun, L.G., & Tedeschi, R.G. (2001). *Posttraumatic growth: The positive lessons of loss.* Washington, D.C.: American Psychological Association.

Callister, L.C. (2006). Perinatal loss: A family perspective. *The Journal of Perinatal and Neonatal Nursing, 20*(3), 227–234.

Carter, D., Misri, S., & Tomfohr, L. (2007). Psychologic aspects of early pregnancy loss. *Clinical Obstetrics and Gynecology, 50*(1), 154–165.

Cassidy, T. (2006). *Birth: The surprising history of how we are born.* New York: Atlantic Monthly Press.

Centers for Disease Control and Prevention. (2012). *Infertility*. Retrieved from http://www.cdc. gov/nchs/fastats/fertile.htm (accessed November 2, 2016).

Choi, P., Henshaw, C., Baker, S., & Tree, J. (2005). Supermum, superwife, supereverything: Performing femininity in the transition to motherhood. *Journal of Reproductive and Infant Psychology, 23*(2), 167–180.

Christiaens, W., Nieuwenhuijze, M.J., & deVries, R. (2013). Trends in the medicalisation of childbirth in Flanders and the Netherlands. *Midwifery, 29*, e1–e8.

Cooklin, A., Rowe, H., & Fisher, J. (2011). Public health implications of paid parental leave: Evidence from a prospective cohort study. *Australian and New Zealand Journal of Public Health, 36*, 249–256.

Cote-Arsenault, D. (2003). Weaving babies lost in pregnancy into the fabric of the family. *Journal of Family Nursing, 9*(1), 23–37.

Cote-Arsenault, D., & Donato, K. (2010). Emotional cushioning in pregnancy after perinatal loss. *Journal of Reproductive and Infant Psychology, 29*(1), 81–92.

Côté-Arsenault, D., Donato, K., & Earl, S.S. (2006). Watching and worrying: Early pregnancy after loss experiences. *The American Journal of Maternal Child Nursing, 31*, 356–363.

Côté-Arsenault, D., & Freije, M.M. (2004). Support groups helping women through pregnancies after loss. *Western Journal of Nursing Research, 26*, 650–670.

Côté-Arsenault, D., & Marshall, R. (2000). One foot in—one foot out: Weathering the storm of pregnancy after perinatal loss. *Research in Nursing and Health, 23*, 473–485.

Davis-Floyd, R. (2004). *Birth as an American rite of passage*. Berkeley: University of California Press.

Dennis, C.L. (2003). The effect of peer support on postpartum depression: a pilot randomized controlled trial. *Canadian Journal of Psychiatry, 48*(2), 115–124.

Dick-Read, G. (1984). *Childbirth without fear: The original approach to natural childbirth*. New York: HarperCollins.

Domar, A.D., Zuttermeister, P.C., & Friedman, R. (1993). The psychological impact of infertility: Comparison with patients with other medical conditions. *Journal of Psychosomatic and Obstetrics and Gynecology, 14*, 45–52.

Dossett, E.C. (2014). The role of reproductive psychiatry in women's mental health. In D.L. Barnes (Ed.), *Women's reproductive mental health across the lifespan* (pp. 301–328). New York: Springer Publishing.

Evans, M., Donelle, L., & Hume-Loveland, L. (2012). Social support and online postpartum depression discussion groups: A content analysis. *Patient Education and Counseling, 87*(3), 405–410.

Feldman, R., Sussman, A.L., & Zigler, E. (2004). Parental leave and work adaptation at the transition to parenthood: Individual, marital, and social correlates. *Applied Developmental Psychology, 25*(4), 459–479.

Field, T., Diego, M., & Hernandez-Reif, M. (2006). Prenatal depression effects on the fetus and newborn: A review. *Infant Behavior and Development, 29*(3), 445–455.

Fonagy, P., Steele, H., & Steele, M. (1991). Maternal representations of attachment during pregnancy predict the organization of infant–mother attachment at one year of age. *Child Development, 62*(5), 891–905.

Friedman, S.H., Heneghan, A., & Rosenthal, M. (2007). Characteristics of women who deny or conceal pregnancy. *Psychosomatics, 48*(2), 117–122.

Galinsky, E., Bond, J.T., & Friedman, D.E. (1996). The role of employers in addressing the needs of employed parents. *Journal of Social Issues, 52*, 111–136.

Gaskin, I.M. (2011). *Birth matters: A midwife's manifesta*. New York: Seven Stories Press.

Gavin, N., Gaynes, N.B., Lohr, K., Meltzer-Brody, S., Gartlehner, G., & Swinson, T. (2005). Perinatal depression: A systematic review of prevalence and incidence. *Obstetrics and Gynecology, 106*(5), 1071–1083.

Geller, P.A., Kerns, D., & Klier, C.M. (2004). Anxiety following miscarriage and the subsequent pregnancy: A review of the literature and future directions. *Journal of Psychosomatic Research, 56*(1), 35–45.

Gissler, M., Hemminki, E., & Lonnqvist, J. (1996). Suicides after pregnancy in Finland, 1987–1994: Register linkage study. *British Medical Journal, 313*, 1431–1434.

Goodman, W., & Crouter, A. (2009). Longitudinal associations between maternal work, stress, negative work–family spillover, and depressive symptoms. *Family Relations, 58*(3), 245–258.

Gove, W.R., & Geerken, M.R. (1977). The effects of children and employment on the mental health of married men and women. *Social Forces, 56*(1), 66–76.

Greil, A.L. (2002). Infertile bodies: Medicalization, metaphor and agency. In M.C. Inhorn, & F. Van Balen (Eds.), *Infertility around the globe: New thinking on childlessness, gender and reproductive technologies: A view from the Social Sciences*. Berkeley, CA: University of California Press.

Hilbrecht, M., Shaw, S.M., Johnson, L.C., & Audrey, J. (2008). 'I'm home for the Kids': Contradictory implications for work–life balance of teleworking mothers. *Gender, Work & Organization, 15*(5), 454–476.

Hock, E., & DeMeis, D.K. (1990). Depression in mothers of infants: The role of maternal employment. *Developmental Psychology, 26*(2), 285–291.

Hock, E., & Schirtzinger, M. (1992). Maternal separation anxiety: Its developmental course and relation to maternal mental health. *Child Development, 63*(1), 93–102.

Hodnett, E. (2002). Pain and women's satisfaction with the experience of childbirth: A systematic review. *American Journal of Obstetrics and Gynecology, 106*(5), S160–S172.

Hsu, H. (2004). Antecedents and consequences of separation anxiety in first-time mothers: Infant, mother and social-contextual characteristics. *Infant Behavior and Development, 27*(2), 113–133.

Ibekwe, P.C., & Achor, J.U. (2008). Psychosocial and cultural aspects of pseudocyesis. *Indian Journal of Pyschiatry, 50*(2), 112–116.

Ismail, M.K., Crome, L., & O'Brien, P.M. (2006). *Psychological disorders in obstetrics and gynecology.* London: Royal College of Obstetrics and Gynecology.

Jaffe, J., & Diamond, M.O. (2011). *Reproductive trauma: Psychotherapy with infertility and pregnancy loss clients.* Washington, D.C.: American Psychological Association.

Katon, W., Russo, J., & Gavin, A. (2014). Predictors of postpartum depression. *Journal of Women's Health, 23*(9), 753–759.

Klaus, M.H., Kennell, J.H., & Klaus, P.H. (1993). *Mothering the mother: How a doula can help you have a shorter, easier, and healthier birth.* Philadelphia: Addison-Wesley Publishing.

Klaus, M.H., Kennell, J.H., & Klaus, P.H. (2012). *The doula book: How a trained labor companion can help you have a shorter, easier and healthier birth.* New York: Merloyd Lawrence.

Kubler-Ross, E. (1969). *On death and dying: What the dying have to teach doctors, nurses, clergy and their own families.* New York: Scribner.

Lamaze, F. (1984). *Painless childbirth: The Lamaze method.* New York: McGraw-Hill.

Lang, A., Fleiszer, A.R., Duhamel, F., Sword, W., Gilbert, KR., & Corsini-Munt, S. (2011). Perinatal loss and parental grief: The challenge of ambiguity and disenfranchised grief. *Journal of Death and Dying, 63*(2), 183–196.

Leavitt, J.W. (1986). *Brought to bed: Child-bearing in America, 1750–1950.* Oxford: Oxford University Press.

Lederman, R., & Weis, K. (2009). *Psychosocial adaptation to pregnancy: Seven dimensions of maternal role development,* 3rd ed. New York: Springer.

Lim, C.E.D., & Cheng, N.C.L. (2011). Clinician's role of psychological support in helping parents and families with pregnancy loss. *Journal of the Australian Traditional Medicine Society, 17*(4), 215–217.

Lok, I.H., & Neugebauer, R. (2007). Psychological morbidity following miscarriage. *Best Practice & Research Clinical Obstetrics & Gynaecology, 21,* 229–247.

Lok, I.H., Yip, A.S., Lee, D.T., Sahota, D., & Chung, T.K. (2010). A 1-year longitudinal study of psychological morbidity after miscarriage. *Fertility and Sterility, 93,* 1966–1975.

Lowe, N. (2002). The nature of labor pain. *American Journal of Obstetrics and Gynecology, 186,* S16–S24.

McCubbin, M.A., & McCubbin, H.L. (1993). Family coping with health crises: The resiliency model of family stress, adjustment, and adaptation. In C. Danielson, B. Hamel-Bissell, & P. Winsted-Frys (Eds.), *Families, health and illness.* New York: Mosby.

MacDorman, M.F., & Gregory, E.C.W. (2015). *Fetal and perinatal mortality, United States, 2013.* National vital statistics reports; vol. 64 no. 8. Hyattsville, MD: National Center for Health Statistics.

McLanahan, S., & Adams, J. (1987). Parenthood and psychological well-being. *Annual Review of Sociology, 13,* 237–257.

Mason, M.A., & Ekman, E.M. (2007). *Mothers on the fast track.* New York: Oxford University Press.

Matthews, T.J., & Hamilton, B.E. (2009). Delayed childbearing: More women are having their first child later in life. *NCHS Data Brief, 21,* 1–8.

Menken, A.E. (2008). A psychodynamic approach to treatment. In S.D. Stone, & A.E. Menken (Eds.), *Perinatal and postpartum mood disorders: Perspectives and treatment guide for the health care practitioner.* New York: Springer.

Meyer, C.L., & Oberman, M. (2001). *Mothers who kill their children: Understanding the acts of moms from Susan Smith to the "prom mom."* New York: New York University Press.

Miles, L.M., Keitel, M., Jackson, M., Harris, A., & Licciardi, F. (2009). Predictors of distress in women being treated for infertility. *Journal of Reproductive and Infant Psychology, 27*(3), 238–257.

Miller, L.J. (2003). Denial of pregnancy. In *Infanticide: Psychosocial and legal perspectives on mothers who kill* (pp. 81–104). Washington, D.C.: American Psychiatric Publishing.

Munk-Olson, T., Larsen, T.M., Pedersen, C.B., Mors, O., & Mortensen, P.B. (2006). New parents and mental disorders: A population-based register study. *Journal of the American Medical Association, 296* (21), 2582–2589.

Nelson, A.M. (2003). Transition to motherhood. *Journal of Obstetric, Gynecologic, and Neonatal Nursing, 32*(4), 465–477.

Nichols, M.R., & Roux, G.M. (2004). Maternal perspectives on postpartum return to the workplace. *Journal of Obstetric, Gynecologic and Neonatal Nursing, 33,* 463–471.

Notman, M.T. (2011). Some thoughts about the psychological issues related to assisted reproductive technology. *Psychoanalytic Inquiry, 31,* 380–391.

O'Boyle, C. (2014). "Being with" while retaining and asserting professional midwifery power and authority in home birth. *Journal of Organizational Ethnography* 3(2), 204–223.

Odent, M. (2012). The doula phenomenon and authentic midwifery. *Midwifery Today, 104,* 9–11.

O'Leary, J. (2004). Grief and its impact on prenatal attachment in the subsequent pregnancy. *Archives of Women's Mental Health, 7,* 7–18.

Ombelet, W., Cooke, I., Dyer, S., Serour, G., & Devroey, P. (2008). Infertility and the provision of infertility medical services in developing countries. *Reproduction Update, 14*(6), 605–621.

Peppers, L.G., & Knapp, R.J. (1980). *Motherhood and mourning: Perinatal death.* New York: Praeger Publishers.

Puryear, L.J. (2007). *Understanding your moods when you're expecting: Emotions, mental health, and happiness – before, during, and after pregnancy.* Boston: Houghton Mifflin.

Quesenberry, J.L., Trauth, E.M., & Morgan, A.J. (2006). Understanding the "Mommy Tracks": A framework for analyzing work–family balance in the IT workforce. *Information Resources Management Journal, 19*(2), 37–53.

Radloff, L.S. (1975). Sex differences in depression: The effects of occupation and marital status. *Sex Roles, 1,* 249–265.

Raphael, D. (1955). *The tender gift.* New York: Shocken Books.

Raphael-Leff, J. (1991). *Psychological processes of childbearing.* New York: Chapman & Hall.

Raphael-Leff, J. (2013). Opening shut doors – The emotional impact of infertility and therapeutic issues. In E. Quagliata (Ed.), *Understanding the experience of miscarriage, premature births, infertility and postnatal depression* (pp. 79–106). London: Karnac Books.

Resnick, P.J. (1969). Child murder by parents: A psychiatric review of filicide. *American Journal of Psychiatry, 26,* 1414–1420.

Robinson, M., Baker, L., & Nackerud, L. (1999). The relationship of attachment theory and perinatal loss. *Death Studies, 23*(3), 257–270.

Romanoff, B., & Terenzio, M. (1998). Rituals and the grieving process. *Death Studies, 22*(8), 697–711.

Rosch, D.S., Sajatovic, M., & Sivec, H. (2003). Behavioral characteristics in delusional pregnancy: A matched control group study. *International Journal of Psychiatry in Medicine, 32*(3), 295–303.

Savs, A.P., Derganc, M., & Licina, M. (2012). P-1477-Pseudocyesis followed by delusions of maternity. *European Psychiatry, 27,* 1.

Schwerdtfeger, K.L., & Shreffler, K.M. (2009). Trauma of pregnancy loss and infertility among mothers and involuntarily childless women in the United States. *Journal of Loss and Trauma, 14,* 211–227.

Selix, N.W., & Goyal, D. (2015). Postpartum depression among working women: A call for practice and policy change. *The Journal for Nurse Practitioners, 11*(9), 897–902.

Shakhar, K., & Fleisig, D. (2014). How to cope with stress and depression in women with recurrent miscarriage. In O.B. Christiansen (Ed.), *Recurrent pregnancy loss.* Hoboken, NJ: John Wiley.

Shreffler, K.M., Greil, A.L., & McQuillan, J. (2011). Pregnancy loss and distress among U.S. Women. *Family Relations, 60,* 342–355.

Simkin, P. (1991). Just another day in a woman's life? Women's long-term perceptions of their first birth experience. Part I. *Birth, 19*(2), 64–81.

Simkin, P. (1992). Just another day in a woman's life? Nature and consistency of women's long-term memories of their first birth experiences. Part II. *Birth, 18*(4), 203–210.

Simkin, P. (2006). What makes a good birth and why does it matter? *International Journal of Childbirth Education, 21*(3), 4–6.

Simkin, P. (2012). Roundtable discussion: The language of birth. *Birth, 39*(2), 156–157.

Smith, J.A. (1999). Identity development during the transition to motherhood: An interpretative phenomenological analysis. *Journal of Reproductive and Infant Psychology, 17*(3), 281–299.

Soares, C.N. (2013). Depression in peri and postmenopausal women: Prevalence, pathophysiology and pharmacologic management. *Drugs and Aging, 30*(9), 677–685.

Spinelli, M.G. (2001). A systematic investigation of 16 cases of neonaticide. *American Journal of Psychiatry, 158*(5), 811–813.

Spinelli, M.G. (2003). Neonaticide: A systematic investigation of 17 cases. In *Infanticide: Psychosocial and legal perspectives on mothers who kill* (pp. 105–118). Washington, D.C.: American Psychiatric Publishing.

Steiner, M., Dunn, E., & Born, L. (2003). Hormones and mood: From menarche to menopause and beyond. *Journal of Affective Disorders, 74*(1), 67–83.

Stern, D.N. (1998). *The motherhood constellation: A unified view of parent–infant psychotherapy.* New York: Basic Books.

Stewart, D.E. Gucciardi, E., & Grace, S.L. (2004). Depression. *BMC Women's Health, 4*(1), 19.

Surkan, P.J., Peterson, K.E., Hughes, M.D., & Gottlieb, B.R. (2006). The role of social networks and support in postpartum women's depression: A multiethnic urban sample. *Maternal and Child Health Journal, 10*(4), 375–383.

Swanson, K.K.M., Chen, H.T.J., Graham, C., Wognar, D.M., & Petras, A. (2009). Resolution of depression and grief during the first year after miscarriage: A randomized controlled clinical trial of couples-focused interventions. *Journal of Women's Health, 18*(8), 1245–1257.

Symonds, A. (1986). *The dynamics of depression in functioning women.* Paper presented at the Neuropsychiatric Society of Central Ohio, Columbus.

Tarin, J.J., Hermenegildo, C., Garcia-Perez, M.A., & Cano, A. (2013). Endocrinology and physiology of pseudocyesis. *Reproductive Biology and Endocrinology, 11*(39), 1186.

Taubman-Ben-Ari, O., Shlomo, S.B., Sivan, S., & Dolizki, M. (2009). The transition to motherhood: A time for growth. *Journal of Social and Clinical Psychology, 28*(8), 943–970.

Tedeschi, R.G., & Calhoun, L.G. (2004). Posttraumatic growth: Conceptual foundations and empirical evidence. *Psychological Inquiry, 15*(1), 1–18.

Turton, P., Hughes, P., Evans, C.D.H., & Fainman, D. (2001). Incidence, correlates and predictors of posttraumatic stress disorder in the pregnancy after stillbirth. *British Journal of Psychiatry, 178*(6), 556–560.

Twomey, T.M. (2009). *Understanding postpartum psychosis: A temporary madness.* Westport, CT: Praeger Publishing.

US Department of Labor: Bureau of Labor Statistics. (2011). *Women in the labor force: A databook.* Washington, D.C.: US Bureau of Labor Force Statistics. Retrieved from: http://www.bls.gov/cps/wlf-databook2011.htm (accessed November 2, 2016).

Usdansky, M.L., Gordon, R.A., Wang, X., & Gluzman, A. (2011). Depression risk among mothers of young children: The role of employment preferences, labor force status and job quality. *Journal of Family and Economic Issues, 33*(1), 83–94.

Valentine, D. (1987). Psychological impact of infertility: Identifying issues and needs. *Social Work Health Care, 11*, 61–69.

Van, P. (2012). Conversations, coping and connectedness: A qualitative study of women who have experienced involuntary pregnancy loss. *Omega, 65*(1), 71–85.

Waldenstrom, U. (2004). Why do some women change their opinion about childbirth over time? *Birth, 31*(2), 102–107.

Wells, J.D., Hobfoll, S.E., & Lavin, J. (1999). When it rains, it pours: The greater impact of resource loss compared to gain on psychological distress. *Personality and Social Psychology Bulletin, 25*(9), 1172–1182.

Wertz, R., & Wertz, D.C. (1977). *Lying in: A history of childbirth in America.* New Haven, CT: Free Press.

Whiffen, V.E., & Johnson, S.M. (1998). An attachment theory framework for the treatment of childbearing depression. *Clinical Psychology: Science and Practice, 5*(4), 478–493.

Winkler, N. (2014). Babies after 40: Is the biological clock really ticking? In D.L. Barnes (Ed.), *Women's reproductive mental health across the lifespan.* New York: Springer Publishing.

Chapter Three
Women at Midlife

*Maria Espinola, helen DeVinney,
and Arlene (Lu) Steinberg*

When I was younger there was much talk about the century of the child . . .

But when, pray, is the century of the adult to begin? (E. Erikson)

Childhood has historically been considered the central period of human development, and adulthood has been perceived as relatively stable, with little change occurring. Perhaps the popular notion of the *midlife crisis* (Jaques, 1965) hinted at a possibility that adulthood wasn't as stable as commonly portrayed. Indeed, the crisis depicts midlife stability as shaken, when individuals question previous decisions, or even change their life course. In this chapter we will focus on women's experience of midlife. Some questions we will address in this chapter include:

- What is the significance of midlife for women, and have societal, medical, and technological advances affected that significance?
- Is the midlife crisis inevitable for all women, or does culture, socioeconomic status, gender identity, or orientation influence it?
- Is menopause a uniformly experienced stressful event in all women's lives?
- Does motherhood positively or negatively impact women's midlife?
- Are there unique midlife issues related to caretaking aging parents?
- In general, is adulthood overall stable, as had been thought, or is it a period marked by transition and change?

While some emphasize stability and little change, others have considered changes that are even personality altering at midlife, such that individuals may differ from their younger self.

Yet what is midlife?

Gail Sheehy (1976), in her landmark book *Passages*, while describing the peak anxiety-ridden years of middle age as 37 to 42, distinguished between marker events, which are real-life events that affect our passages, and developmental stages triggered by marker events that change us from within (Blatt & Blass, 1990). At these junctures Sheehy felt we can move toward growth or stay with the security we know, reflective of Erik Erikson's (1950; Erikson & Erikson, 1997) generativity vs. stagnation stage in his developmental model. She considered the midlife crisis an important juncture, leading to increased assertiveness, responsiveness, and independence. Much of her work seems reflective of Erikson's model.

Joan Erikson, Erik Erikson's wife, described that the midlife stage was almost left out, as with Shakespeare's similar neglect of this stage in the seven stages described in *As You Like It*. Ironically, Erikson initially left out the stage he and his wife were in at that time. Erikson then added generativity vs. stagnation between the then sixth and seventh stage, to be followed by old age. Is his initial neglect of middle age reflective of repression of the unique issues faced by many at this stage? While Freud (1924) believed sexuality was the main issue people repressed, in focusing on *eros*, perhaps his theoretical neglect of *thanatos* reflected other significant issues, as one crosses the midline of life and faces mortality, that can get ignored.

In addition, the commonly described turbulence at midlife and midlife crises (Jaques, 1965) might be exacerbated by cultural surrounds, as we live in an environment valuing physical power and sexuality and portraying retirement as a time to "go fishing," rather than as a period of continued mental agility, creativity, and development (Davidson, 1975). Growth arising from challenge, crises, and turbulence is not of the *zeitgeist* (Wray, 2007). With increased commodification of the body, the female body at midlife has become associated with the maintenance of an "ageless body." This, combined with many women having the possibility of delaying childbearing, has also confused timetables as well as the resulting stresses of these timetables. For others it also has relieved or delayed the pressures and crises, as it's not clear where the midpoint of life resides.

Much of the research in this area seems to be anecdotal, as there has been a general dearth of empirical research exploring midlife (Wray, 2007). Most writing has been theoretical, without sufficient clinical and empirical substantiation. While popular notions have depicted the midlife crisis for women as revolving around women's alienation from their aging body, whatever empirical research there is has instead reflected the diverse meanings midlife has for women, mediated by their ethnic and cultural backgrounds.

Levinson (1978), with ripples of Elliott Jaques (1965), in his study of men, considered midlife to be a period of confronting one's own personal mortality and renouncing one's denial of aging. Indeed, reflecting Becker's (1973) emphasis on the denial of death as a significant human motivator, midlife was defined as the period when the fleeting nature of existence becomes a salient issue both in the intrapsychic and real worlds. Levinson sees adult development as a predictable reaction to physical decline. Yet, Neugarten (1979) and others, while acknowledging some diminishing capacities with age, also propose cognitive developments at these later stages (Hauser & Kates, 1982). Others add that momentous life events, historically associated with younger ages, occur now more at later stages, with individuals becoming not only grandparents but also parents at later years, further adding to the confusion.

Yet, overall, both women and men are faced with an increasing awareness at midlife of the finiteness of personal time and that they will die. Yet, if all goes well, a feeling of both physical and temporal freedom may ensue. An increasing awareness of the preciousness of time and a reordering of one's priorities may begin (Peterson & Duncan, 2007). Neugarten (1979) describes the awakening of a feeling of "time left to live, rather than time since birth." Indeed, one can raise the question as to whether the prominence of treatments like hormone replacement therapy, and the youthful emphasis, can even deprive women of potential growth resulting from the turbulence.

Yalom (2008) states that it's not easy to live every moment aware of death, that it is like "staring at the sun . . . you can stand only so much." The methods we use to cope include projecting ourselves into the future through children, and professional and creative accomplishment. Yalom says, "The physicality of death may destroy us, but the idea can save us," and encourages us toward the creation of an authentic life of engagement. He describes rippling as a way we live on, creating "concentric circles of influence, wisdom, virtue and guidance," that can live on for generations. Sometimes the experience of confronting this period may involve a confrontation with a difficult or traumatic past. That which does not kill us can make us stronger or, as Hemingway (1957) had said, "we become stronger in the broken places." Parental death at this stage can also contribute to the stress. One not only mourns the parent, but also for one's own mortality. Other losses at this stage include loss of one's spouse and emptying of the nest.

For women the passage of time, and time itself, is significant, as their lives are marked by one's monthly menstrual cycle, the span of pregnancy, the biological clock and then menopause, considered a temporal watershed leading to a mourning of the ability to create more time through the creation of new life (Colarusso, 1999). Resolution of this mourning can lead to transformation of the subjective sense of time. No longer bound in the same way by time, women can feel freer to use time in new ways.

Nemiroff and Colarusso (1985) felt that a problematic reaction to menopause was not inevitable —that some may feel freer by it. The temporal freedom can be used for generative purposes, working out the loss and mourning of what could have been, leading to greater awareness of reality as it is, and as it can be. Past is past, distinguished from present and future, thus releasing more affect to be invested in life. Colarusso and Montero (2007) consider the developmental process to be lifelong and continuous and not just restricted to childhood, with midlife a particularly dynamic and conflicted phase in it, rather than a transition or crisis. They see the potential for dramatic changes at midlife, as a result of the interaction between the adult aging body, the psyche, and the ever-changing environment. Thus midlife seems to be considered both traumatic for some, and generative for those same, and for others. Neugarten (1979) considers an increased capacity for increased self-reflection at this stage.

Any speculation as to the incidence of midlife crises is tentative at best. In addition, momentous midlife transition is not a universal phenomenon (Moraglia, 1994). Certain ethnic groups appear to be more reactive than others (Goldstein, 1987). Yet, extending Langer and Rodin's (1976) findings in their study of the elderly, to the extent women not only confront but also take charge of this transition, they may overall fare better.

Cultural Differences

Wray (2007) argues that the meaning of midlife varies among women of diverse ethnic and cultural backgrounds. She states that, in Western society, the intersection of ageism and sexism plays a role in associating physical appearance with women's worth, which leads women to feel more concerned about losing their youth. Indeed, Western views of midlife emphasize menopause, and the loss of a youthful physical appearance, as two of the main sources of stress for women in midlife. Wray (2007) interviewed women of different ethnic backgrounds and found that White British women were more likely than British women of color to endorse concerns associated with appearing older than they felt. Additionally, some of them spoke about feeling like their bodies "mask" their true identities. On the other hand, British Pakistani, Muslim, West Indian, and African Caribbean women seemed more concerned about not having as much energy and physical strength as they did when they were younger.

Studies have indicated that Caucasian women tend to be slightly more dissatisfied with their body images than Hispanic and African American women. Additionally, Caucasian women have been found to have the most distorted views about what body type men find attractive, guessing that men prefer women to be significantly thinner than men's actual preferences (Demarest & Allen, 2000). Aging can present more challenges to women's body images. Jackson et al. (2014) indicated that midlife women who hold negative body images have a higher risk of developing clinical depression.

The media's preference for young and thin women has been blamed for creating unreasonable standards of female beauty. Popular actresses have brought attention to the combination of sexism and ageism that influences movie directors' tendency to pair men with much younger women. At age 37, Maggie Gyllenhaal was told that she was "too old to play the lover of a man who was 55" (Otterson, 2015). Olivia Wilde, 32, was rejected for being too old to be paired with 41-year-old Leonardo Di Caprio (Helligar, 2016). Popular movies that feature men with much younger women include *Pretty Women* (18-year difference), *As Good as it Gets* (27-year difference), *A Perfect Murder* (28-year difference), *Third Person* (32-year difference), and *Something's Gotta Give* (35-year difference). Zoe Saldana has said, "by the time you are 28, you are expired, you are playing mommy roles" (Bertodano, 2014).

In her TED Talk, "Life's Third Act," Jane Fonda (2011) argues against the "old paradigm of age as an arch," where people are seen as declining into "decrepitude." Fonda states that age can be seen as "potential." She points out that studies have shown the majority of people over the age of 50 report feeling better than they did when they were younger. She states that when she was in her late 30s, her first thoughts of the day were mainly negative, which led her to fear that her approach to life was going to worsen with age. Fonda said that, much to her surprise, her outlook on life became more positive with age, and, now in her 70s, she says she has "never been happier." She admits finding happiness came after conducting a life review, which involved changing her relationship with her past by forgiving herself and others. She highlights that changing how we respond to life circumstances is fundamental. Fonda adds that little girls start life by feeling whole and confident, but that confidence erodes during puberty. She proposes that older women, who are the largest demographic group in the world, can go back, redefine themselves, become whole, and lead an example for girls and younger women to follow.

While speaking about aging, the writer Isabel Allende (2014) pointed out that it can be very difficult for women to get older in a culture that values youth. She says, "I feel good, I feel charming, seductive, sexy. Nobody else sees that. I'm invisible." She stresses that she makes a continuous effort to maintain a positive attitude. Allende says, "Unless you are ill or very poor, you have choices. I have chosen to stay passionate, engaged with an open heart." Cameron Diaz has publicly embraced aging and turning 40 by saying, "It's the best age. That's when a woman knows how to work things, or she doesn't care about that any more. You just stop being afraid" (Corriston, 2014).

After interviewing 16,000 women of five ethnic backgrounds, Sommer et al. (1999) found that African American women reported significantly more positive feelings towards menopause than women from other ethnic backgrounds. The authors hypothesized that African American women, who have been discriminated against and oppressed throughout their lives, may perceive changes of midlife as significantly less stressful than the experiences they have already been able to overcome.

Many Latinas embrace turning 50 years old by commemorating the occasion with a celebration called *cincuentañera,* which serves as an empowering ritual to reconnect with feminine cultural roots (Prestbo & Staats-Westover, 2008).

Comas-Diaz and Greene (2013) speak about women of color's reconnection with an individual and social empowerment after menopause. They state that Latinas may choose activism and community education by becoming *promotoras,* and African American women may assume high positions in their churches or places of worship. Older Latinas are often perceived as wiser due to their maturity and life experiences. In the role of *promotoras,* older Latinas can act as community educators, lay health workers, or advocates.

Workplace

Women in midlife face great challenges entering, remaining, and succeeding in the workplace. Some of these challenges include pay inequality, age and gender discrimination, low political power, underrepresentation in leadership positions and high-paying employment, and caregiving demands and penalties (OWL, 2012). Although great progress has been made regarding women's rights in the last 100 years, women's lives are negatively impacted by inequality all around the world.

A study released by the National Economic Bureau of Research shows that age discrimination disproportionately affects women more than men (Neumark, Burn, & Button, 2015). The researchers sent 40,000 job applications for positions in multiple professions. They found no statistically significant discrimination against men before the age of 51. Indeed, men aged 49 to 51 received more calls than younger men when seeking janitor positions. They also found no discrimination at any age against men looking for security positions. On the other hand, high rates of discrimination against women older than 49 was consistent in every industry.

The Institute for Women's Policy Research recommends that promoting gender equality in the United States requires changes at the systemic level, including increasing women's participation in politics, reducing poverty among women, improving women's healthcare quality and access, reducing gender violence, and increasing women's safety (Hess, Milli, Hayes, & Hegewisch, 2015). At the individual level, Facebook COO Sheryl Sandberg (2013) proposes that gender inequality can be reduced by changing the messages women tell themselves, the women around them, and their daughters. She gives three main pieces of advice: (1) Sit at the table; (2) Make your partner a real partner; and (3) Don't leave before you leave (don't reject opportunities or leave your job to have a child before you have to leave to care for your child). Sandberg points out that women underestimate their own abilities and attribute their success to external factors such as luck instead of giving credit to themselves. Sandberg argues that feeling undeserving of success or not understanding the reasons behind their success prevents women from negotiating their salaries or asking for promotions. For instance, only 7% of women negotiate their first salaries, as opposed to 57% of men. Sandberg admits that changing this trend is more complicated than just telling women to be proud of their success and make more demands at work, mainly due to society's sexism.

Motherhood

The gender socialization of girls promotes the idea that the most important role in the life of a woman is being a mother. Many girls learn to provide motherly care for their dolls before they are able to speak properly. Despite how deeply personal the decision to become a mother is, most women have had the experience of being questioned, even by strangers, about their choices regarding when to become a mother and/or how to properly parent their children. Hays (1996) states that the American "public ideology of appropriate child rearing has urged mothers to stay home with their children, thereby ostensibly maintaining consistency in women's nurturing and selfless behavior" (p. 3).

Despite many mothers' desire to spend more time with their children, most mothers in the United States have to struggle to balance work and family responsibilities. The images of ideal mothers that are often portrayed in TV sitcoms conflict with the reality that working mothers must face on a daily basis. This discrepancy can lead mothers to experience negative emotions related to not being able to fulfill personal, familial, and societal expectations of motherhood.

Different studies have looked at the individual experiences of motherhood for women before and during midlife. Gersick and Kram (2002) indicated that women in their 30s struggle with more complicated career–family dilemmas while women in their 40s concentrate more on finding balance between work and family and postponing big new commitments. Winslow (1987) interviewed women aged 35 to 44 who were expecting their first child and identified several factors that impacted these women's decision to become mothers. These factors included: (1) having a serious, committed relationship with their child's father; (2) decreased fertility and concerns about having a child with Down syndrome; (3) a sense of having had numerous accomplishments, economic security, travel opportunities, property acquisitions, and career achievements; (4) desire to have a child (the intensity of this desire was not equal among the women interviewed); and (5) the decision to not reach menopause without having a child.

Several studies have indicated a relationship between depression and parenthood (Evenson & Simon, 2005; Nomaguchi & Milkie, 2003). However, this relationship appeared to be mediated by gender differences (Nomaguchi & Milkie, 2003). There are two theories that highlight gender differences regarding parenting: the *gender role perspective* and the *parental role*. The *gender role perspective* states that gender socialization leads women to perceive their sense of self as more connected to parenthood than men, which then leads them to experience higher psychological costs and rewards associated with motherhood (Simon, 1992). The *parental role perspective* (Scott & Alwin, 1989) states that women's role in raising young children is significantly more consuming than men's role, which leads women to experience higher levels of distress than men (Umberson & Williams, 1999).

Parenting teenagers can present additional stressors for women in midlife. Ballenski and Cook (1982) reported that mothers experienced the highest feelings of inadequacy as parents than at any other time in their children's lives. Koski and Steinberg (1990) found a positive correlation between severe midlife concerns and lower parental satisfaction, which was moderated by psychological health and marital satisfaction.

An increasing number of women in midlife are not having children by choice or circumstances. During the 1970s, one in ten women reached menopause without having children. In 2010, that number increased to one in five women and it is even higher (one in four) for college-educated women. In the study *Shades of Otherhood* (2014), the marketing firm Devries Global sought to understand the perspectives and behaviors of women without children. The study found that 80% of women without children believe they could be happy living a childfree life.

Despite its many challenges, many women report great satisfaction from being mothers (Rogers & White, 1998). Rittenour and Colaner (2012) studied women's motherly, feminist, and generativity identities' relationship to women's life and self-satisfaction. In order to measure mothering identity, the authors modified Johnson, Caughlin, and Huston's (1999) couple identity scale. Items in the modified scale included, "Being a mother helps you feel good about yourself." Generativity identity was measured using the Loyola Generativity Scale (McAdams & de St. Aubin, 1992), a 20-item assessment tool that includes items such as, "I have made and created things that have had an impact on other people." Feminist identity was assessed with the passive acceptance subscale of the Feminist Identity Scale (Downing & Roush, 1985). Results indicated that women with higher generativity identity report higher self and life satisfaction and women with high motherly identities show stronger associations between life satisfaction and generativity. Additionally, this study indicated that women who endorsed a high generativity identity have a tendency to identity as feminists.

Divorce

The majority of divorces are granted to women and men in midlife, between 45 and 54 years old (Kreider & Simmons, 2003). Women in particular file 60% of divorces in midlife (Sakraida, 2005). Hilton and Anderson (2009) applied social exchange theory to understand why women in midlife may choose to pursue a divorce. Social exchange theory is based on the idea that individuals make decisions with the goal of increasing rewards and diminishing losses (White & Klein, 2002). Thus, if a woman perceives that her losses outnumber the rewards she is receiving from a marriage, she may file for divorce. Hilton and Anderson (2009) cite multiple factors that have been found to contribute to instability in the marriage, including: (1) younger age at the time of marriage; (2) short duration of the marriage; (3) women's employment; (4) high economic costs of the divorce; (5) unhappiness; (6) life satisfaction; (7) lack of self-efficacy; (8) lack of mastery; and (9) conservative beliefs about gender roles.

Studies suggest that African American women have higher levels of well-being after divorce than White women. Kitson (1992) indicated that African American women maintain greater inner peace, experience the divorce as less unpleasant, and do not stigmatize divorce as much as women from other cultural backgrounds. McKelvey and McKenry (2000) indicated that Black women report higher levels of economic well-being and personal mastery than White women after going through a marital dissolution. Further, these authors suggested that African American women have culturally based strengths (e.g., independence, self-reliance) that facilitate a better adjustment to divorce.

Case Study: Victoria[1]

Victoria is a biracial 40-year-old Latina woman who sought therapeutic services because she was "having a midlife crisis mixed with a potential divorce mixed with bipolar issues." Victoria was born in the Dominican Republic and immigrated to the United States at age 18. Victoria explained that, one year before seeking services, she found out that her husband of 16 years was having an affair with a 20-year-old White woman. She stated that she became "overwhelmed with every emotion." She felt extreme anger towards him and his lover, anger at herself for not finding out about the affair sooner, sadness about losing her trust towards him, sadness for their children who could potentially have to see them go through a divorce, guilt about not dedicating more time to her relationship with her husband, and shame about what others might say about her.

Victoria, who had worked as a model in the past, began to believe she was "no longer beautiful." She also began to think that her husband, who is White, chose a White woman as a lover because she had the "right skin color, the right hair, the right nose." Victoria is a marriage and family therapist, and felt she was no longer going to be trusted to provide counseling since she "could not even help herself."

Victoria stated that financial issues, her concern about her children, and worries about the impact her divorce might have on her professional image led her to remain in the marriage. She said that even though she verbally forgave him, she still resented him, and could not regulate her anger at times. Victoria began to believe that if she had an affair, she could "make it even" in her mind, and not feel like she "was less than him."

Victoria began a very intense exercise routine, started to go out again with her girlfriends, did "every beauty treatment imaginable," and bought a "whole new closet." She said that she started to flirt with men, who responded to her, and that made her feel "beautiful and sexy again." Victoria, who had never had an affair, never dated a married man, and never dated someone at work, began to see a married colleague. She said her goal was to have a sexual relationship "without feelings," but she found herself falling in love with him in "a way [she] never felt before."

Victoria, who has a history of bipolar II disorder, said the "ridiculous, out-of-control love" she felt precipitated in her a hypomanic episode. She reported insomnia, racing thoughts, rapid speech, grandiosity, hypersexuality, binge drinking, and excessive spending. Her colleague fell in love with her as well, and was ready to leave his wife and three children. Victoria said that hearing he was ready to start a life with her was "amazing on one side, but absolutely horrible on the other side." She said, "I can't live with the guilt of ruining two families." Thus, she decided to end their relationship a month before coming to therapy. Since making her decision, she had daily crying spells, and "felt hopeless, lost, and broken."

Victoria's treatment consisted of 25 individual therapy sessions. A therapeutic approach that integrated multicultural therapy, feminist therapy, and dialectical behavior therapy was utilized. During sessions one to five, the clinician concentrated on developing a warm, trusting, and egalitarian relationship with Victoria. Her case conceptualization and therapeutic approach were discussed openly. The clinician communicated to Victoria that her symptoms were being viewed as specialized coping behaviors rather than manifestations of pathology. Victoria reported she felt empowered to express herself freely without being judged and her feelings of abandonment, isolation, and helplessness were validated. Since Victoria described being "tormented with memories from the past and worries about the future," mindfulness techniques were introduced to help her focus on the present moment and reduce the emotions associated with past and potential future experiences.

During sessions five to ten, issues regarding Victoria's gender socialization, cultural background, and experiences of racism and oppression were explored. Victoria was invited to look at how these issues have influenced her life experiences, and her current world view. Victoria shared that, as a biracial Latina immigrant, she has been exposed to high levels of discrimination and racism. She spoke about feeling "constantly out of place, not considered part of any group, not Black enough, not White enough, not Latina enough." She said these feelings were intensified after reaching midlife, and finding out about her husband's affair because she began to also feel "not young enough, and not pretty enough." Victoria said that she stayed with her husband because she could not tolerate other aspects of her identity (wife, mother, professional) to "fall apart too."

Victoria shared that the messages she received from society had become part of her internal dialogue. Therapy then focused on increasing Victoria's ability to engage in self-compassion and self-validation. These techniques helped Victoria find greater inner peace, and unconditionally appreciate the multiple aspects of her identity.

During sessions ten to 20, dialectical behavioral therapy exercises were included in treatment to help Victoria increase her ability to regulate emotions (particularly sadness, guilt, anger, and shame), and tolerate distress. The technique chain analysis was utilized to increase Victoria's self-awareness and control over her impulsive behaviors. By incorporating the information learned in previous sessions, Victoria was able to identify new, more skillful, behaviors that could replace problem behaviors.

During the termination phase (sessions 20 to 25), Victoria was encouraged to concentrate on the strengths that allowed her to survive many challenges throughout her life. She was asked to recognize and use her sense of personal power to overcome her current struggles. By applying the techniques learned during treatment, Victoria was able to decrease problem behaviors, improve her ability to regulate emotions, tolerate distress, and improve her interpersonal effectiveness. She left her husband, and decided not to enter another relationship for "some time." Victoria said she wanted to dedicate more time to her children, and to the relationship she learned to have with herself during therapy, one in which she could love herself unconditionally, independently of societal norms, standards, or expectations.

Victoria's case highlighted some of the challenges women in midlife often face (concerns about aging, divorce, career, and parenting issues) as well as the additional challenges she specifically encountered due to being a biracial immigrant woman in a bicultural relationship. Victoria's case illustrated the importance of validating the complexity of women's midlife. When clinicians provide therapeutic services to women in midlife, it is fundamental that they look at the multiple factors that may be influencing each woman's unique story and that they provide a supportive, non-judgmental environment where that story can be heard.

Parent Caretaking

Women often report finding it difficult to give voice to the ways that caring for one's parents adds stress to their lives for fear of sounding selfish and uncaring

(Kramer, 2005). Cultural and societal beliefs, gender roles, and lack of access to resources can increase the pressure that women feel to take a leadership role in parent care (Leopold, Raab, & Engelhardt, 2014). Asian women may report acculturative stress, as they can experience a conflict between embracing North American values around independence and self-pursuit while also feeling a sense of cultural obligation to have their aging parents move in with them (Vega, 2014). While in most Western countries, the development of "communities for persons over 50," and assisted-living options, are seen as ways for aging parent to maintain degrees of independence, there are exceptions, such as France, where the law dictates that adult children care for aging parents (Anichkin, 2015). Additionally, in most Asian, African, and Middle Eastern countries, there are strong cultural norms around adult children caring for aging parents. The development of support groups specifically tailored to address the needs and experiences of adult children caring for aging parents has helped many women find their voice and tolerate their ambivalence. These groups have been important in helping develop a societal dialogue in the United States about the ways in which caring for aging parents can be difficult, even when one is eager to be of assistance. While these advances in talking honestly about the more basic challenges of assuming parental caretaking roles are helpful progress, many adult children still struggle to find resources of support that address parent caretaking.

While many women will profess that they take up caretaking for aging parents willingly, many of those same women will also acknowledge privately that taking care of one's parents brings its own unique stress at a time when many women are already feeling overwhelmed (Kramer, 2005). Women report high levels of stress in midlife, and the prospect of taking on the physical, emotional, and financial burdens associated with caring for one's parents weighs heavily (Leopold et al., 2014). Women in midlife may find themselves at critical phases in their careers, in childrearing, and in their marriage or life partnerships at the same time as their parents' needs increase. Middle-aged women who have children may find themselves pulled to care for both their children and parents, leaving them not only exhausted, but feeling unsupported (Kramer, 2005). Women who have taken time off to have children, or whose careers involved graduate school, may find themselves at crucial points of career development and advancement, without the flexibility to take time off to care for aging parents.

In addition to the stresses of financial and career demands, women in midlife also often find themselves negotiating intimate relationships, whether it be understanding how a long-term relationship changes with age, or exploring new romantic relationships that may come, leaving less time and emotional resources for the needs of aging parents. Another internal struggle for many women caring for aging parents is that, as they face menopause, they may be contemplating their own advancing age concurrently with beginning to think about their parents' mortality.

Menopause

In the United States, many women fear the beginning of menopause due to the loss of fertility (and thus the loss of youth), and the possible decline of their physical body and sexuality. Many women feel confused about how to respond to menopause from a medical standpoint due to the controversy over whether a woman needs to pursue hormone replacement therapy or take natural supplements. Women may feel even less support surrounding the profound emotional and psychological effects that the onset of menopause can bring. Many women believe there is one normal or healthy way to go through menopause, which can lead them to feel shame about having specific symptoms. Women who feel liberated by menopause may struggle with feelings of shame related to seeing themselves as selfish, oversexed, or unfeminine. Finally, as the United States becomes more inclusive in its understanding of gender issues, transgender women may also grapple with menopause, and look for outlets and supports to openly explore what menopause means to them.

Many studies have demonstrated that cultural attitudes toward menopause and aging strongly impact women's individual experience of menopause, both in attitude and physical symptoms (Kowalcek, Rotte, Banz, & Diedrich, 2005). A study comparing women in Papua New Guinea and Germany found that women in Papua New Guinea not only had healthier attitudes about menopause, but also experienced fewer physical symptoms (Kowalcek et al., 2005). A similar study in the United States looking at women of different ethnic groups found that the attitudes within a given culture even within the same country have a profound effect on women's individual experience of menopause with regard to both physical symptoms and their anticipation of what menopause will mean for them (Dillaway, Byrnes, Miller, & Rehan, 2008). As Ayers, Forshaw, and Hunter (2010) found, women with more negative attitudes toward menopause experience more difficult transitions to menopause, with higher rates of negative symptoms and emotional distress. One suggestion for women's more successful transition to menopause is to develop a positive postmenopausal identity (Morrison et al., 2014). This development of a new, positive, postmenopausal identity may help many women find a greater degree of possibility as they enter menopause. As the aforementioned studies demonstrate, if women do not hold negative attitudes towards menopause, and if they are able to see menopause as a stage of life symbolic of their own value and empowerment, they may increasingly experience menopause as a time to try new things, further develop as sexual and emotional beings, and claim their roles as elders within their families and communities.

Case Study: Rebecca[1]

As we consider the various changes a woman faces in the middle years of her life, another case example may help illustrate the ways in which, although there are aspects of the experience that may be generalizable, each woman's experience will be specific and unique, an amalgam of her identity, health, and access/privilege. Rebecca is a woman of South Asian ethnicity, who is 54 years of age. She was born to married parents in the United States, and is the youngest of three, with two older brothers. Following her birth, her father left the family and never returned.

Rebecca continues to value certain customs of her ethnic culture, but she was raised to hold organized religion of any faith suspect, and sometimes feels apart from others who often connect over Hinduism or Hindi spoken in the home. She identifies as bisexual, though she has only had sexual relationships with men. Rebecca has had romantic relationships with men and women, though she has not had a romantic relationship for some years, and has never married.

Rebecca was diagnosed with bipolar I disorder while attending undergraduate school. This diagnosis resulted in Rebecca having to delay or forgo many of her life's pursuits, both personal and professional. Rebecca acknowledges that one of her deepest desires was to be a mother, but her father's initial abandonment has made it difficult for her to be emotionally vulnerable with others, resulting in her often keeping potential life partners at arm's length. In recent years, Rebecca has begun to anticipate looking for a potential romantic partner, and she has reported feeling more free to pursue her desire to have a relationship with a woman, though she has expressed anxiety over coming across as a "sexual beginner" with a woman.

Rebecca was 48 years old when she re-entered therapy. At that time, she had been living with her mother for a couple of years, following a period of unusual difficulty in her own life, in which she found herself deeply depressed. Now, at 54, Rebecca's life has changed. She is feeling better than she has in years, has been able to re-establish social relationships, and she even completed a doctoral degree that had been put on hold because of her symptoms years earlier. While she initially moved in with her mother as a way to support herself emotionally and financially, she now finds herself in the role of primary caretaker, as her mother is 90 years of age, and has suffered a number of serious, life-threatening health crises.

Consistent with cultural views, Rebecca and her mother firmly believe that loved ones should be cared for by family. In this case, Rebecca is the only child in close proximity, and so the caretaking falls solely to her. Additionally, her brothers and her mother believe that a female adult child is the more natural or appropriate caregiver over male siblings. Rebecca routinely notes that she would not have it any other way, but that it is indeed a burden. Because of

Rebecca's illness, she is on disability, and so her financial security also becomes dubious after her mother dies. She fears how she will live and make ends meet, but feels compelled to conceal this fear from her mother, as she does not want to cause her undue worry in her final years.

Rebecca has many mixed emotions about her new role as primary caretaker to her mother. She feels angry about the lack of emotional support she experiences from her brothers, resentful that her brothers do not value the services she is providing to their mother, and fearful about what it will mean to lose her mother. She also feels a growing anticipation for a time when she may be able to turn her attention to herself, her own relationships, and her work, as opposed to the role of caretaking; and, she feels guilt for allowing herself the fleeting thought that her mother's passing may ultimately introduce a level of freedom and possibility.

Rebecca is also beginning to experience more unpredictability in her menstrual cycle, another event that brings with it a complex set of emotions. For Rebecca, the end of her menses represents the end of the possibility of a biological child, and a reminder that her youth has passed, and that much of it was spent struggling, as opposed to enjoying. Rebecca also has some fear of how fluctuations in her hormones may trigger unwanted instability in her mood, which has now been stable for several years.

At the same time, Rebecca also sees menopause as an opportunity for more freedom, both in a return to more predictability in her body and increased possibility. Part of what has helped Rebecca has been her membership in a group of older women, most of whom are postmenopausal, who have challenged Rebecca's previously held ideas about the limits associated with menopause. Partially in response to their influence, Rebecca has also expressed viewing menopause as a marker of "life lived," and she is recognizing it as a natural signifier of acquired wisdom and empowerment. This sense of knowing herself and feeling more confident in who she is has contributed to her feeling that this time in her life may be an opportunity for trying things she previously felt incapable of—socially, romantically, and professionally. She sees this time in her life as a moment when she may be able to create a new chapter and to realize things she previously felt would not be possible; thus, she anticipates the coming years with a mix of excitement, anxiety, and stepping into the unknown.

Other case examples include several women in midlife who utilized the emptying of their nest, and the loss of their parents, as opportunities to explore their identities, redefine their career goals, and overall reported feelings marked by increased freedom in their lives, consistent with Jane Fonda's report. Indeed, facing not only the loss of loved ones, but also one's own mortality, à la Yalom, can lead to greater freedom and enhanced self-actualization, perhaps also captured in Erikson's notion of generativity.

Conclusion

While midlife has been a historically neglected area, our current tendency to overfocus on women and midlife, the midlife crisis, and the travails of menopause may similarly neglect the relative position of midlife as one stage within the whole life cycle. Its experience is affected by women's confronting mortality, physiological changes, and ethnic and cultural differences. Some women mourn the loss of their beauty or younger physical selves and others lament feeling depletion in energy or physical strength; yet the same and others feel invigorated by the process, and freer to pursue different goals. In other words, it is difficult to generalize. Some of the challenges women face have to do with their internal struggles, reflecting on their own life choices and life circumstances and the impact that sexism, ageism, and societal assumptions have on their lives. As societal norms have shifted with possibilities for delayed aging and childbearing and the acceptance of more untraditional family constellations, assumptions about norms and stresses for this stage are difficult to make. Additionally, the internal struggles that women in midlife experience are often intensified by the systemic stressors women faced throughout their lives, including gender inequality, poverty, gender violence, lack of political power, and lack of safety. The picture is not uniform and not all women experience greater stress at this phase, and even those who do experience increased stress can also report growth and generativity through the struggle.

Future studies should focus on assisting mental health professionals to understand the differences among women in midlife and develop interventions that can help turn midlife challenges into midlife opportunities. Mental health professionals can empower women in midlife to make changes at the individual level, as suggested by Sandberg, or at the systemic level by promoting social change. Further, it would be fundamental that we all work together towards a celebration of aging and the aged, and not just of youth.

Note

1 All identifying information has been altered to protect confidentiality.

References

Allende, I. (2014, March). *Isabel Allende: How to live passionately, no matter your age* (video file). Retrieved from https://www.ted.com/talks/isabelle_allende_how_to_live_passionately_no_matter_your_age (accessed November 21, 2016).

Anichkin, A. (2015, June 18). Care for the elderly in France. *The Moscow Times.*

Ayers, B., Forshaw, M., & Hunter, M. (2010). The impact of attitudes toward the menopause on women's symptom experience: A systematic review. *Mauritas, 65,* 28–36.

Ballenski, C., & Cook A. (1982). Mother's perceptions of their competence in managing selected parenting tasks. *Family Relations, 31,* 489–494.

Becker, E. (1973). *The denial of death.* New York: Free Press Paperbacks.

Bertodano, H. (2014, July 27). Guardians of the Galaxy's Zoe Saldana: On ageism and sexism in Hollywood. *Telegraph.*

Blatt, S., & Blass, R. (1990). Attachment and separateness: A dialectic model of the products and processes of development throughout the life cycle. *The Psychoanalytic Study of the Child, 45,* 107–127.

Colarusso, C. (1999). The development of the time sense. *Psychoanalytic Quarterly, 68,* 52–83.

Colarusso, C., & Montero, G. (2007). Transience during midlife as an adult psychic organizer: The midlife transition and crisis continuum. *Psychoanalytic Study of the Child, 62,* 329–358.

Comas-Diaz, L., & Greene, B. (Eds.). *Psychological health of women of color: Intersections, challenges, and opportunities* (pp. 57–80). Santa Barbara, CA: Praeger.

Corriston, M. (2014, July 2). Cameron Diaz on loving her 40s, Why she's not having kids. *People.*

Davidson, L. (1975). Preventive attitudes toward midlife crisis. *American Journal of Psychoanalysis, 39,* 165–173.

Demarest, J., & Allen, R. (2000). Body image: Gender, ethnic, and age differences. *Journal of Social Psychology, 140*(4), 465–472.

Devries Global. (2014). *Shades of otherhood.* Retrieved from http://www.devriesglobal.com (accessed November 21, 2016).

Dillaway, H., Byrnes, M., Miller, S., & Rehan, S. (2008). Talking "among us": How women from different racial-ethnic groups define and discuss menopause. *Health Care for Women International, 29,* 766–781.

Downing, N., & Roush, K. (1985). From passive acceptance to active commitment: A model of feminist identity development for women. *The Counseling Psychologist, 13*(4), 695–709.

Erikson, E. (1950). *Childhood and society.* New York: Norton.

Erikson, E., & Erikson, J. (1997). *The life cycle completed.* New York: Norton.

Evenson, R.J., & Simon, R.W. (2005). Clarifying the relationship between parenthood and depression. *Journal of Health and Social Behavior, 46,* 341–358.

Fonda, J. (2011, December). *Jane Fonda: Life's third act* (video file). Retrieved from https://www.ted.com/talks/jane_fonda_life_s_third_act/transcript?language=en#t-38397 (accessed November 2, 2016).

Freud, S. (1924). *Beyond the pleasure principle.* New York: Boni and Liveright.

Gersick, C., & Kram, K. (2002). High-achieving women at midlife: An exploratory study. *Journal of Management Inquiry, 11*(2), 104–127.

Goldstein, M. (1987). Aspects of gender and ethnic identity in menopause: Two Italian-American women. *Journal of American Academy of Psychoanalysis, 15,* 383–394.

Hauser, S.T., & Kates, W.W. (1982). Book essay: Understanding adults. *Psychoanalysis and Contemporary Thought, 5,* 117–146.

Hays, S. (1996). *The cultural contradictions of motherhood.* New Haven, CT: Yale University.

Helligar, J. (2016, March 16). Olivia Wilde, 32, was rejected as 'too old' for Margot Robbie's role in *The Wolf of Wall Street. The Fix.* Retrieved from http://thefix.ninemsn.com.au

Hemingway, E. (1957). *A farewell to arms.* New York: Scribner.

Hess, C., Milli, J., Hayes, J., & Hegewisch, M. (2015). *The status of women in the states: 2015. Institute for Women's Policy Research.* Retrieved from: http://statusofwomendata.org (accessed November 2, 2016).

Hilton, J., & Anderson, T. (2009). Characteristics of women with children who divorce in midlife compared to those who remain married. *Journal of Divorce and Remarriage, 50*(5), 309–329.

Jackson, K., Janssen, I., Appelhans, B.M., Kazlauskaite, R., Karavolos, K., Dugan, S.A., Avery, E.A., Shipp-Johnson, K.J., Powell, L.H., & Kravitz, H.M. (2014). Body image satisfactio and depression in midlife women: The Study of Women's Health Across the Nation (SWAN). *Archives of Women's Mental Health, 17,* 177–187.

Jaques, E. (1965). Death and the midlife crisis. *International Journal of Psychoanalysis. 46,* 502–514.

Johnson, M.P., Caughlin, J.P., & Huston, T.L. (1999). The tripartite nature of marital commitment: Personal, moral, and structural reasons to stay married. *Journal of Marriage and the Family, 61,* 160–177. doi:10.2307/353891

Kitson, G. (1992). *Portrait of divorce: Adjustment to marital breakdown.* New York: Guilford.

Koski, K.J., & Steinberg, L. (1990). Parenting satisfaction of mothers during midlife. *Journal of Youth and Adolescence. 19*(5), 465–474.

Kowalcek, I., Rotte, D., Banz, C., & Diedrich, K. (2005). Women's attitudes and perceptions towards menopause in different cultures: Cross-cultural and intra-cultural comparison of pre-menopausal and post-menopausal women in Germany and Papua New Guinea. *Maturitas, 51*(3), 227–235.

Kramer, M. (2005). Self-characterizations of adult female informal caregivers: Gender identity and the bearing of burden. *Research and Theory for Nursing Practice: An International Journey, 19*(2), 137–161.

Kreider, R.M., & Simmons, T. (2003). *Marital status: 2000, Census 2000 brief.* Washington, DC: U.S. Department of Commerce, U.S. Census Bureau.

Langer, E.J., & Rodin, J. (1976). The effects of choice and enhanced personal responsibility for the aged: A field experiment in an institutional setting. *Journal of Personality and Social Psychology, 34*(2), 191–198.

Leopold, T., Raab, M., & Engelhardt, H. (2014). The transition to parent care: Costs, commitments, and caregiver selection among children. *Journal of Marriage and Family, 76*, 300–318.

Levinson, D. (1978). *Seasons of a man's life.* New York: Ballantine Books.

McAdams, D.P., & de St. Aubin, E. (1992). A theory of generativity and its assessment through self-report, behavioral acts, and narrative themes in autobiography. *Journal of Personality and Social Psychology, 62*, 1003–1015. doi:10.1037/0022-3514.62.6.1003.

McKelvey, M.W., & McKenry, P.C. (2000). The psychosocial well-being of Black mothers and white mothers following marital dissolution. *Psychology of Women Quarterly, 24*, 4–14.

Moraglia, G. (1994). C. G. Jung and the psychology of adult development. *Journal of Analytic Psychology. 39*, 55–75.

Morrison, L.A., Brown, D.E., Sievert, L.L., Reza, A., Rahberg, N., Mills, P., & Goodloe, A. (2014). Voices from the Hilo Women's Health Study: Talking story about menopause. *Health Care for Women International, 35*, 529–548.

Nemiroff, R.A., & Colarusso, C.A. (1985). *The race against time: Psychotherapy and psychoanalysis in the second half of life.* New York: Plenum.

Neugarten, B.I. (1979). Time, age and the life cycle. *American Journal of Psychiatry, 136*, 887–894.

Neumark D., Burn, I., & Button, P. (2015). Is it harder for older workers to find jobs? Working Paper 21669, *National Bureau of Economic Research.* Retrieved from http://www.nber.org/papers/w21669.pdf (accessed November 2, 2016).

Nomaguchi, K.M., & Milkie, M.A. (2003). Costs and rewards of children: The effects of becoming a parent in adults' lives. *Journal of Marriage and Family, 65*, 356–374.

Otterson, J. (2015, May 21). 11 Leading ladies who have spoken out against ageism, sexism in Hollywood. *The Wrap.* Retrieved from https://www.thewrap.com.

OWL. (2012). *OWL 2012 Mother's Day report: Women and the workforce: Challenges and opportunities facing women as they age.* Retrieved from http://www.owl-national.org (accessed November 2, 2016).

Peterson, B., & Duncan, L. (2007). Midlife women's generativity and authoritarianism: Marriage, motherhood, and 10 years of aging. *Psychology and Aging, 3*, 411–419.

Prestbo, D., & Staats-Westover, H. (2008). The goddess has returned! In C. Rayburn & L. Comas-Diaz (Eds.), *WomanSoul: The inner life of women's spirituality* (pp. 19–38). Westport, CT: Praeger.

Rittenour, C.E., & Colaner, C.W. (2012). Finding female fulfillment: Intersecting role-based and morality-based identities of motherhood, feminism, and generativity as predictors of women's self satisfaction and life satisfaction. *Sex Roles, 67*, 351–362.

Rogers, S. J., & White, L.K. (1998). Satisfaction with parenting: The role of marital happiness, family structure, and parents' gender. *Journal of Marriage and the Family, 60*, 293–308.

Sakraida, T.J. (2005). Divorce transition differences of midlife women. *Issues in Mental Health Nursing, 26*, 225–249.

Sandberg, S. (2013). *Lean in: Women, work, and the will to lead.* New York: Alfred A. Knopf.

Scott, J., & Alwin, D.F. (1989). Gender differences in parental strain: Parental role or gender role? *Journal of Family Issues, 10*, 482–503.

Shakespeare, W. (2003). *William Shakespeare's As you like it.* Auburn, CA: Audio Partners.

Sheehy, G. (1976). *Passages: Predictable crises of adult life.* New York: Bantam.

Simon, R.W. (1992). Parental role strains, salience of parental identity, and gender differences in psychological distress. *Journal of Health and Social Behavior, 33*, 25–35.

Sommer, B., Avis, N., Meyer, P., Ory, M., Madden, T., Kagawa-Singer, M., . . . & Adler, S. (1999). Attitudes toward menopause and ageing across ethnic/racial groups. *Psychosomatic Medicine, 61*, 868–875.

Umberson, D., & Williams, K. (1999). Family status and mental health. In C.S. Aneshensel & J.C. Phelan (Eds.), *Handbook of the sociology of mental health* (pp. 225–254). New York: Kluwer Academic.

Vega, T. (2014, January 14). As parents age, Asian-Americans struggle to obey a cultural code. *The New York Times.*

White, J.M., & Klein, D.M. (2002). *Family theories* (2nd ed.). Thousand Oaks, CA:Sage.

Winslow, W. (1987). First pregnancy after 35: What is the experience? *MCN, 12*, 92–96.

Wray, S. (2007). Women making sense of midlife: Ethnic and cultural diversity. *Journal of Aging Studies, 21*, 31–42.

Yalom, I. (2008). *Staring at the sun: Overcoming the terror of death.* San Francisco: Jossey-Bass.

Chapter Four
Older Women's Mental Health

Zhen Cong and Yaolin Pei

Older women are vulnerable to mental health issues because they are both women and older persons, which is usually described as double jeopardy or layered vulnerability (Chrisler, Barney, & Palatino, 2016; Minkler & Stone, 1985; Rodeheaver & Datan, 1988). Older women also show resilience in mental health as a result of acquired coping strategies from being a disadvantaged group and the selection process that favors the survival of more advantageous and healthier ones when people get older (Feinson, 1987; Pachana, McLaughlin, Leung, Byrne, & Dobson, 2012; Skultety & Whitbourne, 2004).

Many risk factors for older women's mental health have been identified, including genetic, behavioral, and physical health, which are also shared by women at other life stages (Bookwala & Lawson, 2011; Brainerd et al., 2013; Choi & DiNitto, 2011; Ganz et al., 2003; Grigoriadis & Erlick Robinson, 2007; Nho et al., 2015). In this chapter focusing on older women, we emphasize the social relationships and life situations that are particularly important to contextualize older women's mental health. We discuss the gender differences concerning mental health status among older adults, theoretical arguments relevant to older women's mental health, and how social relationships and social contexts affect older women's mental health. We also cover topics including the effects of older women's mental health on their health, older women's mental health care utilization, and intervention programs that help promote older women's mental health.

Gender Differences in Mental Health

Women have longer life expectancy than men, and thus the older the population, the higher percentage of women (Davidson, DiGiacomo, & McGrath, 2011; Ortman, Velkoff, & Hogan, 2014; Waldron, 1976). In 2012, 56.4% of older adults aged 65 and above were women, and 66.6% among those 85 years and older were women, though the gap is expected to narrow with a rapid increase in men's life expectancy (Ortman et al., 2014). The aging experience of women is distinctively different from that of men, which underpins their differences in mental health problems and their contributing factors.

Depression

There are no consistent findings of the differences between women and men in old age concerning depression (Beck & Pearson, 1989; Feinson, 1987; Pinquart & Sorensen, 2001). Some studies suggest no significant differences between older men and older women, whereas other studies suggest that older women have a higher prevalence rate of depression than older men (American Psychiatric Association, 2000; Federal Interagency Forum on Age-Related Statistics, 2013). However, the gap between women and men with regard to depressive symptoms decreases with age and the higher prevalence of major depression disorder in women in comparison to men also decreases with age (Barefoot, Mortensen, Helms, Avlund, & Schroll, 2001; Byers, Yaffe, Covinsky, Friedman, & Bruce, 2010). The narrowed gap could be a result of decreased prevalence of depression among older women relative to younger women, and stable or increased prevalence of depression among men over their life course (American Psychiatric Association, 2000; Jeste et al., 1999; Rokke & Klenow, 1998).

Anxiety Disorders and Posttraumatic Stress Disorder

Older women are more likely to have anxiety disorders than older men because of various medical, psychosocial (e.g., living arrangement, social support network), and substance usage factors (Byers et al., 2010; Weissman & dLevine, 2007). In addition, women are more at risk of developing posttraumatic stress disorder symptoms as they are more frequently subjected to the high frequency of trauma in the form of physical and sexual assault (Courtois, 2004; Ellsberg, Jansen, Heise, Watts, & Garcia-Moreno, 2008; Higgins & Follette, 2002; Shmotkin, Blumstein, & Modan, 2003). Older age presents more challenges for older women because older trauma survivors are likely to experience greater severity of trauma symptoms, or have delayed trauma reactions because of the co-occurrence of stressful life events, such as retirement and loss of social supports, and compromised coping capacities (deVries, 1996; Wolkenstein & Sterman, 1998). For example, one study found that re-victimization was a common experience for older women, and older women who experienced multiple types of trauma, including rape, childhood abuse, and domestic violence, had more severe psychological and physiological distress (Higgins & Follette, 2002).

Dementia

Studies suggest that there may not be consistent gender differences in the risks of developing dementia until very advanced age. A study has reported that older women have higher risks of developing Alzheimer's disease relative to older men (Andersen et al., 1999), whereas another study did not find gender differences until the 90s, with women more likely to develop Alzheimer's disease (Ruitenberg, Ott, van Swieten, Hofman, & Breteler, 2001). In addition, older men have higher risks than older women of developing vascular dementia and dementia due to diffuse Lewy body disease (Malatesta, 2007; Ruitenberg et al., 2001). Furthermore, the average age of schizophrenia onset in women is several years older than in men and the majority of later-onset cases (i.e., after age 45) are women (41% vs. 20%) (Lindamer, Lohr, Harris, & Jeste, 1999).

Theoretical Perspectives to Understand Women's Mental Health

The differences in mental health between women and men in old age could be a result of competing advantages and disadvantages of older women relative to older men. Older women are more likely to live in poverty, be widowed, and have poorer health, which suggests more stressors and poorer mental health; on the other hand, older women also display unique resilience factors that counterbalance their disadvantages, such as that women have advantages in using coping strategies (e.g., intrapsychic coping) that are effective to cope with adversities in old age as a consequence of their lifelong disadvantaged situation, and reduced differences in traditional social and gender roles when people get older (Bennett, 1997; Bookwala & Lawson, 2011; Doress-Worters, 1994; Feinson, 1987; Lim & Ng, 2010; Pachana et al., 2012; Pinquart & Sorensen, 2001; Rodeheaver & Datan, 1988; Skultety & Whitbourne, 2004; Tiedje et al., 1990).

Cumulative Advantage/Disadvantage

An important theoretical perspective to understand older women's mental health is the cumulative perspective. Cumulative advantage/disadvantage theory proposes to explain the increased diversities and inequality among older adults concerning socioeconomic situation, and their physical and mental health as the result of interactions among social institutions and individuals' social, cultural, and economic backgrounds over the life course (Crystal & Shea, 1990; Dannefer, 2003). Concerning mental health, this theory argues that women's social, economic, and health disadvantages in income, employment, and caregiving responsibilities accumulate into old age, and therefore could undermine women's mental health. For example, older women are more likely to be in poverty partly because current and earlier caregiving roles have limited their workforce participation, which prevents them from accruing adequate assets, pension, or social security (Davidson et al., 2011; Lowe, Young, Dolja-Gore, & Byles, 2008; Navaie-Waliser, Spriggs, & Feldman, 2002; Wakabayashi & Donato, 2006).

Even though marriages to some extent provide financial protection for women, their own labor force participation is an important factor for financial security in old age (Angel, Jimenez, & Angel, 2007; Gillen & Kim, 2009; Sevak, Weir, & Willis, 2004; Willson & Hardy, 2002). Poverty and financial strain among older women are serious problems, and they are both strong predictors of poor mental health and barriers to mental health utilization (Shippee, Wilkinson, & Ferraro, 2012). Caregiving responsibilities have also impaired older women's health and exposed them to long-term stressful situations (Brazil, Thabane, Foster, & Bedard, 2009; Gibbons et al., 2014; Holtzman, Abbey, Singer, Ross, & Stewart, 2011; Jenkins, 1997; Pinquart & Sorensen, 2006; Stewart et al., 2016). The cumulative effects of these factors are consequential for older women's mental health.

While the cumulative advantage/disadvantage theory focuses on how gendered disadvantages accumulate over time, several other theories direct attention to how social relationships in old age contextualize older women's mental health. For example, the life course perspective brings up how interactions with significant others, in addition to the environment that individuals have been exposed to across the life course, their own choices over the life course, and early life experiences, shape the heterogeneity of aging experiences (Elder & Johnson, 2003). Moreover, as suggested by the socioemotional selectivity theory, when people get older, time is regarded as limited and thus people are more selective about their social relationships and concentrate on important, rewarding, and meaningful ones; consequently, intimate and important relationships such as those with family members are more central to older adults and thus have more psychological consequences (Carstensen, Fung, & Charles, 2003).

Role Changes

Some theories also specifically address how the change of roles in old age affects older women's mental health. Old age is associated with loss of roles and older men and older women experience the loss of roles in different ways (Elwell & Maltbie-Crannell, 1981; Li, Chi, Krochalk, & Xu, 2011; Vo et al., 2015). Because of the life transition, different theoretical perspectives have proposed different challenges for older women's mental health. In the field of gerontology, the activity theory of aging, role enrichment theory, and the successful aging perspective propose that older adults enjoy better mental health by maintaining active social activities (Havinghust, 1961; Rowe & Kahn, 1997). Being actively socially engaged could help older adults to replace the lost roles caused by retirement and widowhood (Byles et al., 2013; Everingham, Warner-Smith, & Byles, 2007; Isherwood, King, & Luszcz, 2012). It also helps older women to maintain social ties that provide social support and reduce isolation, which contributes to better mental health (Kikuzawa, 2006). Specifically, role enrichment perspective argues that having concurrent multiple roles would improve mental health because having different roles provides opportunities for increased social support, a buffer which reduces the negative impacts of stressors, and power and prestige that offer satisfaction and enhanced mental health (Coleman & Antonucci, 1983; Moen, Robison, & Fields, 1994; Pearlin, 1989; Sieber, 1974).

However, the findings are not always consistent with the above perspectives and being engaged in productive roles does not always have beneficial effects (Hinterlong, Morrow-Howell, & Rozario, 2007). An alternative role-strain perspective argues that having multiple roles results in competing demands and reduces the performance for each role, which results in burnout, failure, and stress that compromise individuals' mental health (Smith, 1994). The role of strain is often observed in caregiving situations when caregivers have competing demands of their own work and caregiving responsibilities (Dautzenberg et al., 2000; Gordon, Pruchno, Wilson-Genderson, Murphy, & Rose, 2012; Kim, Ingersoll-Dayton, & Kwak, 2013; Mui, 1992; Wang, Shyu, Chen, & Yang, 2011). Partially consistent with the role-strain perspective, a study in Australia suggests that women at different stages are differently affected by multiple roles: while middle-aged women could benefit from multiple roles, older women who have only one role have the best mental health (Lee & Powers, 2002). But another study in the United States suggests that older American women have better mental health when they occupy different roles related to family, job, and community (Kikuzawa, 2006).

Social Relationships and Older Women's Mental Health

In this section, we discuss several social contexts that are especially important for older women and profoundly affect their mental health. The discussion focuses on the effects of spouses' declined health, widowhood, relationships with children, grandparenting, retirement, and being lesbian.

Spouses' Declining Health

As explained in the life-course perspective, older women's mental health is intertwined with and profoundly affected by the people around them, especially spouses. In old age, declining health in spouses imposes higher risks on older women for poor mental health outcomes due to the caregiving burden caused by providing care to their spouses (Hoppmann, Gerstorf, & Hibbert, 2011; Monserud & Peek, 2014). For example, older women who were caregivers for spouses with dementia reported poorer mental health and sleep quality (Willette-Murphy, Todero, & Yeaworth, 2006).

While among older adults, functional limitations and depression in one spouse are associated with higher levels of depression in the other spouse (Hoppmann et al., 2011; Monserud & Peek, 2014), the effects of spouses' functional limitation and mental health are stronger for wives than for husbands. For example, when both spouses are chronically ill, the number of chronic conditions in husbands is positively related to depressive symptoms in wives, while the relationship between the chronic condition in a wife and depressive symptoms in a husband is weaker and less robust (Thomeer, 2016). Another study found that older women's mental health was negatively affected by their spouses' onset of health problems, whereas it was older men's self-reported health at stake when their wives had health problems (Valle, Weeks, Taylor, & Eberstein, 2013). It was also reported that cancer survivors experienced increased risks of depression when their spouses displayed depressed mood and poor quality of life because of health-related reasons and the effects were stronger for survivors who were women (Litzelman & Yabroff, 2015).

Widowhood

Widowhood is a remarkable experience in old age, starts a significant transition in life and loss of roles with accompanying stressors, and has important mental health consequences (Bennett, 1997; Carr, 2004). Older women are more likely to be widowed than older men because of longer life expectancy (Lee, Willetts, & Seccombe, 1998; Li et al., 2011). In 2012, older women were less likely to be married than older men (45% vs. 72%), and there were more than four times as many widows as widowers (8.5 million vs. 2.1 million) (Administration on Aging, 2012).

Studies are not always consistent with respect to the effect of widowhood on older women. Some studies found no effect and some studies found more profound influences (Bennett, 1997; Umberson, Wortman, & Kessler, 1992). Other studies indicated a resilience pattern that recently widowed women suffered most in their mental health, but in the longer term widows could even have improved mental health over time (Feldman, Byles, & Beaumont, 2000; Wilcox et al., 2003). Another study found that older widows who were emotionally dependent on their husbands changed from having the lowest levels of self-esteem when married to having the highest levels of self-esteem after being widowed, suggesting a strong tendency of resilience among older women.

It has been consistently shown that widowhood affects older men and women in different ways. Generally speaking, widowhood imposes a heavier toll on men than women, which could be attributed to men's shorter time in experiencing widowhood, difficulties in dealing with household tasks, and lower levels of social engagement and social support, such as attending church or assisting children (Lee, DeMaris, Bavin, & Sullivan, 2001; Umberson et al., 1992). In contrast, financial strain is a major problem for widowed women and an important reason for higher levels of depression among widows (Angel et al., 2007; Gillen & Kim, 2009; Umberson et al., 1992). Widowhood also has an indirect negative effect on women's mental health through the increased likelihood of living alone (Bennett, 1997).

Relationships with Children

Relationships and interactions with children have been prominent factors that affect older adults' mental health (Katz, 2009; Lin & Wu, 2011; Silverstein & Bengtson, 1994; Silverstein, Chen, & Heller, 1996; Silverstein, Cong, & Li, 2006; Whitbeck, Hoyt, & Tyler, 2001). Interactions and relationships with adult children are summarized as including six dimensions in the intergenerational solidarity model: (1) associational solidarity such as contact; (2) affectual solidarity such as emotional attachment; (3) consensual solidarity such as agreement; (4) functional solidarity such as intergenerational exchanges of support; (5) normative solidarity, such as familism; and (6) structural solidarity indicating opportunity structure for family interaction (Bengtson & Roberts, 1991).

Studies have shown differences concerning the patterns of intergenerational interactions between older women and older men (Buber & Engelhardt, 2008; Li, Song, & Feldman, 2009; Okamoto & Tanaka, 2004). For example, relative to older men, older women are more likely to have stronger ties with their adult children, such as they are more likely to coreside with children, have more contact, and exchange more support, which are usually effective in reducing depression and promote mental health (Bengtson, Giarrusso, Mabry, & Silverstein, 2002; Buber & Engelhardt, 2008).

In addition to differences in intergenerational interactions and access to intergenerational support, the effects of intergenerational relationships on older women are also different from those on older men. For example, it was found that the frequency of contact with children was more beneficial to older fathers' than to older mothers' psychological consequences, whereas strained relationships and parental dissatisfaction were more detrimental to older mothers than older fathers (Umberson, 1992). In contrast, it was reported in Singapore that the benefits of receiving children's support on reducing depression were stronger among older mothers than among older fathers, suggesting the more prominent role of children in the older women's lives because of their more active roles in maintaining ties among kin and higher levels of reliance on family support (Ang & Malhotra, 2016). In addition, a study based on older couples in the British Household Panel Survey showed that coresiding with adult children impaired husbands' mental health but was a protective factor for wives' mental health (Read & Grundy, 2011). Those findings reveal that different effects of intergenerational relationships on older women's and older men's psychological consequences are highly dependent on specific dimensions of relationships and cultural contexts.

Intergenerational support sometimes may suggest negative psychological consequences, such as in the situation when too much support was provided to cause a loss of self-autonomy and self-control (Lin & Wu, 2011; Silverstein et al., 1996). It was also reported in Europe that instrumental support from children was more influential on older women's depression than on older men's, and women have a higher threshold than men for too much instrumental support to deteriorate their mental health (Djundeva, Mills, Wittek, & Steverink, 2014). This could be because intergenerational relationships are more central to older women than older men due to socialization and cultural reasons.

Grandparenting

Taking care of grandchildren is an important part of older adults' lives and its mental health consequences have attracted many researchers' attention, especially when increased life expectancy has elevated the opportunities for grandparents and grandchildren to have shared lives, and improved health of older adults has enabled them to take care of grandchildren (Baker & Silverstein, 2008; Bengtson & Lowerstein, 2003; Doley, Bell, Watt, & Simpson, 2015; Uhlenberg, 2009). Older women are much more likely to be involved in taking care of grandchildren than older men because of traditional caregiving roles, closer relationships with their children, especially daughters, and possible stronger genetic motivations to invest in grandchildren caused by maternal certainty of grandchildren (Chan & Elder, 2000; Cox, 2007; Danielsbacka, Tanskanen, & Rotkirch, 2015).

Studies have consistently shown that older women's mental health is affected by their involvement in grandparenting, but the effects are highly contextual. Grandmothers' involvement in taking care of grandchildren could be dramatically different, ranging from light to heavily involved, and highly involved grandmothers could be coparenting or surrogate parents (Goodman & Silverstein, 2002). Variations in the involvement usually reflect social and cultural differences. For example, for grandparents in White families, intimacy at a distance has been regarded as the norm, but grandparents in African American, Hispanic, and Asian American families are more likely to be involved in the intensive care of their grandchildren (Arber & Timonen, 2012;

Lee, Ensminger, & Laveist, 2005). Especially, African American grandmothers are more likely to coreside with their grandchildren, and even substitute the roles of their daughters to be the surrogate parents for their grandchildren as a response to teen pregnancy, single motherhood, substance abuse, and family disruptions (Gibson, 2002; Lee et al., 2005).

Custodial grandmothers usually have more mental health problems, such as depression and anxiety, than other grandmothers because of higher levels of stressors in their lives as a result of competing obligations (Baker & Silverstein, 2008). Risk factors for higher levels of mental health problems among those grandparents, especially grandmothers, include higher levels of stress, poverty, shorter time after stepping into the primary caregiver roles, poor health, and lack of social support (Burnette, 1999; Caputo, 2001; Ehrle, Geen, & Clark, 2001; Kelley, Whitley, Sipe, & Yorker, 2000; Letiecq, Bailey, & Kurtz, 2007; Minkler, Fuller-Thomson, Miller, & Driver, 1997; Waldrop & Weber, 2001).

The mental health implications of grandparenting also depend on support available and family environment. Social support reduces levels of depression among grandparents who raise grandchildren (Doley et al., 2015). In addition, taking the custodian grandparenting role is not always a stressor. When grandmothers assume grandparenting roles not under stress, such as in the situation when reasons for them to step into taking care of grandchildren are not family disruptions, grandparenting could help improve older women's mental health, such as in some Hispanic families (Goodman & Silverstein, 2005). Particularly, lower levels of acculturation of Hispanic caregiving grandmothers predict higher levels of life satisfaction and lower negative affect among them because of social resources available to this group of grandmothers (Goodman & Silverstein, 2005). In addition, a study in Chile found that grandmothers who provided more care experienced lower levels of depression (Grundy et al., 2012). Those findings suggest that the effect of grandparenting on older women depends on their social and cultural backgrounds and situations when grandparenting occurs.

Retirement

Retirement typically happens in later life and is an important transition that could tremendously change individuals' social roles, financial security, lifestyle, and support system, and thus has noticeable mental health implications (Angel et al., 2007). Gender has profoundly shaped the retirement experience from the life-course perspective, as women and men are different concerning their occupation, timing and duration of employment, and reasons for retirement, which in turn affect the social resources they have access to and challenges they are facing (Dow & Meyer, 2010; Jefferson, 2005; Noone, Alpass, & Stephens, 2010; Warner-Smith, Powers, & Hampson, 2008). Consequently, there are substantial gender differences concerning the effect of retirement on mental health among older adults.

Relative to men, women tend to retire earlier and are more likely to retire to be caregivers (Dow & Meyer, 2010; Jefferson, 2005; Noone et al., 2010; Warner-Smith et al., 2008); both are risk factors for poor mental health outcomes (Butterworth et al., 2006). However, studies have shown that retirement, especially early retirement, has more prominent effects on men than on women (Loretto & Vickerstaff, 2013; Olesen, Butterworth, & Rodgers, 2012). It is suggested that women may not feel a sharp transition into retirement because many retired women shoulder caregiving responsibilities and other unpaid work, such as volunteer work, but retired men, particularly those who retire early, could experience substantial distress because work achievements are central to men's identity, and men are usually expected to be the financial providers for the family (Butterworth et al., 2006; Byles et al., 2013; Everingham et al., 2007; Syzdek & Addis, 2010).

Older Lesbians

For older women who are lesbians, there are special challenges in their lives and their identity is an important factor to consider in mental health (D'augelli & Grossman, 2001; Fredriksen-Goldsen & Muraco, 2010). Generally speaking, older lesbians evaluate their mental health very positively (Averett & Jenkins, 2012; Berger, 1984). Actually, some studies suggest that older lesbians could be more resilient than heterosexual older women in the face of stressors due to their developed coping skills because of oppression, discrimination, victimization, and marginalization (Jones & Nystrom, 2002). Older lesbians have learned to adapt to adversities and create opportunities out of barriers and they also have strong social networks and social support from partners, ex-partners, and lesbian communities (Hall & Fine, 2005). Relative to older gay men, older lesbians have lower income, and thus financial security is a concern of older lesbians that could relate to poor mental health outcomes (Averett & Jenkins, 2012; Grossman, D'Augelli, & Hershberger, 2000; Quam & Whitford, 1992).

Effects of Mental Health on Health Among Older Women

Mental health problems, especially depression, are closely related to mortality, morbidity, and functional decline among older women. For example, depression was associated with higher risk of mortality (Teng, Yeh, Lee, Lin, & Lai, 2013), self-rated health (Han, 2002), cardiovascular disease (Windle & Windle, 2013), diabetes (Windle & Windle, 2013), fracture (Biderman, Cwikel, Fried, & Galinsky, 2002; Whooley et al., 1999), and other dimensions of functioning, such as negative attitudes of aging, and self-rated success in aging

(Vahia et al., 2010). The effect may depend on the types of depression (recurrent vs. single episode) or severity of depression (minor vs. major) as well as types of mortality (i.e., cancer vs. non-cancer) (Teng et al., 2013; Whooley & Browner, 1998; Windle & Windle, 2013). The risks of depression on mortality, morbidity, and functional decline could be the result of risky behaviors, such as reduced physical activities and social interactions, higher risks of indulging behaviors such as smoking, compromised sleep quality, and persistent fatigue (Kivelä & Pahkala, 2001; McHugh, Casey, & Lawlor, 2011; Penninx, Leveille, Ferrucci, Van Eijk, & Guralnik, 1999). It could also be the result of mental stress that is closely related to risk factors associated with mortality, such as hypertension, autonomic dysfunction, and increased circulating platelets (Ariyo et al., 2000; Whooley & Browner, 1998).

Studies on gender differences are not always consistent, but findings suggest that older women were more robust to minor and incident depression, and only major and chronic depression would contribute to increased risks of mortality. For instance, no gender difference was reported concerning the effect of depression on self-rated health among older adults (Han, 2002). Concerning mortality, it was found that both minor and major depression were risk factors for older men but only major depression predicted mortality in older women (Penninx, Geerlings, et al., 1999). A study in Taiwan also identified that only chronic depression was associated with a higher risk of mortality for older women whereas incident depression could contribute to higher risks of mortality for older men (Teng et al., 2013).

Older Women's Mental Health Care Use

Older adults are substantially underrepresented in mental health service use, in spite of recent estimates that almost 20% of older adults met criteria for a mental disorder (Ahn, Tai-Seale, Huber, Smith, & Ory, 2011; Gould, Coulson, & Howard, 2012; Karel, Gatz, & Smyer, 2012; Mackenzie, Scott, Mather, & Sareen, 2008; Wang et al., 2005). A study reported that older adults were three times less likely to use mental health services than their younger counterparts (Karlin, Duffy, & Gleaves, 2008). Many barriers to their use of mental health services have been identified, including the lack of perceived need to seek help, poverty, and enabling resources such as access to properly trained geriatric mental health professionals, and the belief of the effectiveness of psychological therapy (Byers, Arean, & Yaffe, 2012; Karlin et al., 2008; Klap, Unroe, & Unutzer, 2003; Mackenzie, Gekoski, & Knox, 2006; Mackenzie et al., 2008; Wuthrich & Frei, 2015).

Relative to older men, older women are more likely to be undertreated because of their greater tendency to be in poverty, higher likelihood of being widowed, and inadequate retirement plans and health insurance resulting from lifelong caregiving responsibilities and sporadic labor force participation (Smith, 2007). In addition, there are substantial racial differences concerning mental health utilization among older women, with racial-ethnic minority older adults less likely to use mental health services because of their reluctance to discuss personal problems with health care professionals, the belief that depression is a sign of personal weakness, other misconceptions, and cultural stigma regarding mental disorders (Byers et al., 2012; Jang, Chiriboga, & Okazaki, 2009). For example, a study found that African American women across different age groups used prayers and counseling to cope with mental illness, but mistrusted the effectiveness of medications; the barriers for them to seek treatment included lack of awareness of mental health problems, limited access to mental health services, and perceived stigma (Ward & Heidrich, 2009). Similarly, in a focus group study, where 85% of participants were African American older women, misconceptions about mental health problems and culturally sanctioned coping strategies were also identified as barriers to the use of mental health care (Conner et al., 2010).

In addition, older women were more likely to be exposed to abuse, particularly domestic violence, relative to older men (Pillemer & Finkelhor, 1988; Zink, Fisher, Regan, & Pabst, 2005; Zink, Jeffrey Jacobson Jr, Regan, & Pabst, 2004). A study on community-dwelling older women found about half of women experienced some kinds of abuse, such as emotional, physical, or sexual, and many experienced multiple types of abuse repeatedly (Fisher & Regan, 2006). Another study showed that the lifetime partner violence prevalence for older women (65 years older and over) was 26.5%; about 18.4% of them experienced physical or sexual abuse or both, and 21.9% experienced non-physical abuse (Bonomi et al., 2007).

Older women who were exposed to previous domestic violence reported various health- and mental health-related problems, such as depression, anxiety, and alcohol dependence (Fisher & Regan, 2006; Wolkenstein & Sterman, 1998). However, older women who experience partner violence are at greater risk of not receiving necessary mental health services because they are reluctant to seek help or initiate talks with their health providers about domestic violence, which imposes barriers on their access to mental health care (Lipsky & Caetano, 2007; Zink et al., 2004). The reluctance to seek help is attributed to unsupportive responses from the family and community, feelings of powerlessness and hopelessness, self-blame, and intention of keeping their trauma experience from others (Beaulaurier, Seff, Newman, & Dunlop, 2006; Zink et al., 2004). In addition, older women with unmet needs for mental health services related to previous domestic violence are more likely to report financial difficulties and inadequate support from peers and family members, which further reduces their access to mental health care (Wolkenstein & Sterman, 1998).

Effective Interventions

Various intervention programs have been developed to promote older women's mental health. As expected, physical activities and exercise are effective in decreasing mental health problems among older women (Lucas et al., 2011). Particularly, age-appropriate walking could be an effective intervention to help with older women's mental health. For example, a study found that, for older women aged 60 to 74 with mild depression, breaking one hour of walking into three to five sessions in a week was more effective in decreasing depression than walking one hour once a week, possibly because higher frequencies of exercise might result in stronger cumulative effects on increasing positive affect, and reducing negative thoughts and ruminative processes (Legrand & Mille, 2009).

Other programs that provide social interactions and social support have also been effective in reducing mental health problems among older women with special needs. A friendship enrichment program showed reduced loneliness, improved friendship quality, and improved subjective well-being among older women (Martina & Stevens, 2006). Programs that target African American grandmothers raising grandchildren could also help to reduce their psychological distress and improve their mental health by providing home visits by registered nurses, social workers, legal assistance, and monthly support in the form of group meetings (Kelley, Whitley, & Sipe, 2007; Kelley, Yorker, Whitley, & Sipe, 2001). The effectiveness of those interventions is related to participants' increased confidence in their abilities to care for their grandchildren, increased security caused by group support, and reduced anger toward the caregiving situations (Kelley et al., 2001, 2007).

Other interventions that focus on older adults, but with the majority of the participants as older women, have also shown the importance of enhanced social interactions on older women's mental health. The Kate Mills Snider Geriatric Psychiatry Outreach Program is an example of providing psychological services for older adults (with 74% older women) who were unable to get to an office-based intervention (Johnston et al., 2010). Patients in the program received a mean of 4.2 home visits and a mean of 30.2 additional contacts (mainly phone calls) and gained psychological benefits. Additionally, in an intergenerational program, older volunteers read picture books to children in a school setting and had reduced social isolation and loneliness as a result of a greater sense of meaningfulness (Murayama et al., 2015). It was also proposed that group interventions that targets specific groups of people with shared needs are particularly effective in reducing social isolation and loneliness, and thus have positive psychological benefits for older adults, especially older women (Cattan, White, Bond, & Learmouth, 2005).

Interventions utilizing special techniques have also been applied to older women and showed significant psychological benefits. For example, reminiscence therapy is a cost-effective intervention in reducing depression and increasing self-transcendence among institutionalized as well as community-dwelling older women (Stinson & Kirk, 2006). Reminiscence is an interpersonal or communicative psychosocial process "using the recall of past events, feelings, and thoughts to facilitate adaptation to present circumstances" (p. 285), and reminiscence therapy is regarded as therapeutic, social, and recreational, and consequently is particularly effective in improving older women's mental health (Jones & Beck-Little, 2002). In addition, Memory Bank is a community life story development intervention program that involves five key elements, namely, life story development, communication, social support, brain exercise, and legacy building (Zanjani, Downer, Hosier, & Watkins, 2014). It was effective in reducing distress and burden related to age and also resulted in significant improvement in depression, mood disturbance, and cognitive performance among older participants, among whom 72% were women (Zanjani et al., 2014).

Conclusion

Women in their older age are facing special challenges as a result of accumulated social, economic, and health disadvantages over the life course. But older women also show resilience because of developed coping skills and better-developed social networks and family engagement due to kin-keeping and caregiving roles. This chapter focused on women's mental health and discussed empirical evidence, relevant theoretical perspectives, special social contexts relevant to older women, influences of mental health on health, their mental health utilization, and effective intervention programs. In spite of coexistence of conflicting evidence, the current literature generally shows that older women experience resilience in mental health relative to older men regardless of life-long disadvantages; however, the resilience has to be understood in the broader social context of vulnerability, especially cumulative disadvantages that could exacerbate among the disadvantaged subgroups among older women, such as those who are of lower socioeconomic status, minority status, and with traumatic experiences. Cumulative advantage/disadvantage theory and role theory are particularly useful to understand the heterogeneity among older women and exacerbated vulnerability among disadvantaged groups. Although older women are overrepresented in the older population, studies on older women's mental health are still limited. Guided by current theories in women studies and gerontology, additional efforts should be made to examine older women's mental health from a life-course perspective with emphasis on social connections, social positions, and heterogeneity among older women to better meet their mental health needs.

References

Administration on Aging, Administration for Country Living, U.S. Department of Health and Human Services. (2012). *A profile of older Americans: 2012*. Retrieved from http://www.aoa. gov/Aging_Statistics/Profile/2012/docs/2012profile.pdf (accessed November 2, 2016).

Ahn, S. N., Tai-Seale, M., Huber Jr, C., Smith, M. L., & Ory, M. G. (2011). Psychotropic medication discussions in older adults' primary care office visits: So much to do, so little time. *Aging and Mental Health, 15*(5), 618–629. doi:10.1080/13607863.2010.548055.

American Psychiatric Association. (2000). *DSM-IV-TR: Diagnostic and statistical manual of mental disorders (4th edition), text revision*. Arlington, VA: American Psychiatric Association.

Andersen, K., Launer, L. J., Dewey, M. E., Letenneur, L., Ott, A., Copeland, J. R. M., . . . & Brayne, C. (1999). Gender differences in the incidence of AD and vascular dementia. The EURODEM Studies. *Neurology, 53*(9), 1992–1992. doi:10.1212/WNL.53.9.1992.

Ang, S., & Malhotra, R. (2016). Association of received social support with depressive symptoms among older males and females in Singapore: Is personal mastery an inconsistent mediator? *Social Science and Medicine, 153*, 165–173. doi:10.1016/j.socscimed.2016.02.019.

Angel, J. L., Jimenez, M. A., & Angel, R. J. (2007). The economic consequences of widowhood for older minority women. *The Gerontologist, 47*(2), 224–234. doi:10.1093/geront/47.2.224.

Arber, S., & Timonen, V. (2012). Grandparenting in the 21st century: New directions. In S. Arber & V. Timonen (Eds.), *Contemporary grandparenting: Changing family relationships in global contexts* (pp. 247–264). Bristol: The Policy Press.

Ariyo, A. A., Haan, M., Tangen, C. M., Rutledge, J. C., Cushman, M., Dobs, A., & Furberg, C. D. (2000). Depressive symptoms and risks of coronary heart disease and mortality in elderly Americans. *Circulation, 102*(15), 1773–1779. doi:10.1161/01.CIR.102.15.1773.

Averett, P., & Jenkins, C. (2012). Review of the literature on older lesbians: Implications for education, practice, and research. *Journal of Applied Gerontology, 31*(4), 537–561. doi:10.1177/0733464810392555.

Baker, L. A., & Silverstein, M. (2008). Depressive symptoms among grandparents raising grandchildren: The impact of participation in multiple roles. *Journal of Intergenerational Relationships, 6*(3), 285–304. doi:10.1080/15350770802157802.

Barefoot, J. C., Mortensen, E. L., Helms, M. J., Avlund, K., & Schroll, M. (2001). A longitudinal study of gender differences in depressive symptoms from age 50 to 80. *Psychology and Aging, 16*(2), 342–345. doi:10.1037/0882-7974.16.2.342.

Beaulaurier, R. L., Seff, L. R., Newman, F. L., & Dunlop, B. (2006). Internal barriers to help seeking for middle-aged and older women who experience intimate partner violence. *Journal of Elder Abuse and Neglect, 17*(3), 53–74. doi:10.1300/J084v17n03_04.

Beck, C. M., & Pearson, B. P. (1989). Mental health of elderly women. *Journal of Women and Aging, 1*(1–3), 175–193. doi:10.1300/J074v01n01_09.

Bengtson, V., Giarrusso, R., Mabry, J. B., & Silverstein, M. (2002). Solidarity, conflict, and ambivalence: Complementary or competing perspectives on intergenerational relationships? *Journal of Marriage and Family, 64*(3), 568–576.

Bengtson, V. L., & Lowerstein, A. (Eds.). (2003). *Global aging and the challenge to families*. New York: Walter de Gruyter.

Bengtson, V. L., & Roberts, R. L. (1991). Intergenerational solidarity in aging families: An example of formal theory construction. *Journal of Marriage and the Family, 53*(4), 856–870. doi:10.2307/352993.

Bennett, K. M. (1997). Widowhood in elderly women: The medium- and long-term effects on mental and physical health. *Mortality, 2*(2), 137–148. doi:10.1080/713685857.

Berger, R. M. (1984). Realities of gay and lesbian aging. *Social Work, 29*(1), 57–62. doi:10.1093/sw/29.1.57.

Biderman, A., Cwikel, J., Fried, A. V., & Galinsky, D. (2002). Depression and falls among community dwelling elderly people: A search for common risk factors. *Journal of Epidemiology and Community Health, 56*(8), 631–636. doi:10.1136/jech.56.8.631.

Bonomi, A. E., Anderson, M. L., Reid, R. J., Carrell, D., Fishman, P. A., Rivara, F. P., & Thompson, R. S. (2007). Intimate partner violence in older women. *The Gerontologist, 47*(1), 34–41. doi:10.1093/geront/47.1.34.

Bookwala, J., & Lawson, B. (2011). Poor vision, functioning, and depressive symptoms: A test of the activity restriction model. *The Gerontologist, 51*(6), 798–808. doi:10.1093/geront/gnr051.

Brainerd, C. J., Reyna, V. F., Petersen, R. C., Smith, G. E., Kenney, A. E., Gross, C. J., . . . & Fisher, G. G. (2013). The apolipoprotein E genotype predicts longitudinal transitions to mild cognitive impairment but not to Alzheimer's dementia: Findings from a nationally representative study. *Neuropsychology, 27*(1), 86–94. doi:10.1037/a0030855.

Brazil, K., Thabane, L., Foster, G., & Bedard, M. (2009). Gender differences among Canadian spousal caregivers at the end of life. *Health and Social Care in the Community, 17*(2), 159–166. doi:10.1111/j.1365-2524.2008.00813.x.

Buber, I., & Engelhardt, H. (2008). Children's impact on the mental health of their older mothers and fathers: Findings from the survey of health, ageing and retirement in Europe. *European Journal of Ageing, 5*(1), 31–45. doi:10.1007/s10433-008-0074-8.

Burnette, D. (1999). Social relationships of Latino grandparent caregivers: A role theory perspective. *The Gerontologist, 39*(1), 49–58. doi:10.1093/geront/39.1.49.

Butterworth, P., Gill, S. C., Rodgers, B., Anstey, K. J., Villamil, E., & Melzer, D. (2006). Retirement and mental health: Analysis of the Australian national survey of mental health and well-being. *Social Science and Medicine, 62*(5), 1179–1191. doi:10.1016/j.socscimed.2005.07.013.

Byers, A. L., Arean, P. A., & Yaffe, K. (2012). Low use of mental health services among older Americans with mood and anxiety disorders. *Psychiatric Services, 63*(1), 66–72. doi:10.1176/appi.ps.201100121.

Byers, A. L., Yaffe, K., Covinsky, K. E., Friedman, M. B., & Bruce, M. L. (2010). High occurrence of mood and anxiety disorders among older adults: The National Comorbidity Survey Replication. *Archives of General Psychiatry, 67*(5), 489–496. doi:10.1001/archgenpsychiatry.2010.35.

Byles, J., Tavener, M., Robinson, I., Parkinson, L., Smith, P. W., Stevenson, D., . . . & Curryer, C. (2013). Transforming retirement: New definitions of life after work. *Journal of Women and Aging, 25*(1), 24–44. doi:10.1080/08952841.2012.717855.

Caputo, R. (2001). Depression and health among grandmothers co-residing with grandchildren in two cohorts of women. *Families in Society: The Journal of Contemporary Social Services, 82*(5), 473–483. doi:10.1606/1044-3894.166.

Carr, D. (2004). Gender, preloss marital dependence, and older adults' adjustment to widowhood. *Journal of Marriage and Family, 66*(1), 220–235. doi:10.1111/j.0022-2445.2004.00016.x.

Carstensen, L. L., Fung, H. H., & Charles, S. T. (2003). Socioemotional selectivity theory and the regulation of emotion in the second half of life. *Motivation and Emotion, 27*(2), 103–123.

Cattan, M., White, M., Bond, J., & Learmouth, A. (2005). Preventing social isolation and loneliness among older people: A systematic review of health promotion interventions. *Ageing and Society, 25*(01), 41–67.

Chan, C. G., & Elder, G. H. J. (2000). Matrilineal advantage in grandchild–grandparent relations. *The Gerontologist, 40*(2), 179–190.

Choi, N. G., & DiNitto, D. M. (2011). Drinking, smoking, and psychological distress in middle and late life. *Aging and Mental Health, 15*(6), 720–731. doi:10.1080/13607863.2010.551343.

Chrisler, J. C., Barney, A., & Palatino, B. (2016). Ageism can be hazardous to women's health: Ageism, sexism, and stereotypes of older women in the healthcare system. *Journal of Social Issues, 72*(1), 86–104. doi:10.1111/josi.12157.

Coleman, L. M., & Antonucci, T. C. (1983). Impact of work on women at midlife. *Developmental Psychology, 19*(2), 290–294. doi:10.1037/0012-1649.19.2.290.

Conner, K. O., Lee, B., Mayers, V., Robinson, D., Reynolds, C. F., Albert, S., & Brown, C. (2010). Attitudes and beliefs about mental health among African American older adults suffering from depression. *Journal of Aging Studies, 24*(4), 266–277. doi:10.1016/j.jaging.2010.05.007.

Courtois, C. A. (2004). Complex trauma, complex reactions: Assessment and treatment. *Psychotherapy: Theory, Research, Practice, Training, 41*(4), 412–425. doi:10.1037/0033-3204.41.4.412.

Cox, D. (2007). Biological basics and the economics of the family. *Journal of Economic Perspectives, 21*(2), 91–108.

Crystal, S., & Shea, D. (1990). Cumulative advantage, cumulative disadvantage, and inequality among elderly people. *The Gerontologist, 30*(4), 437–443. doi:10.1093/geront/30.4.437.

Danielsbacka, M., Tanskanen, A. O., & Rotkirch, A. (2015). Impact of genetic relatedness and emotional closeness on intergenerational relations. *Journal of Marriage and Family, 77*(4), 889–907.

Dannefer, D. (2003). Cumulative advantage/disadvantage and the life course: Cross-fertilizing age and social science theory. *The Journals of Gerontology Series B: Psychological Sciences and Social Sciences, 58*(6), S327–S337.

D'augelli, A. R., & Grossman, A. H. (2001). Disclosure of sexual orientation, victimization, and mental health among lesbian, gay, and bisexual older adults. *Journal of Interpersonal Violence, 16*(10), 1008–1027. doi:10.1177/088626001016010003.

Dautzenberg, M. G. H., Diederiks, J. P. M., Philipsen, H., Stevens, F. C. J., Tan, F. E. S., & Vernooij-Dassen, M. J. F. J. (2000). The competing demands of paid work and parent care middle-aged daughters providing assistance to elderly parents. *Research on Aging, 22*(2), 165–187. doi:10.1177/0164027500222004.

Davidson, P. M., DiGiacomo, M., & McGrath, S. J. (2011). The feminization of aging: How will this impact on health outcomes and services? *Health Care for Women International, 32*(12), 1031–1045. doi:10.1080/07399332.2011.610539.

deVries, M. W. (1996). Trauma in cultural perspective. In B. van der Kolk, A. McFarlance, & L. Weisaeth (Eds.), *Traumatic stress: The effects of overwhelming experience on mind, body and society* (pp. 398–413). New York: Guilford Press.

Djundeva, M., Mills, M., Wittek, R., & Steverink, N. (2014). Receiving instrumental support in late parent–child relationships and parental depression. *The Journals of Gerontology Series B: Psychological Sciences and Social Sciences, 70*(6), 981–994. doi:10.1093/geronb/gbu136.

Doley, R., Bell, R., Watt, B., & Simpson, H. (2015). Grandparents raising grandchildren: Investigating factors associated with distress among custodial grandparent. *Journal of Family Studies, 21*(2), 101–119. doi:10.1080/13229400.2015.1015215.

Doress-Worters, P. B. (1994). Adding elder care to women's multiple roles: A critical review of the caregiver stress and multiple roles literatures. *Sex Roles, 31*(9–10), 597–616. doi:10.1007/BF01544282.

Dow, B., & Meyer, C. (2010). Caring and retirement: Crossroads and consequences. *International Journal of Health Services, 40*(4), 645–665. doi:10.2190/HS.40.4.e.

Ehrle, J., Geen, R., & Clark, R. (2001). *Children cared for by relatives: Who are they and how are they faring?* New Federalism: National Survey of America's Families: Series Number B-28). Washington, DC: The Urban Institute.

Elder, G. H. J., & Johnson, M. K. (2003). The life course and aging: Challenges, lessons and new directions. In R. A. Settersten, Jr. (Ed.), *Invitation to the life course: Toward a new understanding of later life* (pp. 49–81). Amityville, NY: Baywood.

Ellsberg, M., Jansen, H. A., Heise, L., Watts, C. H., & Garcia-Moreno, C. (2008). Intimate partner violence and women's physical and mental health in the WHO multi-country study on women's health and domestic violence: an observational study. *The Lancet, 371*(9619), 1165–1172.

Elwell, F., & Maltbie-Crannell, A. D. (1981). The impact of role loss upon coping resources and life satisfaction of the elderly. *Journal of Gerontology, 36*(2), 223–232. doi:10.1093/geronj/36.2.223.

Everingham, C., Warner-Smith, P., & Byles, J. (2007). Transforming retirement: Re-thinking models of retirement to accommodate the experiences of women. *Women's Studies International Forum, 30*(6), 512–522. doi:10.1016/j.wsif.2007.09.006.

Federal Interagency Forum on Age-Related Statistics. (2013). Older Americans 2012: Key indicators of well-being. Retrieved from http://www.aarp.org/content/dam/aarp/livable-communities/learn/demographics/older-americans-2012-key-indicators-of-well-being-aarp.pdf (accessed November 21, 2016).

Feinson, M. C. (1987). Mental health and aging: Are there gender differences? *The Gerontologist, 27*(6), 703–711. doi:10.1093/geront/27.6.703.

Feldman, S., Byles, J. E., & Beaumont, R. (2000). 'Is anybody listening?' The experiences of widowhood for older Australian women. *Journal of Women and Aging, 12*(3–4), 155–176. doi:10.1300/J074v12n03_10.

Fisher, B. S., & Regan, S. L. (2006). The extent and frequency of abuse in the lives of older women and their relationship with health outcomes. *The Gerontologist, 46*(2), 200–209. doi:10.1093/geront/46.2.200.

Fredriksen-Goldsen, K. I., & Muraco, A. (2010). Aging and sexual orientation: A 25-year review of the literature. *Research on Aging, 32*(3), 372–413. doi:10.1177/0164027509360355.

Ganz, P. A., Guadagnoli, E., Landrum, M. B., Lash, T. L., Rakowski, W., & Silliman, R. A. (2003). Breast cancer in older women: Quality of life and psychosocial adjustment in the 15 months after diagnosis. *Journal of Clinical Oncology, 21*(21), 4027–4033. doi:10.1200/JCO.2003.08.097.

Gibbons, C., Creese, J., Tran, M., Brazil, K., Chambers, L., Weaver, B., & Bedard, M. (2014). The psychological and health consequences of caring for a spouse with dementia: A critical comparison of husbands and wives. *Journal of Women and Aging, 26*(1), 3–21. doi:10.1080/08952841.2014.854571.

Gibson, P. (2002). African American grandmothers as caregivers: Answering the call to help their grandchildren. *Families in Society: The Journal of Contemporary Social Services, 83*(1), 35–43.

Gillen, M., & Kim, H. (2009). Older women and poverty transition: Consequences of income source changes from widowhood. *Journal of Applied Gerontology, 28*(3), 320–341. doi:10.1177/0733464808326953.

Goodman, C., & Silverstein, M. (2002). Grandmothers raising grandchildren family structure and well-being in culturally diverse families. *The Gerontologist, 42*(5), 676–689. doi:10.1093/geront/42.5.676.

Goodman, C. C., & Silverstein, M. (2005). Latina grandmothers raising grandchildren: Acculturation and psychological well-being. *The International Journal of Aging and Human Development, 60*(4), 305–316. doi:10.2190/NQ2P-4ABR-3U1F-W6G0.

Gordon, J. R., Pruchno, R. A., Wilson-Genderson, M., Murphy, W. M., & Rose, M. (2012). Balancing caregiving and work: Role conflict and role strain dynamics. *Journal of Family Issues, 33*(5), 662–689. doi:10.1177/0192513X11425322.

Gould, R. L., Coulson, M. C., & Howard, R. J. (2012). Cognitive behavioral therapy for depression in older people: A meta-analysis and meta-regression of randomized controlled trials. *Journal of the American Geriatrics Society, 60*(10), 1817–1830. doi:10.1111/j.1532-5415.2012.04166.x.

Grigoriadis, S., & Erlick Robinson, G. (2007). Gender issues in depression. *Annals of Clinical Psychiatry, 19*(4), 247–255. doi:10.3109/10401230701653294.

Grossman, A. H., D'Augelli, A. R., & Hershberger, S. L. (2000). Social support networks of lesbian, gay, and bisexual adults 60 years of age and older. *The Journals of Gerontology Series B: Psychological Sciences and Social Sciences, 55*(3), P171–P179. doi:10.1093/geronb/55.3.P171.

Grundy, E. M., Albala, C., Allen, E., Dangour, A. D., Elbourne, D., & Uauy, R. (2012). Grandparenting and psychosocial health among older Chileans: A longitudinal analysis. *Aging and Mental Health, 16*(8), 1047–1057. doi:10.1080/13607863.2012.692766.

Hall, R. L., & Fine, M. (2005). The stories we tell: The lives and friendship of two older black lesbians. *Psychology of Women Quarterly, 29*(2), 177–187. doi:10.1111/j.1471-6402.2005.00180.x.

Han, B. (2002). Depressive symptoms and self-rated health in community-dwelling older adults: A longitudinal study. *Journal of the American Geriatrics Society, 50*(9), 1549–1556. doi:10.1046/j.1532-5415.2002.50411.x.

Havinghust, R. J. (1961). Successful aging. *The Gerontologist, 1*(1), 8–13. doi:10.1093/geront/1.1.8.

Higgins, A. B., & Follette, V. M. (2002). Frequency and impact of interpersonal trauma in older women. *Journal of Clinical Geropsychology, 8*(3), 215–226. doi:10.1023/A:1015948328291.

Hinterlong, J. E., Morrow-Howell, N., & Rozario, P. A. (2007). Productive engagement and late life physical and mental health findings from a nationally representative panel study. *Research on Aging, 29*(4), 348–370. doi:10.1177/0164027507300806.

Holtzman, S., Abbey, S. E., Singer, L. G., Ross, H. J., & Stewart, D. E. (2011). Both patient and caregiver gender impact depressive symptoms among organ transplant caregivers: Who is at risk and why? *Journal of Health Psychology, 16*(5), 843–856. doi:10.1177/1359105310393542.

Hoppmann, C. A., Gerstorf, D., & Hibbert, A. (2011). Spousal associations between functional limitation and depressive symptom trajectories: Longitudinal findings from the study of Asset and Health Dynamics Among the Oldest Old (AHEAD). *Health Psychology, 30*(2), 153. doi:10.1037/a0022094.

Isherwood, L. M., King, D. S., & Luszcz, M. A. (2012). A longitudinal analysis of social engagement in late-life widowhood. *The International Journal of Aging and Human Development, 74*(3), 211–229. doi:10.2190/AG.74.3.c.

Jang, Y., Chiriboga, D. A., & Okazaki, S. (2009). Attitudes toward mental health services: Age-group differences in Korean American adults. *Aging and Mental Health, 13*(1), 127–134. doi:10.1080/13607860802591070.

Jefferson, T. (2005). Women and retirement incomes in Australia: A review. *Economic Record, 81*(254), 273–291. doi:10.1111/j.1475-4932.2005.00261.x.

Jenkins, C. L. (1997). Women, work, and caregiving: How do these roles affect women's well-being? *Journal of Women and Aging, 9*(3), 27–45. doi:10.1300/J074v09n03_03.

Jeste, D. V., Alexopoulos, G. S., Bartels, S. J., Cummings, J. L., Gallo, J. J., Gottlieb, G. L., . . . & Reynolds, C. F. (1999). Consensus statement on the upcoming crisis in geriatric mental health: Research agenda for the next 2 decades. *Archives of General Psychiatry, 56*(9), 848–853. doi:10.1001/archpsyc.56.9.848.

Johnston, D., Smith, M., Beard-Byrd, K., Albert, A., Legault, C., McCall, W. V., . . . & Reifler, B. (2010). A new home-based mental health program for older adults: Description of the first 100 cases. *The American Journal of Geriatric Psychiatry, 18*(12), 1141–1145. doi:10.1097/JGP.0b013e3181dd1c64.

Jones, E. D., & Beck-Little, R. (2002). The use of reminiscence therapy for the treatment of depression in rural-dwelling older adults. *Issues in Mental Health Nursing, 23*(3), 279–290. doi:10.1080/016128402753543018.

Jones, T. C., & Nystrom, N. M. (2002). Looking back . . . looking forward: Addressing the lives of lesbians 55 and older. *Journal of Women and Aging, 14*(3–4), 59–76. doi:10.1300/J074v14n03_05.

Karel, M. J., Gatz, M., & Smyer, M. A. (2012). Aging and mental health in the decade ahead: What psychologists need to know. *American Psychologist, 67*(3), 184. doi:10.1037/a0025393.

Karlin, B. E., Duffy, M., & Gleaves, D. H. (2008). Patterns and predictors of mental health service use and mental illness among older and younger adults in the United States. *Psychological Services, 5*(3), 275. doi:10.1037/1541-1559.5.3.275.

Katz, R. (2009). Intergenerational family relations and subjective well-being in old age: A cross-national study. *European Journal of Ageing, 6*(2), 79–90. doi:10.1007/s10433-009-0113-0.

Kelley, S. J., Whitley, D., & Sipe, T. A. (2007). Results of an interdisciplinary intervention to improve the psychosocial well-being and physical functioning of African American grandmothers raising grandchildren. *Journal of Intergenerational Relationships, 5*(3), 45–64. doi:10.1300/J194v05n03_04.

Kelley, S. J., Whitley, D., Sipe, T. A., & Yorker, B. C. (2000). Psychological distress in grandmother kinship care providers: the role of resources, social support, and physical health. *Child Abuse and Neglect, 24*(3), 311–321.

Kelley, S. J., Yorker, B. C., Whitley, D. M., & Sipe, T. A. (2001). A multimodal intervention for grandparents raising grandchildren: Results of an exploratory study. *Child Welfare, 80*(1), 27.

Kikuzawa, S. (2006). Multiple roles and mental health in cross-cultural perspective: The elderly in the United States and Japan. *Journal of Health and Social Behavior, 47*(1), 62–76. doi:10.1177/002214650604700105.

Kim, J., Ingersoll-Dayton, B., & Kwak, M. (2013). Balancing eldercare and employment: The role of work interruptions and supportive employers. *Journal of Applied Gerontology, 32*(3), 347–369. doi:10.1177/0733464811423647.

Kivelä, S. L., & Pahkala, K. (2001). Depressive disorder as a predictor of physical disability in old age. *Journal of the American Geriatrics Society, 49*(3), 290–296. doi:10.1046/j.1532-5415.2001.4930290.x.

Klap, R., Unroe, K. T., & Unutzer, J. (2003). Caring for mental illness in the United States: A focus on older adults. *The American Journal of Geriatric Psychiatry, 11*(5), 517–524. doi:10.1097/00019442-200309000-00006.

Lee, C., & Powers, J. R. (2002). Number of social roles, health, and well-being in three generations of Australian women. *International Journal of Behavioral Medicine, 9*(3), 195–215.

Lee, G. R., DeMaris, A., Bavin, S., & Sullivan, R. (2001). Gender differences in the depressive effect of widowhood in later life. *The Journals of Gerontology Series B: Psychological Sciences and Social Sciences, 56*(1), S56–S61. doi:10.1093/geronb/56.1.S56.

Lee, G. R., Willetts, M. C., & Seccombe, K. (1998). Widowhood and depression: Gender differences. *Research on Aging, 20*(5), 611–630. doi:10.1177/0164027598205004.

Lee, R. D., Ensminger, M. E., & Laveist, T. A. (2005). The responsibility continuum: Never primary, coresident and caregiver—heterogeneity in the African-American grandmother experience. *The International Journal of Aging and Human Development, 60*(4), 295–304.

Legrand, F. D., & Mille, C. R. (2009). The effects of 60 minutes of supervised weekly walking (in a single vs. 3-5 session format) on depressive symptoms among older women: Findings from a pilot randomized trial. *Mental Health and Physical Activity, 2*(2), 71–75. doi:10.1016/j.mhpa.2009.09.002.

Letiecq, B. L., Bailey, S. J., & Kurtz, M. A. (2007). Depression among rural Native American and European American grandparents rearing their grandchildren. *Journal of Family Issues, 29*(3), 334–356. doi:10.1177/0192513X07308393.

Li, S., Song, L., & Feldman, M. W. (2009). Intergenerational support and subjective health of older people in rural China: A gende-based longitudinal study. *Australasian Journal on Ageing, 28*(2), 81–86. doi:10.1111/j.1741-6612.2009.00364.x.

Li, Y., Chi, I., Krochalk, P. C., & Xu, L. (2011). Widowhood, family support, and self-rated health among older adults in China. *International Journal of Social Welfare, 20*(s1), S72–S85. doi:10.1111/j.1468-2397.2011.00818.x.

Lim, L. L., & Ng, T. P. (2010). Living alone, lack of a confidant and psychological well-being of elderly women in Singapore: The mediating role of loneliness. *Asiaâ-Pacific Psychiatry, 2*(1), 33–40. doi:10.1111/j.1758-5872.2009.00049.x.

Lin, I.-F., & Wu, H.-S. (2011). Does informal care attenuate the cycle of ADL/IADL disability and depressive symptoms in late life? *Journal of Gerontology: Social Sciences, 66*(5), 585–594.

Lindamer, L. A., Lohr, J. B., Harris, M. J., & Jeste, D. V. (1999). Gender-related clinical differences in older patients with schizophrenia. *The Journal of Clinical Psychiatry, 60*(1), 1,478–467. doi:10.4088/JCP.v60n0114.

Lipsky, S., & Caetano, R. (2007). Impact of intimate partner violence on unmet need for mental health care: Results from the NSDUH. *Psychiatric Services, 58*(6), 822–829.

Litzelman, K., & Yabroff, K. R. (2015). How are spousal depressed mood, distress, and quality of life associated with risk of depressed mood in cancer survivors? Longitudinal findings from a national sample. *Cancer Epidemiology, Biomarkers and Prevention, 24*(6), 969–977. doi:10.1158/1055-9965.EPI-14-1420.

Loretto, W., & Vickerstaff, S. (2013). The domestic and gendered context for retirement. *Human Relations, 66*(1), 65–86. doi:10.1177/0018726712455832.

Lowe, J., Young, A. F., Dolja-Gore, X., & Byles, J. (2008). Cost of medications for older women. *Australian and New Zealand Journal of Public Health, 32*(1), 89–89. doi:10.1111/j.1753-6405.2008.00174.x.

Lucas, M., Mekary, R., Pan, A., Mirzaei, F., O'Reilly, É. J., Willett, W. C., . . . & Ascherio, A. (2011). Relation between clinical depression risk and physical activity and time spent watching television in older women: A 10-year prospective follow-up study. *American Journal of Epidemiology, 174*(9), 1017–1027.

McHugh, J. E., Casey, A. M., & Lawlor, B. A. (2011). Psychosocial correlates of aspects of sleep quality in community-dwelling Irish older adults. *Aging and Mental Health, 15*(6), 749–755. doi:10.1080/13607863.2011.562180.

Mackenzie, C. S., Gekoski, W. L., & Knox, V. J. (2006). Age, gender, and the underutilization of mental health services: The influence of help-seeking attitudes. *Aging and Mental Health, 10*(6), 574–582. doi:10.1080/13607860600641200.

Mackenzie, C. S., Scott, T., Mather, A., & Sareen, J. (2008). Older adults' help-seeking attitudes and treatment beliefs concerning mental health problems. *The American Journal of Geriatric Psychiatry, 16*(12), 1010–1019. doi:10.1097/JGP.0b013e31818cd3be.

Malatesta, V. J. (2007). Introduction: The need to address older women's mental health issues. *Journal of Women and Aging, 19*(1–2), 1–12. doi:10.1300/J074v19n01_01.

Martina, C. M. S., & Stevens, N. L. (2006). Breaking the cycle of loneliness? Psychological effects of a friendship enrichment program for older women. *Aging and Mental Health, 10*(5), 467–475. doi:10.1080/13607860600637893.

Minkler, M., Fuller-Thomson, E., Miller, D., & Driver, D. (1997). Depression in grandparents raising grandchildren: Results of a national longitudinal study. *Archives of Family Medicine, 6*(5), 445–452.

Minkler, M., & Stone, R. (1985). The feminization of poverty and older women. *The Gerontologist, 25*(4), 351–357. doi:10.1093/geront/25.4.351.

Moen, P., Robison, J., & Fields, V. (1994). Women's work and caregiving roles: A life course approach. *Journal of Gerontology:, 49*(4), S176–S186. doi:10.1093/geronj/49.4.S176.

Monserud, M. A., & Peek, M. K. (2014). Functional limitations and depressive symptoms: A longitudinal analysis of older Mexican American couples. *The Journals of Gerontology Series B: Psychological Sciences and Social Sciences, 69*(5), 743–762. doi:10.1093/geronb/gbu039.

Mui, A. C. (1992). Caregiver strain among black and white daughter caregivers: A role theory perspective. *The Gerontologist, 32*(2), 203–212. doi:10.1093/geront/32.2.203.

Murayama, Y., Ohba, H., Yasunaga, M., Nonaka, K., Takeuchi, R., Nishi, M., . . . & Fujiwara, Y. (2015). The effect of intergenerational programs on the mental health of elderly adults. *Aging and Mental Health, 19*(4), 306–314. doi:10.1080/13607863.2014.933309.

Navaie-Waliser, M., Spriggs, A., & Feldman, P. H. (2002). Informal caregiving: Differential experiences by gender. *Medical Care, 40*(12), 1249–1259. doi:10.1097/01.MLR.0000036408.76220.

Nho, K., Ramanan, V. K., Horgusluoglu, E., Kim, S., Inlow, M. H., Risacher, S. L., . . . & Gao, S. (2015). Comprehensive gene- and pathway-based analysis of depressive symptoms in older adults. *Journal of Alzheimer's Disease, 45*(4), 1197–1206. doi:10.3233/JAD-148009.

Noone, J., Alpass, F., & Stephens, C. (2010). Do men and women differ in their retirement planning? Testing a theoretical model of gendered pathways to retirement preparation. *Research on Aging, 32*(6), 715–738. doi:10.1177/0164027510383531.

Okamoto, K., & Tanaka, Y. (2004). Gender differences in the relationship between social support and subjective health among elderly persons in Japan. *Preventive Medicine, 38*(3), 318–322.

Olesen, S. C., Butterworth, P., & Rodgers, B. (2012). Is poor mental health a risk factor for retirement? Findings from a longitudinal population survey. *Social Psychiatry and Psychiatric Epidemiology, 47*(5), 735–744. doi:10.1007/s00127-011-0375-7.

Ortman, J. M., Velkoff, V. A., & Hogan, H. (2014). *An aging nation: The older population in the United States.* Retrieved from https://www.census.gov/prod/2014pubs/p25-1140.pdf (accessed November 2, 2016).

Pachana, N. A., McLaughlin, D., Leung, J., Byrne, G., & Dobson, A. (2012). Anxiety and depression in adults in their eighties: Do gender differences remain? *International Psychogeriatrics, 24*(01), 145–150. doi:10.1017/S1041610211001372.

Pearlin, L. I. (1989). The sociological study of stress. *Journal of Health and Social Behavior, 30*(3), 241–256.

Penninx, B. W., Geerlings, S. W., Deeg, D. J. H., van Eijk, J. T. M., van Tilburg, W., & Beekman, A. T. F. (1999). Minor and major depression and the risk of death in older persons. *Archives of General Psychiatry, 56*(10), 889–895. doi:10.1001/archpsyc.56.10.889.

Penninx, B. W., Leveille, S., Ferrucci, L., Van Eijk, J., & Guralnik, J. M. (1999). Exploring the effect of depression on physical disability: Longitudinal evidence from the established populations for epidemiologic studies of the elderly. *American Journal of Public Health, 89*(9), 1346–1352. doi:10.2105/AJPH.89.9.1346.

Pillemer, K., & Finkelhor, D. (1988). The prevalence of elder abuse: A random sample survey. *The Gerontologist, 28*(1), 51–57. doi:10.1093/geront/28.1.51.

Pinquart, M., & Sorensen, S. (2001). Gender differences in self-concept and psychological well-being in old age: A meta-analysis. *The Journals of Gerontology Series B: Psychological Sciences and Social Sciences, 56*(4), P195–P213. doi:10.1093/geronb/56.4.P195.

Pinquart, M., & Sorensen, S. (2006). Gender differences in caregiver stressors, social resources, and health: An updated meta-analysis. *The Journals of Gerontology Series B: Psychological Sciences and Social Sciences, 61*(1), P33–P45. doi:10.1093/geronb/61.1.P33.

Quam, J. K., & Whitford, G. S. (1992). Adaptation and age-related expectations of older gay and lesbian adults. *The Gerontologist, 32*(3), 367–374. doi:10.1093/geront/32.3.367.

Read, S., & Grundy, E. (2011). Mental health among older married couples: The role of gender and family life. *Social Psychiatry and Psychiatric Epidemiology, 46*(4), 331–341. doi:10.1007/s00127-010-0205-3.

Rodeheaver, D., & Datan, N. (1988). The challenge of double jeopardy: Toward a mental health agenda for aging women. *American Psychologist, 43*(8), 648. doi:10.1037/0003-066X.43.8.648.

Rokke, P. D., & Klenow, D. J. (1998). Prevalence of depressive symptoms among rural elderly: Examining the need for mental health services. *Psychotherapy: Theory, Research, Practice, Training, 35*(4), 545–558. doi:10.1037/h0087683.

Rowe, J. W., & Kahn, R., L. (1997). Successful aging. *The Gerontologist, 37*(4), 433–440. doi:10.1093/geront/37.4.433.

Ruitenberg, A., Ott, A., van Swieten, J. C., Hofman, A., & Breteler, M. M. B. (2001). Incidence of dementia: Does gender make a difference? *Neurobiology of Aging, 22*(4), 575–580. doi:10.1016/S0197-4580(01)00231-7.

Sevak, P., Weir, D. R., & Willis, R. J. (2004). The economic consequences of a husband's death: Evidence from the HRS and AHEAD. *Social Security Bulletin, 65*(3), 31.

Shippee, T. P., Wilkinson, L. R., & Ferraro, K. F. (2012). Accumulated financial strain and women's health over three decades. *The Journals of Gerontology Series B: Psychological Sciences and Social Sciences, 67*(5), 585–594. doi:10.1093/geronb/gbs056.

Shmotkin, D., Blumstein, T., & Modan, B. (2003). Tracing long-term effects of early trauma: A broad-scope view of Holocaust survivors in late life. *Journal of Consulting and Clinical Psychology, 71*(2), 223–234. doi:10.1037/0022-006X.71.2.223.

Sieber, S. D. (1974). Toward a theory of role accumulation. *American Sociological Review, 39*(4), 567–578.

Silverstein, M., & Bengtson, V. L. (1994). Does intergenerational social support influence the psychological well-being of older parents? The contingencies of declining health and widowhood. *Social Science & Medicine, 38*(7), 943–957. doi:10.1016/0277-9536(94)90427-8.

Silverstein, M., Chen, X., & Heller, K. (1996). Too much of a good thing? Intergenerational social support and the psychological well-being of older parents. *Journal of Marriage and the Family, 58*(4), 970–982.

Silverstein, M., Cong, Z., & Li, S. (2006). Intergenerational transfers and living arrangements of older people in rural China: Consequences for psychological well-being. *The Journals of Gerontology Series B: Psychological Sciences and Social Sciences, 61*(5), S256–S266. doi:10.1093/geronb/61.5.S256.

Skultety, K. M., & Whitbourne, S. K. (2004). Gender differences in identity processes and self-esteem in middle and later adulthood. *Journal of Women and Aging, 16*(1–2), 175–188. doi:10.1300/J074v16n01_12.

Smith, D. H. (1994). Determinants of voluntary association participation and volunteering: A literature review. *Nonprofit and Voluntary Sector Quarterly, 23*(3), 243–263. doi:10.1177/089976409402300305.

Smith, H. M. (2007). Psychological service needs of older women. *Psychological Services, 4*(4), 277. doi:10.1037/1541-1559.4.4.277.

Stewart, N. J., Morgan, D. G., Karunanayake, C. P., Wickenhauser, J. P., Cammer, A., Minish, D., . . . & Hayduk, L. A. (2016). Rural caregivers for a family member with dementia models of burden and distress differ for women and men. *Journal of Applied Gerontology, 35*(2), 150–178. doi:10.1177/0733464813517547.

Stinson, C. K., & Kirk, E. (2006). Structured reminiscence: An intervention to decrease depression and increase self-transcendence in older women. *Journal of Clinical Nursing, 15*(2), 208–218. doi:10.1111/j.1365-2702.2006.01292.x.

Syzdek, M. R., & Addis, M. E. (2010). Adherence to masculine norms and attributional processes predict depressive symptoms in recently unemployed men. *Cognitive Therapy and Research, 34*(6), 533–543. doi:10.1007/s10608-009-9290-6.

Teng, P., Yeh, C., Lee, M., Lin, H., & Lai, T. (2013). Change in depressive status and mortality in elderly persons: Results of a national longitudinal study. *Archives of Gerontology and Geriatrics, 56*(1), 244–249. doi:10.1016/j.archger.2012.08.006.

Thomeer, M. B. (2016). Multiple chronic conditions, spouse's depressive symptoms, and gender within marriage. *Journal of Health and Social Behavior, 57*(1), 59–76. doi:10.1177/002214651 6628179.

Tiedje, L. B., Wortman, C. B., Downey, G., Emmons, C., Biernat, M., & Lang, E. (1990). Women with multiple roles: Role-compatibility perceptions, satisfaction, and mental health. *Journal of Marriage and the Family*, 63–72. doi:10.2307/352838.

Uhlenberg, P. (2009). Children in an aging society. *Journal of Gerontology: Social Sciences, 64B*(4), 489–496.

Umberson, D. (1992). Relationships between adult children and their parents: Psychological consequences for both generations. *Journal of Marriage and the Family, 54*(3), 664–674.

Umberson, D., Wortman, C. B., & Kessler, R. C. (1992). Widowhood and depression: Explaining long-term gender differences in vulnerability. *Journal of Health and Social Behavior, 33*(1), 10–24.

Vahia, I. V., Meeks, T. W., Thompson, W. K., Depp, C. A., Zisook, S., Allison, M., . . . & Jeste, D. V. (2010). Subthreshold depression and successful aging in older women. *The American Journal of Geriatric Psychiatry, 18*(3), 212–220. doi:10.1097/JGP.0b013e3181b7f10e.

Valle, G., Weeks, J. A., Taylor, M. G., & Eberstein, I. W. (2013). Mental and physical health consequences of spousal health shocks among older adults. *Journal of Aging and Health, 25*(7), 1121–1142. doi:10.1177/0898264313494800.

Vo, K., Forder, P. M., Tavener, M., Rodgers, B., Banks, E., Bauman, A., & Byles, J. E. (2015). Retirement, age, gender and mental health: Findings from the 45 and Up Study. *Aging and Mental Health, 19*(7), 647–657. doi:10.1080/13607863.2014.962002.

Wakabayashi, C., & Donato, K. M. (2006). Does caregiving increase poverty among women in later life? Evidence from the Health and Retirement Survey. *Journal of Health and Social Behavior, 47*(3), 258–274. doi:10.1177/002214650604700305.

Waldron, I. (1976). Why do women live longer than men? *Social Science and Medicine (1967), 10*(7), 349–362. doi:10.1016/0037-7856(76)90090-1.

Waldrop, D., & Weber, J. (2001). From grandparent to caregiver: The stress and satisfaction of raising grandchildren. *Families in Society: The Journal of Contemporary Social Services, 82*(5), 461–472. doi:10.1606/1044-3894.177.

Wang, P. S., Lane, M., Olfson, M., Pincus, H. A., Wells, K. B., & Kessler, R. C. (2005). Twelve-month use of mental health services in the United States: Results from the National Comorbidity Survey Replication. *Archives of General Psychiatry, 62*(6), 629–640. doi:10.1001/archpsyc.62.6.629.

Wang, Y. N., Shyu, Y. I. L., Chen, M. C., & Yang, P. S. (2011). Reconciling work and family caregiving among adult–child family caregivers of older people with dementia: Effects on role strain and depressive symptoms. *Journal of Advanced Nursing, 67*(4), 829–840. doi:10.1111/j.1365-2648.2010.05505.x.

Ward, E. C., & Heidrich, S. (2009). African American women's beliefs, coping behaviors, and barriers to seeking mental health services. *Qualitative Health Research, 19*(11), 1589–1601. doi:10.1177/1049732309350686.

Warner-Smith, P., Powers, J., & Hampson, A. (2008). Women's experiences of paid work and planning for retirement (Report to the Office for Women). *Women's Health Australia*. Retrieved from https://www.dss.gov.au/sites/default/files/documents/05_2012/womens_experiences_of_paid_work_final_report_survey.pdf (accessed November 2, 2016).

Weissman, J., & dLevine, S. (2007). Anxiety disorders and older women. *Journal of Women and Aging, 19*(1–2), 79–101. doi:10.1300/J074v19n01_06.

Whitbeck, L. B., Hoyt, D. R., & Tyler, K. A. (2001). Family relationship histories, intergenerational relationship quality, and depressive affect among rural elderly people. *Journal of Applied Gerontology, 20*(2), 214–229. doi:10.1177/073346480102000206.

Whooley, M. A., & Browner, W. S. (1998). Association between depressive symptoms and mortality in older women. *Archives of Internal Medicine, 158*(19), 2129–2135. doi:10.1001/archinte.158.19.2129.

Whooley, M. A., Kip, K. E., Cauley, J. A., Ensrud, K. E., Nevitt, M. C., & Browner, W. S. (1999). Depression, falls, and risk of fracture in older women. *Archives of Internal Medicine, 159*(5), 484–490. doi:10.1001/archinte.159.5.484.

Wilcox, S., Evenson, K. R., Aragaki, A., Wassertheil-Smoller, S., Mouton, C. P., & Loevinger, B. L. (2003). The effects of widowhood on physical and mental health, health behaviors, and health outcomes: The Women's Health Initiative. *Health Psychology, 22*(5), 513. doi:10.1037/0278-6133.22.5.513.

Willette-Murphy, K., Todero, C., & Yeaworth, R. (2006). Mental health and sleep of older wife caregivers for spouses with Alzheimer's disease and related disorders. *Issues in Mental Health Nursing, 27*(8), 837–852. doi:10.1080/01612840600840711.

Willson, A. E., & Hardy, M. A. (2002). Racial disparities in income security for a cohort of aging American women. *Social Forces, 80*(4), 1283–1306. doi:10.1353/sof.2002.0036.

Windle, M., & Windle, R. C. (2013). Recurrent depression, cardiovascular disease, and diabetes among middle-aged and older adult women. *Journal of Affective Disorders, 150*(3), 895–902. doi:10.1016/j.jad.2013.05.008.

Wolkenstein, B. H., & Sterman, L. (1998). Unmet needs of older women in a clinic population: The discovery of possible long-term sequelae of domestic violence. *Professional Psychology: Research and Practice, 29*(4), 341–348. doi:10.1037/0735-7028.29.4.341.

Wuthrich, V. M., & Frei, J. (2015). Barriers to treatment for older adults seeking psychological therapy. *International Psychogeriatrics, 27*(07), 1227–1236. doi:10.1017/S1041610215000241.

Zanjani, F., Downer, B. G., Hosier, A. F., & Watkins, J. D. (2014). Memory banking: A life story intervention for aging preparation and mental health promotion. *Journal of Aging and Health, 27*(2), 355–376. doi:10.1177/0898264314551170.

Zink, T., Fisher, B. S., Regan, S., & Pabst, S. (2005). The prevalence and incidence of intimate partner violence in older women in primary care practices. *Journal of General Internal Medicine, 20*(10), 884–888. doi:10.1111/j.1525-1497.2005.0191.x.

Zink, T., Jeffrey Jacobson Jr, C., Regan, S., & Pabst, S. (2004). Hidden victims: The healthcare needs and experiences of older women in abusive relationships. *Journal of Women's Health, 13*(8), 898–908. doi:10.1089/jwh.2004.13.898.

Part II

Diversity Issues in Women's Mental Health

Chapter Five
Racial/Ethnic Disparities in Women's Mental Health

Linda Cedeno and Lesia M. Ruglass

The U.S. Surgeon General's supplement report provided a critical illustration of the state of racial/ethnic-minority mental health, predicated on extant empirical literature (U.S. Department of Health and Human Services, 2001). The report noted that racial/ethnic-minority groups contend with greater social and ecological disparities that significantly increase the likelihood of psychological dysfunction. Furthermore, racial/ethnic-minority mental health needs go largely unmet, services are underutilized, disorders tend to be more severe, and racial/ethnic groups continue to be largely underrepresented in research. This has led to an increase in mental health research focusing on underrepresented populations (C. Brown, Abe-Kim, & Barrio, 2003; Chin, Walters, Cook, & Huang, 2007; Greer, 2011; Rosenfield & Mouzon, 2013).

The body of literature investigating mental health disparities and service use has grown since the dissemination of the U.S. Surgeon General's report, but examinations of how race *and* gender contribute to variations in the population are limited. This chapter will provide an overview of research examining racial/ethnic differences in women's mental health, risk factors that likely render racial/ethnic groups more vulnerable to higher rates of pathology, barriers to treatment, such as language, trust, racism, and fear of stigma, and strategies for reducing these disparities. And we will consider the research challenges in ascertaining an accurate picture of disparities in women's mental health.

Social Stress Theory

The predominant theoretical framework for research examining the association between social status and mental health outcomes is the social stress model (Horwitz, 2013; Pearlin, 1989). The perspective outlines how a person's or group's location in the social hierarchy differentially dictates access to valuable resources. Individuals with a lower social standing are subjected to more stressful environmental conditions and less access to resources with which to cope.

In addition to contending with such stressors as inferior schools, limited employment opportunities, poverty, and violence, racial/ethnic minorities may experience overt and subtle racism that adds a significant source of stress over and beyond other stressors (Williams & Mohammed, 2009). For example, racial differences are observed at every level of income, highlighting the unique contribution of race to health outcomes, partially mediated by racism (Williams & Mohammed, 2009). This elevated level of stress is postulated to translate into worse mental health through a myriad of processes affecting physical and psychological well-being, behavior, and attitudes. On average, lower-status groups will experience worse health outcomes than advantaged groups. These disparities should be understood as attributable to the disadvantage itself, created by the stratification of individuals, as opposed to something inherent in particular groups (Schwartz & Meyer, 2010).

Empirical Findings for the Impact of Racism on Mental Health

Racism refers to a complex system of power in which individuals are grouped into a hierarchy according to the construct of race to privilege certain groups with access to resources and freedoms from which racial/ethnic minorities are largely excluded (Essed, 1991). Underlying institutional racism is an ideology of cultural racism relegating the culture of certain groups to an inferior status while elevating the others to a superior status (Jones, 1997). Racism may also occur at an individual or personal level (e.g., a negative racial slight or slur). A substantive body of evidence indicates that racism is deeply entrenched in society in a plethora of contexts, including the criminal justice system, housing, medical care, and education (Blank, Dabady, & Citro, 2004)

Paradigms that detail the impact of racism on health tend to draw on Lazarus and Folkman's (1984) transactional model of stress, defined as a "relationship between the person and environment that is appraised by the person as taxing or exceeding his or her resources and endangering his or her resources or well-being" (p. 19).

Similarly, race-related stress is conceptualized as transactions between individuals and the environment that are appraised as explicit or implicit forms of racism, and that strain one's health by exceeding coping resources (Harrell, 2000). Extant empirical findings show that discrimination is related to pathology. Racial/ethnic minorities who report greater experiences of racism/discrimination have poorer levels of psychological functioning expressed by symptoms such as increased anxiety, obsessive-compulsive, and depressive symptoms; substance use; and HIV risk behavior (Bynum, Burton, & Best, 2007; Chae et al., 2010; Schulz et al., 2006; Williams & Mohammed, 2009).

In a recent meta-analysis, greater exposure to and perception of racist events were positively associated with psychiatric symptoms, including depression, anxiety, posttraumatic stress disorder (PTSD), and somatization, irrespective of the population sampled and measurements of racism utilized, adding to the burgeoning evidence suggesting relationships between racist and discriminatory experiences and trauma-related symptoms (Pieterse, Todd, Neville, & Carter, 2012).

The internalization of racism or broader negative stereotypes about one's marginalized group may also affect health outcomes, including psychological and somatic functioning, and academic performance (R. T. Carter, 2007; Steele, 1997; S. Sue, Yan Cheng, Saad, & Chu, 2012), though the effect of this process may go undetected. For example, the internalization of controlling images by Black women (e.g., matriarch, Black lady overachiever, Jezebel) may lead to the obsolescence of the self whereby experiences that deviate from circumscribed images (e.g., vulnerability, distress, dependency) may be disowned, leading to underreporting and detection of symptoms (Taylor, 1999).

Despite the mounting evidence showing a consistent correlation between racism and mental health, more research is required to expand the complexities of the connection and its implication in mental health disparities. For example, in a review and critique of the racial disparities and health literature, Williams and Mohammed (2009) noted that one difficulty in ascertaining the effects of racism on health is the unconscious and conscious efforts to deny the occurrence of painful race-related events. Furthermore, within-group variability in exposure to and recognition of discrimination influenced by factors including appearance, class, residential context, personality, and culture can confound analyses examining the link between discrimination and mental health outcomes (Schwartz & Meyer, 2010). Some argue that subtle and "covert" forms of racism, or microaggressions, defined as "brief and commonplace daily verbal, behavioral, or environmental indignities, whether intentional or unintentional, that communicate hostile, derogatory or negative racial slights and insults toward people of color" (D. W. Sue et al., 2007, p. 271), must also be accounted for to deepen our understanding of the impact of discrimination on health (R. T. Carter, 2007).

The failure to racialize surveys examining stress ranging from daily hassles, ubiquitous stressors, life events, and psychological outcomes likely yields outcomes and deductions that would limit generalizability if minority participants were included (T. N. Brown, 2008). Thus, current findings presumably underestimate the impact of racism on psychological health. Likewise, examinations of Whiteness are virtually absent from the literature, obscuring whether Whites experience advantages, or disadvantages, to being racist, or avoiding being antiracist, perhaps reflecting the power and privilege of a majority White discipline that benefits from the avoidance of such empirical examinations (T. N. Brown, 2008).

Racial Ethnic Differences in Mental Health Outcomes

In contrast to within-group analyses that show a consistent link between greater exposure to and perception of race-related stress, and more psychiatric symptoms, between-group analyses diverge from expected outcomes. Epidemiological research, including meta-analytic and large-scale studies, demonstrates similar or better mental health for racial/ethnic groups compared with non-Hispanic White women (C. Brown et al., 2003; Onoye, Goebert, Morland, Matsu, & Wright, 2009; Rosenfield & Mouzon, 2013; Wei, Greaver, Marson, Herndon, & Rogers, 2008). These results are perplexing given that marginalized groups, such as Blacks, Hispanics, and American Indians/Native Americans, are consistently worse off on numerous physical health indicators (Williams & Mohammed, 2009), experience greater trauma (e.g., Bryant-Davis, Chung, Tillman, & Belcourt, 2009; Ghafoori, Barragan, Tohidian, & Palinkas, 2012), and are disproportionately affected by structural inequalities, including racism and poverty (U.S. Department of Health and Human Services, 2001; Williams & Mohammed, 2009). This phenomenon is referred to as the epidemiological paradox.

A paucity of research investigating female mental health disparities goes beyond Black and White comparisons to include multiple racial groups, but few racial differences have been found. For example, in a study exploring sexual identity, stressors (e.g., trauma, discrimination), harmful behaviors (e.g., alcohol use), and mental health (e.g., depression, anxiety) in a group of young adult sexual-minority women, trauma exposure, mental health, and health behaviors were similar across African American, Latina/Hispanic, Asian, and White women, though African American women reported more childhood sexual assault relative to White participants, and Asian women reported less (Balsam et al., 2015).

In a meta-analytic review focusing specifically on body dissatisfaction and psychological sequelae among Black, Hispanic, Asian American, and White women, White participants reported significantly more body dissatisfaction compared with Black participants, though the effect was modest, and Asian American and Hispanic women were just as dissatisfied as White women, challenging stereotypes that racial-ethnic groups are inoculated from the Eurocentric thin aesthetic (Grabe & Hyde, 2006). However, for racial/ethnic-minority groups, body dissatisfaction and pursuit of a thin standard may be an attempt to avoid further discrimination (Hesse-Biber, Livingstone, Ramirez, Barko, & Johnson, 2010).

Conversely, other aspects of body dissatisfaction might be more germane for racial/ethnic minorities, such as skin color, features, and hair. In a qualitative analysis sampling Black women pursuing advanced degrees, and those in possession of college and graduate degrees, Black women's body image self-evaluations included hair, skin color, shape, and attitude, which were (positively and negatively) related to social worth, including experiences of oppression (e.g., invisibility, racism), and media depictions (Capodilupo & Kim, 2014).

Some findings reveal worse psychological outcomes for racial and ethnic minorities, particularly when examining older, Native American/American Indian, Pacific Islander, Native Alaskan, Asian subgroups, and sexual-minority women (Harris, Edlund, & Larson, 2015; Spence, Adkins, & Dupre, 2011; S. Sue et al., 2012; Wei et al., 2008). In a study assessing racial/ethnic differences in depressive symptoms in a sample of middle-aged women, Hispanic and African American women reported elevated symptoms relative to White, Japanese, and Chinese women, the latter two groups expressing the lowest levels. Stress, and poor physical health, had main effects on depressive symptoms. The authors postulated that race might be conceived of as an important risk factor for Black/Latina women because they experience higher rates of physical health issues and psychosocial stressors that may mediate or precipitate depression (Bromberger, Harlow, Avis, Kravitz, & Cordal, 2004). The higher prevalence of poor physical health conditions in racial/ethnic minorities increases risk for mental health disorders given the "mind–body connection," as well as concomitant challenges (U.S. Department of Health and Human Services, 2001).

Alternative Explanations

Protective Factors

Given the significant physical health disparities between Whites and racial/ethnic-minority groups, and underutilization of services by marginalized groups, more research is required to understand similar mental health standing across groups overall. It has been hypothesized that racial/ethnic-minority women may utilize certain culturally based coping strategies or resources that bolster their sense of well-being, or serve as protective factors against the effects of stressors or traumas. Among racial/ethnic-minority women, there are several salient coping strategies and protective factors that have been theorized to mitigate the negative impact of actual or perceived stressors on mental health functioning, including social support, spirituality/religiosity, and ethnic identity.

Decades of research have shown a link between the utilization of social support and improved psychological and physical well-being, mediated by its impact on the stress-response system (Charney et al., 2007; Thoits, 2011). Social support refers to the perception that one's interpersonal relationships are available to provide help during times of need. Studies suggest racial/ethnic minorities are less likely to seek out or utilize professional supports during times of stress (Alegría, Chatterji, & Wells, 2008; Substance Abuse and Mental Health Services Administration, 2015), thus social support is often viewed as a culturally relevant coping strategy that provides a buffer against the adverse effects of stressful life events among this population. Indeed, studies have shown that certain racial/ethnic-minority groups (e.g., African Americans, Hispanic/Latinos) may be more likely to seek out and utilize social support as a way of coping with stress compared with White individuals (Knouse, 1991; Short et al., 2000). In contrast, studies show that Asians or Asian Americans are less likely than Caucasian Americans to seek out social support due to concerns about the impact on their relationships and/or due to the belief that one should independently solve one's problems (Kim, Sherman, & Taylor, 2008). Very few studies, however, have tested the interactive effect of race and gender on the buffering effects of social support, and the findings to date have been mixed.

On the one hand, studies confirm the importance of social support among racial/ethnic-minority women (Campos et al., 2008; Fowler & Hill, 2004). For example, in a sample of African American women with a history of partner abuse, Fowler and Hill (2004) found that those with higher levels of functional support had lower levels of self-reported depression symptoms. And, in a sample of 246 pregnant women, Campos et al. (2008) found that Latina women had higher levels of family orientation than Caucasian women, and the strength of the association between a family orientation and social support was stronger for Latina women than Caucasian women.

On the other hand, Mouzon (2013) conducted a secondary analysis of data from the National Survey of American Life and found that, while African Americans reported better mental health status with lower odds of psychiatric disorders than Whites, these findings were not mediated by various forms of social support. Mouzon (2013) speculated that African Americans may cope with stress by utilizing other self-regulation strategies that might protect against mental health problems. The author also considered the possibility that the mental health paradox may be a function of culturally biased measurements of mental health (Mouzon, 2013).

Spirituality and religious coping have also been shown to be associated with reduced psychological distress and psychological well-being among many individuals (Ano & Vasconcelles, 2005; Gillum, Sullivan, & Bybee, 2006). Religion/spirituality may enhance well-being through various means by providing a sense of purpose during challenging times; enhancing self-efficacy and control over stressful life events; or providing a sense of support during times of distress (Fiori, Brown, Cortina, & Antonucci, 2006). Religiosity, however, can have both positive and negative components (Chatters, Taylor, Jackson,

& Lincoln, 2008; Fiori et al., 2006). For example, negative beliefs about being punished, or feeling abandoned by God during one's time of need, have been associated with poorer outcomes during times of distress (Pargament, Smith, Koenig, & Perez, 1998). Moreover, religious beliefs that promote exclusive support or treatment by religious leaders instead of the utilization of professional mental health or medical treatment during times of need may delay the timely receipt of essential treatment for mental health disorders (Chatters et al., 2008).

Previous studies indicate women and racial/ethnic minorities are more likely to utilize spirituality and religious coping to deal with stressful life events than men and non-Hispanic Whites (Ahrens, Abeling, Ahmad, & Hinman, 2010; Chatters et al., 2008; Dunn & Horgas, 2000; Fiori et al., 2006). Given a history of oppression and restricted opportunities, it has been speculated that the greater utilization of religion and spirituality among women and racial/ethnic minorities may reflect an attempt to maintain or increase a sense of personal control in the midst of distressing life events (Dunn & Horgas, 2000; Fiori et al., 2006). For example, El-Khoury et al. (2004) examined the use of religious coping among African American and Caucasian survivors of interpersonal partner violence and found that African American women were more likely to use prayer as a coping strategy and found it more helpful than Caucasian women.

Racial/ethnic identity is a multidimensional construct, often described as one's sense of affiliation with and connection to one's racial/ethnic group (Phinney & Ong, 2007; Smith & Silva, 2011). Studies suggest racial/ethnic identity may either have a direct effect on psychological well-being or an indirect effect as a protective mechanism that buffers the impact of experiences of discrimination (Mossakowski, 2003; Smith & Silva, 2011). Some scholars have theorized and found that holding a strong positive racial/ethnic identity, in the face of derogatory views or stereotypes about one's racial/ethnic group, may prevent the internalization of negative attitudes about one's racial/ethnic group (Mossakowski, 2003).

Others, in contrast, have hypothesized and found that a strong ethnic identity may actually exacerbate discrimination-related distress because one's difference from the majority group is highlighted, which may threaten the sense of self and exacerbate minority stress (Quintana, 2007; Yip, Gee, & Takeuchi, 2008). Smith and Silva (2011) conducted a meta-analysis of 184 studies and found only a modest positive association between ethnic identity and psychological well-being among various racial/ethnic-minority groups. And, this association did not differ by gender, suggesting that racial/ethnic-minority women were no more or less likely to benefit from their ethnic identity than their male counterparts. The authors argued that, despite the salience of ethnic identity for racial/ethnic minorities, its small effect on positive outcomes suggests other variables may be more instrumental in racial/ethnic minorities' mental health and well-being.

In sum, although theoreticians hypothesize that racial/ethnic minorities are more likely to utilize culturally relevant coping strategies to counter the deleterious effects of racism and discrimination, the empirical literature has been mixed in regard to their actual impact on psychological well-being. Moreover, Schwartz and Meyer (2010) discount the idea that disadvantaged groups may possess, on average, higher rates of coping that mitigate/mute the effects of group status in that social stress theorists postulate disparities in the distribution of exposure to stressors, as well as resources, including coping.

Research/Clinical Issues

Some research suggests that racial/ethnic differences in the experience of distress, symptom expression, prevalence, and culture-bound disorders should be expected (U.S. Department of Health and Human Services, 2001). However, poor knowledge and detection of culturally bound disorders, risk factors, and cultural differences likely shroud findings (C. Brown et al., 2003; U.S. Department of Health and Human Services, 2001).

A substantive body of work suggests that experiences of distress are informed by circumscribed expressions of distress, and beliefs and attitudes about the etiology of distress (U.S. Department of Health and Human Services, 2001). For example, African American women tend to emphasize somatic symptoms of distress and physical functioning, which may account for purported lower levels of psychopathology (see C. Brown et al., 2003, for a review). Neurasthenia, a culture-bound disorder found in Chinese Americans, is characterized by mental and physical exhaustion, pain, irritability, and anxiety. *Hwa-byung,* a syndrome (commonly found) in Korean American women, emphasizes physical, emotional, and interpersonal elements, though psychological features may become more prominent with acculturation (C. Brown et al., 2003).

Mental health professionals drawing on standardized classification systems of mental health disorders are likely to miss indications of distress. Another cultural factor garnering increasing attention in the literature is referred to as the strong Black woman (SBW) race–gender schema, whereby African American females cope by demonstrating self-reliance, strength, and self-silencing in the face of adversity. Higher rates of identification with the schema predict psychological distress, and a possible link with underutilization of care (Watson & Hunter, 2015). Cultural demands/schemas, such as saving face (consistent with Asian values) and SBW, might mitigate endorsements of emotional distress that might be better captured by somatic or interpersonal prompts (Watson & Hunter, 2015). Thus, bias may be introduced in between-group estimates when symptoms of distress and disorders go unrecognized.

Another research challenge that can skew the representation of mental health is sampling bias. Healthier Blacks, for example, are oversampled in between-group comparisons, given the difficulties in sampling marginalized populations due to disproportionate rates of incarceration, homelessness and impoverishment (Choldin, 1994). Studies that sample a greater percentage of foreign-born participants may also dilute research findings as immigrants may have a lower prevalence of psychiatric disorders (Sue et al., 2012; Williams & Mohammed, 2009). Untangling the complexities of racial groups also requires an assessment of such factors as nativity and acculturation.

The heterogeneity within racial/ethnic groups is primarily ignored in extant research (Brown, 2008). For example, the conflation of race and ethnicity whereby a racial category such as "Asian" or "Black" is comprised of multiple ethnic groups likely confounds conclusions by categorizing them together. Recent work suggests the benefit of a more refined approach to categorization (Sue et al., 2012). For example, Williams et al. (2007) examined mental health variation with African American and Caribbean Black populations and found ethnicity, immigration, language, and generation were associated with risk for psychiatric disorders. African American women had greater risks for anxiety and substance use disorders relative to Caribbean women, and women from the Spanish Caribbean had elevated levels of mood and anxiety disorders relative to English-speaking Caribbean women. Black Caribbean who were primarily socialized in their majority Black birthplace were conferred a mental health advantage relative to those who immigrated before young adulthood. The authors suggested that increases in pathology are likely related to societal stressors and "downward social mobility associated with being Black in America" (p. 52). The degree to which participants identified with their ethnicity relative to the dominant culture was not assessed, but such an individual variable would likely enhance findings examining racial/ethnic mental health disparities, as much within-group variation exists in racial identification.

Mental Health Services Utilization

Although the data suggests racial/ethnic minorities may have lower or equivalent rates of mental or substance use disorders compared to Whites, evidence suggests that, once developed, these disorders tend to be more persistent and disabling for racial/ethnic minorities, enhancing the need for and duration of care required among these populations (Bailey, Blackmon, & Stevens, 2010). Yet, despite the need, evidence suggests disparities in access, utilization, and quality of care that have worsened over time (Alegría et al., 2008; Cook, McGuire, & Miranda, 2007; Wells, Klap, Koike, & Sherbourne, 2001).

Lower Access and Quality of Care

Alegría et al. (2008), examining a sample of 8,862 adults, found that among those with depressive disorders, racial/ethnic minorities were less likely to access care than Whites, even after controlling for socioeconomic factors. Among those with depression who did access care, African Americans reported receiving less quality care than Whites. Aggregated data from the 2008–2012 National Surveys on Drug Use and Health (Substance Abuse and Mental Health Services Administration, 2015) revealed similar trends. While 16.6% of Whites utilized some mental health services in the past year, only 8.6%, 7.3%, and 4.9% of Blacks, Latinas, and Asians, respectively, utilized these same services in the past year. Utilization rates also differed by gender. White females had the highest rate (21.5%) of any mental health service utilization compared to Black females (10.3%), Latina females (9.2%), and Asian females (5.3%). These differential patterns remained after adjusting for age, poverty status, and insurance status.

After entering treatment, racial/ethnic minorities are more likely to receive unequal treatment: i.e., they are less likely to receive evidence-based treatments for depression and anxiety (Alegría et al., 2008; Wang et al., 2005); and are less likely to be prescribed newer medications with fewer side-effects (Melfi, Croghan, & Hanna, 2000). Moreover, they are more likely to miss appointments and terminate treatment prematurely (Chu & Sue, 2011; Olfson et al., 2009; Wang, 2007), potentially worsening treatment outcomes. Overall, these trends are alarming and call for a greater understanding of the factors contributing to these disparities.

Reasons for Disparities in Mental Health Care

The mechanisms underlying racial/ethnic disparities in mental health care are multifaceted and include the intersections of socioeconomic, provider, and individual factors. In comparison to Whites, racial/ethnic minorities are more likely to struggle with financial barriers that make it difficult to purchase health insurance and pay for mental health services, and are more likely to live in geographic regions characterized by fewer and poorer-quality mental health services (McGuire & Miranda, 2008). They may struggle with other logistical issues, such as transportation problems, inflexible work schedules, or inadequate childcare options, making it difficult to seek and receive help (Smedley, Stith, & Nelson, 2003). Even when insurance coverage and other economic factors are similar across groups, racial/ethnic minorities are still less likely to seek or utilize mental health services care, suggesting other factors are at play in the decisions around seeking mental health care (Nadeem et al., 2007).

The public and internalized stigma associated with mental illness may be salient barriers to help seeking among racial/ethnic minorities (Gary, 2005;

Nadeem et al., 2007; Ojeda & McGuire, 2006). Stigma may hinder access to treatment due to concerns about being perceived or treated negatively because of having a mental illness (public stigma) or feelings of shame/guilt about needing mental health treatment (internalized stigma) (Corrigan, 2004), thus individuals may avoid the mental health care system because of its association with perceived threats to the self (Burgess, Ding, Hargreaves, van Ryn, & Phelan, 2008).

Although stigma concerns are prevalent across individuals with mental illnesses, studies indicate African American and Latina women, and in particular immigrant women of color, are more likely to endorse stigma concerns regarding seeking mental health treatment compared to White females (Menke & Flynn, 2009; Nadeem et al., 2007; Watson & Hunter, 2015). Gary (2005) coined the term "double stigma" to highlight the greater burden racial/ethnic minorities endure from having to deal with the stress associated with both their racial/ethnic-minority status and mental illness. Research regarding the association between stigma concerns and mental health service utilization among racial/ethnic minorities, however, has been mixed (Brown et al., 2010; Snowden & Yamada, 2005).

For example, in a subsample of African American adults, Brown et al. (2010) found a direct association between internalized stigma, use of mental health services, and attitudes towards mental health treatment. In contrast, in a study of 15,383 low-income women, Nadeem et al. (2007) found that, while United States-born Black and immigrant Latina women were less likely to be in treatment than their United States-born White counterparts, stigma-related concern was not a significant predictor of being in treatment. And, in a study of 1,103 African American and White primary care patients, Menke and Flynn (2009) found that the association between perceived stigma and depression treatment use was fully mediated by the severity level of depression, suggesting symptom severity may override stigma in determining when and how one seeks help.

Other barriers to seeking help may include cultural beliefs and attitudes about mental illness, type of treatment needed, and whether mental health treatment is likely to be effective in improving one's psychological problems (Anglin, Alberti, Link, & Phelan, 2008; Watson & Hunter, 2015). Anglin et al. (2008) conducted a study of Caucasian and African American adults to examine racial differences in perceptions of mental illness and need for treatment and found that, although African Americans were more likely to perceive mental health treatment as effective than White Americans, they were also more likely to believe that mental health problems would resolve on their own.

Among African American women in particular, the SBW schema has been shown to be a double-edged sword that contributes to discomfort with asking for help or seeking out professional mental health services (Watson & Hunter, 2015).

Likewise, Asian cultural values that emphasize emotional inhibition, "saving face," and maintaining family honor and privacy may provide strong prohibitions against seeking professional mental health services due to the high stigmatization placed on mental illnesses in this culture (Shea & Yeh, 2008), although these associations may be moderated by degree of enculturation or acculturation (Chu & Sue, 2011). Further, scholars have suggested that racial/ethnic minorities may be more likely to utilize the primary care system rather than mental health services due to somatization of their psychological concerns and may also prefer alternative and complementary medicine options (Snowden & Yamada, 2005). Limited English proficiency may also serve as a barrier to accessing formal mental health treatment. Language barriers may contribute to lack of knowledge of available mental health services, as well as communication difficulties between client and providers given the dearth of bilingual and bicultural mental health providers in most agencies (Chu & Sue, 2011; Sentell, Shumway, & Snowden, 2007; Spencer, Chen, Gee, Fabian, & Takeuchi, 2010).

Another formidable barrier to treatment among racial/ethnic minorities is lack of trust in the mental health system and service providers. Given a long history of, and ongoing experiences with, prejudice, discrimination, and systemic racism, racial/ethnic minorities may have strong feelings of mistrust of White service providers (Benkert, Peters, Clark, & Keves-Foster, 2006; Whaley, 2001), which may negatively influence help seeking and adherence to treatment recommendations. The Tuskegee syphilis experiment from 1932–1972, and the mass involuntary sterilization of racial/ethnic-minority women during the eugenics movement of 1929–1974, are two of the most prominent reasons cited for the mistrust of the health care system among African Americans (Benkert et al., 2006; Whaley, 2001). However, contemporary experiences with stereotyping/discrimination by service providers may also fuel feelings of distrust among racial/ethnic minorities. Studies consistently show that racial/ethnic minorities are more likely to report perceived discrimination within the health care system, and as a consequence may have lower levels of trust and satisfaction with the care received (Benkert et al., 2006) or avoid utilization of needed care altogether (Burgess et al., 2008).

Research also consistently demonstrates that there are significant differences in the way mental health care providers interact with and treat racial/ethnic-minority clients that contribute to racial/ethnic disparities. Mental health providers are more likely to underdetect or misdiagnose mental health disorders among racial/ethnic minorities compared to Whites (Atdjian & Vega, 2005; Bailey et al., 2010; Suite, La Bril, Primm, & Harrison-Ross, 2007). They may exert less effort and fail to communicate appropriately with their racial/ethnic-minority clients about treatment options or provide poorer-quality care than that provided to Caucasian clients (McGuire & Miranda, 2008).

These differential behaviors are often attributed to medical uncertainty or conscious/unconscious biases that contribute to stereotyping and discrimination (McGuire & Miranda, 2008; Schraufnagel, Wagner, Miranda, & Roy-Byrne, 2006). Taken together, these factors all combine to make it less likely that racial/ethnic minorities will seek and remain in treatment, potentially increasing morbidity, mortality, and decreasing psychological well-being.

Treatment Outcomes

Although empirically supported treatments exist for most mood and anxiety disorders, a majority of the clinical trials conducted to date have been primarily with Caucasian clients, with racial/ethnic minorities typically underrepresented compared to their representation in the larger population. Few studies have examined racial/ethnic differences in treatment process and outcomes. Those that have often fail to account for confounding factors such as socioeconomic status, immigration status, and level of acculturation, thus rendering findings inconclusive. At present, it remains inconclusive whether evidence-based treatment strategies are generalizable across all racial/ethnic groups or need to be tailored to specific cultural groups.

A meta-analysis of 17 studies of cognitive-behavioral therapy (CBT) for substance use disorder found that, although standard cognitive-behavioral therapy was as effective in samples that were predominantly African Americans/Hispanics, the effect was stronger among predominantly Caucasian samples when examining pre–post substance use outcomes (Windsor, Jemal, & Alessi, 2015). A main limitation of this analysis, however, was that the predominantly African African/Hispanic samples also included Caucasian participants, thus limiting the authors' ability to examine the interaction between race/ethnicity and treatment outcomes.

Lambert et al. (2006) conducted an archival study of four racial/ethnic-minority groups, who were matched to Caucasian clients by level of psychological disturbance (as assessed by the Outcomes Questionnaire-45) and various sociodemographic factors (e.g., age, gender, marital status), and received therapy from a university counseling center. They found no differences in treatment outcomes across racial/groups (Lambert et al., 2006). Similarly, Ince et al. (2014) conducted a meta-analysis of 56 randomized controlled trials of psychotherapy treatments for adults with depression and found that the proportion of racial/ethnic minorities in a study was not a significant moderator of the effectiveness of the treatments, suggesting psychotherapy was equally effective for racial/ethnic minorities and non-minorities, and thus generalizable across groups (Ince et al., 2014). Lastly, Carter, Mitchell, and Sbrocco (2012) examined the PTSD treatment outcome literature completed over the past 30 years for adults and concluded that racial/ethnic-minority groups benefitted equally to Caucasians when provided with PTSD treatment. Although given methodological limitations with some of the studies reviewed, the lack of difference in outcomes should be taken with caution.

Summary and Conclusion

Decades of research have shown that experiences of racism and discrimination can have detrimental effects on the physical and psychological functioning of racial/ethnic minorities, and would suggest increased rates of mental illness compared to Whites. Yet, despite greater exposures to adversities, research suggests similar or better mental health functioning among racial/ethnic-minority women compared with non-Hispanic White women—a phenomenon referred to as the mental health paradox. Theorists argue that racial/ethnic-minority women may utilize certain coping strategies, such as social support and religiosity/spirituality, which buffer the effects of stressors and traumas. Yet, the empirical literature has been mixed in regard to the actual impact of these coping strategies on mental health functioning.

Others have argued that the mental health paradox may be a function of methodological challenges: underdetection of mental health problems among racial/ethnic minorities secondary to biased measurement tools, cultural differences in expressions of distress, and the oversampling of healthier racial/ethnic minorities in epidemiological studies. Brown (2008) proposes that groups define mental health and pathology within their respective communities. Thus, culturally valid and reliable measures will inform predictions of whether or which mental disorders may be more prevalent between social groups and in what context. Nevertheless, data indicate that, once developed, mental disorders tend to be more persistent and disabling for racial/ethnic minorities.

Despite need for care, there are significant racial/ethnic disparities in access, utilization, and quality of care received. Reasons for these disparities are multifaceted and include the intersections of socioeconomic factors, stigma, cultural mistrust, language barriers, and stereotyping and discrimination by the mental health system/providers. Strategies to reduce these disparities include reducing unconscious bias, and increasing multicultural competence among service providers, development of culturally congruent or culturally sensitive treatments, increasing the diversity of the mental health workforce, incorporating interpreter services in mental health agencies, and improving the quality of care provided to racial/ethnic-minority women (McGuire & Miranda, 2008).

Once in treatment, preliminary evidence suggests that the benefits of evidence-based treatments cut across racial/ethnic-minority groups. However, given the methodological limitations of existing trials, it remains inconclusive whether current evidence-based treatment strategies will meet the needs of racial/ethnic groups or need to be modified or adapted for different racial/ethnic-minority groups in general and for women in particular.

Overall, more studies are needed that analyze group members' experiences at multiple intersections, including gender, sexuality, race, and racial identification. This will help elucidate our understanding of health disparities by unveiling cultural variations in meaning and manifestations of psychological health and illness. Research is also needed to examine the impact of the differential histories and stereotypes of minorities, such as Native American/American Indian, Pacific Islanders, Latino, and Asian Americans, and their impact on mental health (Okazaki, 2009). Finally, further studies are warranted that test the differential impact of traditional empirically supported treatment versus culturally adapted treatments on racial/ethnic-minority mental health needs.

References

Ahrens, C. E., Abeling, S., Ahmad, S., & Hinman, J. (2010). Spirituality and well-being: The relationship between religious coping and recovery from sexual assault. *Journal of Interpersonal Violence*, 25(7), 1242–1263. doi:10.1177/0886260509340533.

Alegría, M., Chatterji, P., & Wells, K. (2008). Disparity in depression treatment among racial and ethnic minority populations in the United States. *Psychiatric Services*, 59(11), 1264–1272. doi:10.1176/appi.ps.59.11.1264.Disparity.

Anglin, D. M., Alberti, P. M., Link, B. G., & Phelan, J. C. (2008). Racial differences in beliefs about the effectiveness and necessity of mental health treatment. *American Journal of Community Psychology*, 42(1–2), 17–24.

Ano, G. G., & Vasconcelles, E. B. (2005). Religious coping and psychological adjustment to stress: A meta-analysis. *Journal of Clinical Psychology*, 61(4), 461–480.

Atdjian, S., & Vega, W. A. (2005). Disparities in mental health treatment in US racial and ethnic minority groups: Implications for psychiatrists. *Psychiatric Services*, 56(12), 1600–1602. doi: 10.1176/appi.ps.56.12.1600.

Bailey, R. K., Blackmon, H. L., & Stevens, F. L. (2010). Major depressive disorder: Meeting the challenges of stigma, misdiagnosis, and treatment disparities. *Handbook of African American Health*, 101(11), 419–430.

Balsam, K. F., Molina, Y., Blayney, J. A., Dillworth, T., Zimmerman, L., & Kaysen, D. (2015). Racial/ethnic differences in identity and mental health outcomes among young sexual minority women. *Cultural Diversity and Ethnic Minority Psychology*, 21(3), 380–390. doi:10.1037/a0038680.

Benkert, R., Peters, R. M., Clark, R., & Keves-Foster, K. (2006). Effects of perceived racism, cultural mistrust and trust in providers on satisfaction with care. *Journal of the National Medical Association*, 98(9), 1532–1540. doi:papers://C3698B6B-F8F3-45D6-B063-32DC323FE3E0/Paper/p1944.

Blank, R. M., Dabady, M., & Citro, C. F. (2004). *Measuring racial discrimination*. Washington, DC: National Academies Press.

Bromberger, J. T., Harlow, S., Avis, N., Kravitz, H. M., & Cordal, A. (2004). Racial/ethnic differences in the prevalence of depressive symptoms among middle-aged women: The Study of Women's Health Across the Nation (SWAN). *American Journal of Public Health*, 94(8), 1378–1385.

Brown, C., Abe-Kim, J. S., & Barrio, C. (2003). Depression in ethnically diverse women: Implications for treatment in primary care settings. *Professional Psychology: Research and Practice*, 34(1), 10–19.

Brown, C., Conner, K. O., Copeland, V. C., Grote, N., Beach, S., Battista, D., & Reynolds, C. F. (2010). Depression stigma, race, and treatment seeking behavior and attitudes. *Journal of Community Psychology*, 38(3), 350–368.

Brown, T. N. (2008). Race, racism, and mental health: Elaboration of critical race theory's contribution to the sociology of mental health. *Contemporary Justice Review*, 11(February 2015), 53–62. doi:10.1080/10282580701850405.

Bryant-Davis, T., Chung, H., Tillman, S., & Belcourt, A. (2009). From the margins to the center: Ethnic minority women and the mental health effects of sexual assault. *Trauma, Violence and Abuse, 10*(4), 330–357. doi:10.1177/1524838009339755.

Burgess, D. J., Ding, Y., Hargreaves, M., van Ryn, M., & Phelan, S. (2008). The association between perceived discrimination and underutilization of needed medical and mental health care in a multi-ethnic community sample. *Journal of Health Care for the Poor and Underserved, 19*(3), 894–911.

Bynum, M. S., Burton, E. T., & Best, C. (2007). Racism experiences and psychological functioning in African American college freshmen: Is racial socialization a buffer? *Cultural Diversity and Ethnic Minority Psychology, 13*(1), 64–71.

Campos, B., Schetter, C. D., Abdou, C. M., Hobel, C. J., Glynn, L. M., & Sandman, C. A. (2008). Familialism, social support, and stress: Positive implications for pregnant Latinas. *Cultural Diversity and Ethnic Minority Psychology, 14*(2), 155.

Capodilupo, C. M., & Kim, S. (2014). Gender and race matter: The importance of considering intersections in Black women's body image. *Journal of Counseling Psychology, 61*(1), 37–49.

Carter, M. M., Mitchell, F. E., & Sbrocco, T. (2012). Treating ethnic minority adults with anxiety disorders: Current status and future recommendations. *Journal of Anxiety Disorders, 26*(4), 488–501. doi:10.1016/j.janxdis.2012.02.002.

Carter, R. T. (2007). Racism and psychological and emotional Injury: Recognizing and assessing race-based traumatic stress. *The Counseling Psychologist, 35*(1), 13–105. doi:10.1177/001100000 6292033.

Chae, D. H., Krieger, N., Bennett, G. G., Lindsey, J. C., Stoddard, A. M., & Barbeau, E. M. (2010). Implications of discrimination based on sexuality, gender, and race/ethnicity for psychological distress among working-class sexual minorities: The United for Health Study, 2003–2004. *International Journal of Health Services : Planning, Administration, Evaluation, 40*(4), 589–608. doi:10.2190/HS.40.4.b.

Charney, D., Southwick, S., Ozbay, F., Johnson, D. C., Dimoulas, E., Morgan, C. A., . . . & Southwick, S. (2007). Social support and resilience to stress. *Psychiatry, 4*(5), 35–40.

Chatters, L. M., Taylor, R. J., Jackson, J. S., & Lincoln, K. D. (2008). Religious coping among African Americans, Caribbean Blacks and Non-Hispanic Whites. *Journal of Community Psychology, 36*(3), 371–386.

Chin, M. H., Walters, A. E., Cook, S. C., & Huang, E. S. (2007). Interventions to reduce racial and ethnic disparities in health care. *Medical Care Research and Review, 64*(5), 7s–28s. doi: 10.1177/1077558707305413.

Choldin, H. M. (1994). *Looking for the last percent: The controversy over census undercounts*. New Brunswick, New Jersey: Rutgers University Press.

Chu, J. P., & Sue, S. (2011). Asian American mental health: What we know and what we don't know. *Online Readings in Psychology and Culture, 3*(1), 4. doi:10.9707/2307-0919.1026.

Cook, B. L., McGuire, T., & Miranda, J. (2007). Measuring trends in mental health care disparities, 2000–2004. *Psychiatric Services, 58*(12), 1533–1540. doi:10.1176/appi.ps.58.12.1533.

Corrigan, P. (2004). How stigma interferes with mental health care. *American Psychologist, 59*(7), 614–625. doi:10.1037/0003-066X.59.7.614.

Dunn, K. S., & Horgas, A. L. (2000). The prevalence of prayer as a spiritual self-care modality in elders. *Journal of Holistic Nursing, 18*(4), 337–351.

El-Khoury, M. Y., Dutton, M. A., Goodman, L. A., Engel, L., Belamaric, R. J., & Murphy, M. (2004). Ethnic differences in battered women's formal help-seeking strategies: A focus on health, mental health, and spirituality. *Cultural Diversity and Ethnic Minority Psychology, 10*(4), 383–393. doi:10.1037/1099-9809.10.4.383.

Essed, P. (1991). *Understanding everyday racism: An interdisciplinary theory* (Vol. 2). Newbury Park, CA: Sage.

Fiori, K. L., Brown, E. E., Cortina, K. S., & Antonucci, T. C. (2006). Locus of control as a mediator of the relationship between religiosity and life satisfaction: Age, race, and gender differences. *Mental Health, Religion and Culture, 9*(03), 239–263. doi:10.1080/13694670600615482.

Fowler, D. N., & Hill, H. M. (2004). Social support and spirituality as culturally relevant factors in coping among African American women survivors of partner abuse. *Violence Against Women, 10*(11), 1267–1282. doi:10.1177/1077801204269001.

Gary, F. A. (2005). Stigma: Barrier to mental health care among ethnic minorities. *Issues in Mental Health Nursing, 26*(10), 979–999. doi:10.1080/01612840500280638.

Ghafoori, B., Barragan, B., Tohidian, N., & Palinkas, L. (2012). Racial and ethnic differences in symptom severity of PTSD, GAD, and depression in trauma-exposed, urban, treatment-seeking adults. *Journal of Traumatic Stress, 25*(1), 106–110. doi:10.1002/jts.21663.

Gillum, T. L., Sullivan, C. M., & Bybee, D. I. (2006). The importance of spirituality in the lives of domestic violence survivors. *Violence Against Women, 12*(3), 240–250. doi:10.1177/1077801206286224.

Grabe, S., & Hyde, J. S. (2006). Ethnicity and body dissatisfaction among women in the United States: A meta-analysis. *Psychological Bulletin, 132*(4), 622–640. doi:10.1037/0033-2909.132.4.622.

Greer, T. M. (2011). Coping strategies as moderators of the relation between individual race-related stress and mental health symptoms for African American women. *Psychology of Women Quarterly, 35*(2), 215–226. doi:10.1177/0361684311399388.

Harrell, S. P. (2000). A multidimensional conceptualization of racism-related stress: Implications for the well-being of people of color. *American Journal of Orthopsychiatry, 70*(1), 42–57. doi:10.1037/h0087722.

Harris, K. M., Edlund, M. J., & Larson, S. (2015). Racial and ethnic differences in the mental health problems and use of mental health care. *Medical Care, 43*(8), 775–784.

Hesse-Biber, S., Livingstone, S., Ramirez, D., Barko, E. B., & Johnson, A. L. (2010). Racial identity and body image among Black female college students attending predominately White colleges. *Sex Roles, 63*(9-10), 697–711.

Horwitz, A. (2013). The sociological study of mental illness: A critique and synthesis of four perspectives. In C. S. Aneshensel, J. C. Phelan, & A. Bierman (Eds.), *Handbook of the sociology of mental health* (2nd ed., pp. 95–112). New York: Kluwer Academic/Plenum Publishers.

Ince, B. Ü., Sc, M., Riper, H., PhD., van't Hof, E., & Cuijpers, P. (2014). The effects of psychotherapy on depression among racial-ethnic minority groups: A metaregression analysis. *Psychiatric Services, 65*(5), 612–617. doi:10.1176/appi.ps.201300165.

Jones, J. M. (1997). *Prejudice and racism*. New York, NY: McGraw-Hill.

Kim, H. S., Sherman, D. K., & Taylor, S. E. (2008). Culture and social support. *American Psychologist, 63*(6), 518. doi:10.1037/0003-066X.

Knouse, S. B. (1991). Social support for Hispanics in the military. *International Journal of Intercultural Relations, 15*(4), 427–444.

Lambert, M. J., Smart, D. W., Campbell, M. P., Hawkins, E. J., Harmon, C., & Slade, K. L. (2006). Psychotherapy outcome, as measured by the OQ-45, in African American, Asian/Pacific Islander, Latino/a, and Native American clients compared with matched Caucasian clients. *Journal of College Student Psychotherapy, 20*(4), 17–29.

Lazarus, R. S., & Folkman, S. (1984). *Stress, appraisal, and coping*. New York: Springer.

McGuire, T. G., & Miranda, J. (2008). New evidence regarding racial and ethnic disparities in mental health: Policy implications. *Health Affairs, 27*(2), 393–403. doi:10.1377/hlthaff.27.2.393.

Melfi, C. A., Croghan, T. W., & Hanna, M. P. (2000). Racial variation in antidepressant treatment in a Medicaid population. *Journal of Clinical Psychiatry, 61*, 16–21.

Menke, R., & Flynn, H. (2009). Relationships between stigma, depression, and treatment in white and African American primary care patients. *Journal of Nervous and Mental Disease, 197*(6), 407–411.

Mossakowski, K. N. (2003). Coping with perceived discrimination: Does ethnic identity protect mental health? *Journal of Health and Social Behavior, 44*(3), 318–331.

Mouzon, D. M. (2013). Can family relationships explain the race paradox in mental health? *Journal of Marriage and Family, 75*(2), 470–485. doi:10.1111/jomf.12006.

Nadeem, E., Lange, J. M., Edge, D., Fongwa, M., Belin, T., & Miranda, J. (2007). Does stigma keep poor young immigrant and US-born black and Latina women from seeking mental health care? *Psychiatric Services, 58*(12), 1547–1554.

Ojeda, V. D., & McGuire, T. G. (2006). Gender and racial/ethnic differences in use of outpatient mental health and substance use services by depressed adults. *Psychiatric Quarterly, 77*(3), 211–222. doi:10.1007/s11126-006-9008-9.

Okazaki, S. (2009). Impact of racism on ethnic minority mental health. *Perspectives on Psychological Science, 4*(1), 103–107. doi:10.1111/j.1745-6924.2009.01099.x.

Olfson, M., Mojtabai, R., Sampson, N. A., Hwang, I., Druss, B., Wang, P. S., ... & Kessler, R. C. (2009). Dropout from outpatient mental health care in the United States. *Psychiatric Services, 60*(7), 898–907.

Onoye, J. M., Goebert, D., Morland, L., Matsu, C., & Wright, T. (2009). PTSD and postpartum mental health in a sample of Caucasian, Asian, and Pacific Islander women. *Archives of Women's Mental Health, 12*(6), 393–400. doi:10.1007/s00737-009-0087-0.

Pargament, K. I., Smith, B. W., Koenig, H. G., & Perez, L. (1998). Patterns of positive and negative religious coping with major life stressors. *Journal for the Scientific Study of Religion*, 710–724.

Pearlin, L. I. (1989). The sociological study of stress. *Journal of Health and Social Behavior, 30*(3), 241–256.

Phinney, J. S., & Ong, A. D. (2007). Conceptualization and measurement of ethnic identity: Current status and future directions. *Journal of Counseling Psychology*, *54*(3), 271.

Pieterse, A. L., Todd, N. R., Neville, H. A., & Carter, R. T. (2012). Perceived racism and mental health among Black American adults: A meta-analytic review. *Journal of Counseling Psychology*, *59*(1), 1–9. doi:10.1037/a0026208.

Quintana, S. M. (2007). Racial and ethnic identity: Developmental perspectives and research. *Journal of Counseling Psychology*, *54*(3), 259. doi:10.1037/0022-0167.54.3.259.

Rosenfield, S., & Mouzon, D. (2013). Gender and mental health. In *Handbook of the sociology of mental health* (pp. 277–296). Dordrecht: Springer.

Schraufnagel, T. J., Wagner, A. W., Miranda, J., & Roy-Byrne, P. P. (2006). Treating minority patients with depression and anxiety: what does the evidence tell us? *General Hospital Psychiatry*, *28*(1), 27–36. doi:10.1016/j.genhosppsych.2005.07.002.

Schulz, A. J., Gravlee, C. C., Williams, D. R., Israel, B. A., Mentz, G., & Rowe, Z. (2006). Discrimination, symptoms of depression, and self-rated health among African American women in Detroit: Results from a longitudinal analysis. *American Journal of Public Health*, *96*(7), 1265–1270. doi:10.2105/AJPH.2005.064543.

Schwartz, S., & Meyer, I. H. (2010). Mental health disparities research: The impact of within and between group analyses on tests of social stress hypotheses. *Social Science and Medicine (1982)*, *70*(8), 1111–1118. doi:10.1016/j.socscimed.2009.11.032.

Sentell, T., Shumway, M., & Snowden, L. (2007). Access to mental health treatment by English language proficiency and race/ethnicity. *Journal of General Internal Medicine*, *22*(2), 289–293.

Shea, M., & Yeh, C. J. (2008). Asian American students' cultural values, stigma, and relational self-construal: Correlates of attitudes toward professional help seeking. *Journal of Mental Health Counseling*, *30*(2), 157.

Short, L. M., McMahon, P. M., Chervin, D. D., Shelley, G. A., Lezin, N., Sloop, K. S., & Dawkins, N. (2000). Survivors' identification of protective factors and early warning signs for intimate partner violence. *Violence Against Women*, *6*(3), 272–285.

Smedley, B. D., Stith, A. Y., & Nelson, A. R. (2003). Committee on understanding and eliminating racial and ethnic disparities in health care. Unequal treatment: confronting racial and ethnic disparities in health care. In *National Academy of Science* (Vol. 180, p. 191). Washington, DC: National Academies Press.

Smith, T. B., & Silva, L. (2011). Ethnic identity and personal well-being of people of color: A meta-analysis. *Journal of Counseling Psychology*, *58*(1), 42. doi:10.1037/a0021528.

Snowden, L. R., & Yamada, A.-M. (2005). Cultural differences in access to care. *Annual Review of Clinical Psychology*, *1*, 143–166. doi:10.1146/annurev.clinpsy.1.102803.143846.

Spence, N. J., Adkins, D. E., & Dupre, M. E. (2011). Racial differences in depression trajectories among older women: Socioeconomic, family, and health influences. *Journal of Health and Social Behavior*, *52*(4), 444–459. doi:10.1177/0022146511410432.

Spencer, M. S., Chen, J., Gee, G. C., Fabian, C. G., & Takeuchi, D. T. (2010). Discrimination and mental health-related service use in a national study of Asian Americans. *American Journal of Public Health*, *100*(12), 2410–2417.

Steele, C. M. (1997). A threat in the air: How stereotypes shape intellectual identity and performance. *American Psychologist*, *52*(6), 613–629.

Substance Abuse and Mental Health Services Administration. (2015). *Racial/ethnic differences in mental health service use among adults*. Rockville, MD: Substance Abuse and Mental Health Services Administration.

Sue, D. W., Capodilupo, C. M., Torino, G. C., Bucceri, J. M., Holder, A., Nadal, K. L., & Esquilin, M. (2007). Racial microaggressions in everyday life: Implications for clinical practice. *American Psychologist*, *62*(4), 271–286.

Sue, S., Yan Cheng, J. K., Saad, C. S., & Chu, J. P. (2012). Asian American mental health: A call to action. *American Psychologist*, *67*(7), 532–544. doi:10.1037/a0028900.

Suite, D. H., La Bril, R., Primm, A., & Harrison-Ross, P. (2007). Beyond misdiagnosis, misunderstanding and mistrust: relevance of the historical perspective in the medical and mental health treatment of people of color. *Journal of the National Medical Association*, *99*(8), 879.

Taylor, J. (1999). Colonizing images and diagnostic labels: Oppressive mechanisms for African American women's health. *Advances in Nursing Science*, *21*(3), 32–45.

Thoits, P. (2011). Mechanisms linking social ties and support to physical and mental health. *Journal of Health and Social Behavior*, *52*(2), 145–161. doi:10.1177/0022146510395592.

U.S. Department of Health and Human Services. (2001). *Mental health: Culture, race, and ethnicity – A supplement to mental health. A report of the Surgeon General*. DHHS Publication No. SMA-01-3613. Rockville, MD: Author.

Wang, T. (2007). Mental health treatment dropout and its correlates in a general population sample. *Medical Care, 45*(3), 224–229.

Wang, P. S., Lane, M., Olfson, M., Pincus, H. A., Wells, K. B., & Kessler, R. C. (2005). Twelve-month use of mental health services in the United States: Results from the National Comorbidity Survey Replication. *Archives of General Psychiatry, 62*(6), 629–640.

Watson, N. N., & Hunter, C. D. (2015). Anxiety and depression among African American women: The costs of strength and negative attitudes toward psychological help-seeking. *Cultural Diversity and Ethnic Minority Psychology, 21*(4), 604–612.

Wei, G., Greaver, L. B., Marson, S. M., Herndon, C. H., & Rogers, J. (2008). Postpartum depression: Racial differences and ethnic disparities in a tri-racial and bi-ethnic population. *Maternal and Child Health Journal, 12*(6), 699–707. doi:10.1007/s10995-007-0287-z.

Wells, K., Klap, R., Koike, A., & Sherbourne, C. (2001). Ethnic disparities in unmet need for alcoholism, drug abuse, and mental health care. *American Journal of Psychiatry, 158*(12), 2027–2032. doi:10.1176/appi.ajp.158.12.2027.

Whaley, A. L. (2001). Cultural mistrust and mental health services for African Americans: A review and meta-analysis. *Counseling Psychologist, 29*(4), 513–531.

Williams, D. R., Haile, R., González, H. M., Neighbors, H., Baser, R., & Jackson, J. S. (2007). The mental health of Black Caribbean immigrants: Results from the National Survey of American Life. *American Journal of Public Health, 97*(1), 52–59. doi:10.2105/AJPH.2006.088211.

Williams, D. R., & Mohammed, S. A. (2009). Discrimination and racial disparities in health: Evidence and needed research. *Journal of Behavioral Medicine, 32*(1), 20–47. doi:10.1007/s10865-008-9185-0.

Windsor, L. C., Jemal, A., & Alessi, E. J. (2015). Cognitive behavioral therapy: A meta-analysis of race and substance use outcomes. *Cultural Diversity and Ethnic Minority Psychology, 21*(2), 300–313. doi:10.1007/s12671-013-0269-8.Moving.

Yip, T., Gee, G. C., & Takeuchi, D. T. (2008). Racial discrimination and psychological distress: The impact of ethnic identity and age among immigrant and United States-born Asian adults. *Developmental Psychology, 44*(3), 787.

Chapter Six
The Impact of Sexual and Gender Diversity on Women's Mental Health

Jessica Punzo

The mental health of sexual- and gender-minority women is of upmost importance, yet has not always had a dedicated and expansive space in the women's health literature. There have been a few books (Hughes, Smith, & Dan, 2003; Mathy & Kerr, 2003) specifically dedicated to the mental health issues of sexual-minority women. However, these are outdated, and unfortunately, do not include the mental health needs of transgender women. Therefore, this chapter provides an updated and comprehensive review of the literature on mental health concerns and strengths within sexual- and gender-minority women.

As this chapter is included in a larger volume of women's mental health concerns, the author will provide a brief overview on what types of individuals may fall within the umbrella term of gender and sexual minorities, as well as some standard definitions. It is important to recognize how diverse this community is, as well as acknowledge the vast levels of intersectionalities that may be present for sexual- and gender-minority women. Due to these complexities, the author will separate the chapter by first addressing specific issues for sexual-minority women, and then addressing specific issues for gender-minority women.

Overview of Terminology

The term sexual minority is typically an umbrella term to describe individuals whose sexual orientation is anything but heterosexual (i.e., lesbian, bisexual, gay, queer, etc.). In contrast, gender minority can be used as an umbrella term to refer to individuals whose gender identity does not conform to social-majority categories of gender (i.e., transgender and genderqueer). It should be noted that the definitions presented in this chapter may not apply to all people and tend to vary and change over time. Moreover, there may be individual variability within certain terms. It is always helpful to ask individuals what is meant by the term they use to identify themselves, instead of assuming.

Based on the above information, a sexual-minority woman may identify her sexual orientation in various different ways. We will present some of the more common orientations and their working definitions. Most people are familiar with the term lesbian, which has typically been used to describe women who are emotionally, romantically, and/or sexually attracted to other women. However, the term gay may also be used to describe a woman who is attracted to another woman. The term bisexual has typically been used to describe a person who is emotionally, romantically, and/or sexually attracted to more than one gender, though not necessarily simultaneously or to the same degree. The term queer has been used by individuals to describe a more fluid sexual orientation, or by those who do not feel other sexual orientation labels fit their experience. It is important to note the change in the use of, and meaning of, the word queer. Historically, the word queer was often used as an insult toward non-heterosexual individuals. However, many LGBT people started to reclaim the word queer in the late 1980s as it felt like a more accurate reflection of their identity. It is always important to mirror terminology that people use for themselves. For example, if someone self-identifies as queer, you may use that label. However, it is not appropriate to label individuals as queer if they have not done so themselves. Finally, the term asexual refers to a person who generally does not have any sexual attraction to others.

It is important to understand that sexual orientation is distinctly different to gender identity. Gender identity refers to people's internal experience of their gender. This identity may or may not be aligned with the person's sex assigned at birth. The term used to describe someone whose sex assigned at birth is aligned with that person's gender identity is cisgender. This is contrasted with the term transgender, which is typically used to describe individuals whose sex assigned at birth does not align with their gender identity. Moreover, some individuals identify as genderqueer, which may describe a more fluid gender identity. Individuals who identify as genderqueer may identify themselves as neither male nor female, being both male and female, or as somewhere outside these gender categories. As this is a book dedicated to women's mental health, the section on gender minority will focus mainly on transgender women. It should be noted that some transgender men or genderqueer individuals may have similar mental health concerns as other transgender or cisgender women, but this will not be addressed in this chapter.

Challenges and Limitations

Before reviewing and discussing recent research, the challenges and limitations of conducting sexual- and gender-minority research must be noted. These are discussed here, so that readers may interpret results with a critical eye as well as understand some of the limitations of the findings that will be presented. In 1999, the Institute of Medicine's Committee on Lesbian Health Research Priorities addressed both the methodological challenges and contextual barriers to conducting lesbian-centered research. They noted one of the biggest challenges to be inconsistencies in the way sexual orientation is defined, which leads to difficulty comparing findings across studies (Solarz, 1999). This challenge has also been cited as a broader issue for LGBT research, in general (Institute of Medicine, 2011). Without a clear and unified understanding of sexual orientation, we cannot create measures to accurately capture this population either, which can lead to erroneous or overgeneralized results. For example, if a researcher defined sexual orientation solely based on behavior, versus identity, a person who identified as bisexual may be grouped into a heterosexual or lesbian/gay identity, depending on his or her current partner. On the other hand, an individual may have sex with more than one gender, although not identify as bisexual, but may be placed in a bisexual category by researchers.

Another common challenge to studying sexual and gender minorities includes the lack of high-quality probability samples. Many studies conducted on lesbian health have relied on convenience samples, which tend to be unrepresentative of the lesbian community as a whole, which then makes generalizability difficult (Solarz, 1999). It has also been cited that studies have grouped both lesbian and bisexual women together in order to achieve a higher sample size and achieve statistical power (Bostwick, 2012). This as well contributes to erroneous findings and inability to generalize findings. Another issue that relates to sampling is lack of an appropriate control or comparison group.

Lastly, a common difficulty in conducting research on sexual and gender minorities is the lack of trust or reluctance to disclose their identities to researchers (Institute of Medicine, 2011; Solarz, 1999). Individuals may be concerned about the anonymity of their responses depending on the collection method, as disclosing sexual or gender identity may have negative consequences. Moreover, individuals may also decline to answer, or intentionally give inaccurate responses on these types of questions, due to the stigma associated with being a gender or sexual minority. Again, much of this can contribute to the lack of clear and accurate data.

Sexual-Minority Women

Research on sexual-minority women has largely focused on lesbian-identified women. Fewer studies have focused on bisexual women, and even less on queer-identified women. Studies that used the term "queer women" in their title often used the term to encompass more than one sexual orientation, rather than identifying it as its own distinct orientation. However, the trend appears to be changing, as those studies in which queer was identified as its own orientation were all dated within the past year six years, appearing more frequently in the past year or two. As many other articles suggest, this is indeed demonstrating a need for more research focused on women who identify as bisexual and queer.

It is beyond the scope of this chapter to provide an exhaustive review of all literature pertaining to the various mental health issues that sexual-minority women face. Therefore, the author has chosen to focus on a select number of issues that have more robust research and seem more common amongst this population. These areas include substance use, trauma, bias and discrimination, and engagement in therapy.

Substance Abuse

When searching the literature on mental health and sexual minorities, one will most often come across research highlighting substance use, more specifically alcohol use, in this population. When comparing sexual-minority women to their heterosexual counterparts, studies consistently show that sexual-minority women have higher rates of lifetime and recent substance use, and are at greater risk for substance abuse (Bloomfield, 1993; Bradford, Ryan, & Rothblum, 1994; McKirnan & Peterson, 1989; Scheer et al., 2003; Skinner & Otis, 1992). When taking a closer look at between-group differences in substance use, we also consistently see bisexuals endorsing the highest rates of substance use and substance use-related problems compared to other sexual-minority women (Green & Feinstein, 2012; McCabe, Hughes, Bostwick, West, & Boyd, 2009; Scheer et al., 2003). These findings on increased levels of substance use (both between and within groups) appear to amplify when focusing on young sexual-minority women, in particular (Kerr, Ding, Burke, & Ott-Walter, 2015; Kerr, Ding, & Chaya, 2014; Lehavot, Williams, Millard, Bradley, & Simpson, 2016; McCabe, Hughes, & Boyd, 2004). One study connected increased rates of substance use in lesbian women to the use of bars as social resources (Bradford et al., 1994). They also found that less frequent involvement with the lesbian and gay community and decreased openness about their identity may have led to a reliance on substances to combat isolation and loneliness. Other studies have linked psychological distress to increases in substance use in sexual-minority women (Newcomb, Heinz, & Mustanski, 2012), and some report that lesbians may use alcohol to regulate negative emotions (Cooper, Frone, Russell, & Mudar, 1995). Furthermore, researchers have explored the link between sexual-minority stress and substance use, finding the impact of sexual-minority stress contributing to hazardous substance use (Lewis, Milletich, Kelly, & Woody, 2012; Mason, Lewis, Gargurevich, & Kelly, 2016).

Trauma

Trauma is another common mental health issue among sexual-minority women. Trauma exposure is very common among all women, regardless of sexual orientation, and women are twice as likely to develop posttraumatic stress disorder following a traumatic event when compared to men (Stoltenborgh, van Ijzendoorn, Euser, & Bakermans-Kranenburg, 2011). However, the literature focusing on traumatic victimization in sexual-minority women has not been as robust. Balsam (2003) suggests some potential reason as to why this may be, including homophobia, heterosexism, and the myth of sexual abuse "causing" a person to become attracted to the same gender. Some other potential reasons may include some of the broader research challenges that were mentioned earlier, such as distrust, inadequate sampling techniques, and unclear definitions of sexual orientation and/or gender.

Despite some of these challenges, the research that has been conducted on sexual-minority women suggests that they are at the same, if not greater, risk for trauma exposure as their heterosexual counterparts (Austin et al., 2008; Corliss, Cochran, & Mays, 2002; Lehavot & Simpson, 2014; Mattocks et al., 2013; Stoddard, Dibble, & Fineman, 2009). Some studies have even looked at within-group differences in trauma experiences in sexual-minority women. Although some literature has not found any significant differences between sexual-minority women (Austin et al., 2008; Hughes et al., 2010; Scheer et al., 2003), more recent data have suggested that bisexual women, in particular, have the highest rates of trauma exposure. The most recent report from the National Coalition of Anti-Violence Programs (NCAVP) (2015) found that people who identified as bisexual were about two times more likely to experience sexual violence than people who did not identify as bisexual. Moreover, Ford and Soto-Marquez (2016) found that, "bisexual women were the most vulnerable to sexual assault in college, as nearly two out of every five bisexual female college students had experienced sexual assault after four years in college" (p. 1). This elevated risk may be due to the high levels of discrimination bisexuals experience from both gay and straight communities coupled with a larger problem of bi-invisibility and bierasure.

Bias and Discrimination

In addition to higher rates of interpersonal trauma, sexual-minority women are often the targets of bias-related violence and discrimination. On top of experiencing sexism, they may also experience biphobia, homophobia, and/ or racism. Balsam (2003) cited the terms "insidious trauma" coined by Root (1992), and "cultural victimization" by Neisen (1993), as examples of this compounded trauma experience. This is important to consider when working with sexual-minority women, as their experiences may present differently than heterosexual counterparts, and thus, approaches to treatment may need to be altered.

Treatment Utilization

It has been found that sexual-minority women often face barriers in obtaining quality health care (Bradford & White, 2000), and this is likely the case when it comes to mental health specifically (Bradford et al., 1994; Razzano, Cook, Hamilton, Hughes, & Matthews, 2006). Unfortunately, it has also been cited that medical and mental health care providers have reported negative attitudes toward sexual-minority women, as well as lack of knowledge about the specific needs and concerns of this population (Bradford, Ryan, Honnold, & Rothblum, 2001). Additionally, research has shown that overt heterosexism (Bowers, Plummer, & Minichiello, 2005; Green, 2007; Israel, Gorcheva, Walther, Sulzner, & Cohen, 2008), as well as sexual-orientation microaggressions (Shelton & Delgado-Romero, 2013) from therapists, exist, and have detrimental effects on clients. Unfortunately, there has not been a dedicated resource for "best practices" for sexual-minority women. They often get pooled into guidelines for the larger LGBT community, which is quite a disservice, as research has shown that this population has unique needs.

Moreover, studies have found high utilization of mental health services among sexual-minority women. A study done in 2002 examined the medical charts of both lesbian and bisexual women at a community LGBT center, and found that about 83% of lesbians, and 81% of bisexual women, reported prior use of outpatient mental health services (Rogers, Emanuel, & Bradford, 2002). A later study in 2006 compared treatment utilization in lesbian and heterosexual women and found that lesbians were one-half times as likely to report using mental health services than heterosexual women, even when controlling for factors shown to influence treatment utilization in the literature (Razzano et al., 2006). These findings should be taken into account when thinking about the long-standing history of heterosexism that has been present in psychology and psychiatry. For example, homosexuality was considered a mental health disorder up until 1973 in psychiatry (American Psychiatric Association (APA), 1973), and it was not until 2009 that the American Psychological Association released a statement advising psychologists not to practice conversion or reparative therapy (Anton, 2010).

Strengths of Sexual-Minority Women

Despite the adversity and concerns that sexual-minority women face, they do have inherent strengths. However, as with much of the other research on sexual identity, few studies have focused specifically on women only. We will briefly cover literature on resilience and strengths within the larger LGB community, and then highlight a few studies that have looked specifically at resilience in sexual-minority women.

A qualitative analysis of an online survey questioning the positive aspects of being a sexual minority revealed 11 themes, including: belonging to a community, creating families of choice, forging strong connections with others, serving as positive role models, developing empathy and compassion, living authentically and honestly, gaining personal insight and sense of self, involvement in social justice and activism, freedom from gender-specific roles, exploring sexuality and relationships, and enjoying egalitarian relationships (lesbian participants only) (Riggle, Whitman, Olson, Rostosky, & Strong, 2008). It should be noted that the authors compiled bisexual and queer-identified women into the label as "lesbian" when presenting findings and completing data analysis. This is noted because the experiences of bisexual and queer women may not be similar to lesbian women, most notably for the lack of community and visibility of these communities. This point is further supported by a later study done by Rostosky, Riggle, Pascale-Hague, and McCants (2010) which found that bisexuals found strength in a *bisexual community* versus the larger gay/lesbian or heterosexual community. Participants also noted the difficulty in identifying with this community due to invisibility.

Kwon (2013) also acknowledged the importance of social support as a resilience factor for LGB people, connecting it with its ability to lower reactivity to prejudice. Moreover, he noted that emotional openness, along with hope and optimism, can serve as factors that increase psychological well-being in LGB individuals. Conceptualizing LGB strengths has also been framed within the minority stress model, and other forms of positive psychology, stating that response to stressors can increase character strengths and growth (Lytle, Vaughan, Rodriguez, & Shmerler, 2014; Meyer, 2003).

Similarly, in regards to sexual-minority women specifically, Balsam (2003) stated that this population often has to deal with "cultural victimization" on a daily basis by finding ways to manage the conflict between their own feelings and societal norms. As a result, they can develop a larger set of coping skills to deal with other types of difficulty in their lives. Other studies have highlighted the importance of social support and acceptance as key factors in resiliency in bisexual and lesbian women (Cooperman, Simoni, & Lockhart, 2003; D'Augelli, 2003). Bowleg, Huang, Brooks, Black, and Burkholder (2003) identified internal strategies (e.g., "uniqueness," "freedom of living authentically," and "labeling sources of oppression") of Black lesbian women that aided in resiliency and strength. Moreover, one study found that lesbian and bisexual women who had high involvement in feminist activities were able to defend against the negative effects of sexism, but only when these sexist events were infrequent (Szymanski & Owens, 2009).

Gender-Minority Women

As with sexual-minority women, gender-minority women face a unique set of issues, and have their own barriers to accessing affirming and competent care. As noted earlier, this section will focus on male-to-female transgender individuals, here on out referred to as trans women. Furthermore, it should be noted that many studies on transgender people do not delineate trans women from trans men, so some of the findings presented may reflect the trans community as a whole, rather than trans women specifically. Similar to the previous section, we will outline the common mental health issues that trans women face along with the strengths of this community.

It seems necessary to provide a brief history of the evolution of trans identities in the mental health field. Like homosexuality, the diagnoses "transsexualism," "gender identity disorder of childhood," and "gender identity disorder" (GID) all appeared in the *Diagnostic and Statistical Manual of Mental Disorders* (DSM) of the APA up until the most recent revision in 2013 (APA, 2013a). In the latest revision to DSM, gender identity disorder was changed to gender dysphoria (GD) (APA, 2013b). According to APA, removal of the word "disorder" was intentional to "avoid stigma and ensure clinical care for individuals who see and feel themselves to be a different gender than their assigned gender" (APA, 2013b, para. 3). They note the most important criterion of the diagnosis was the "presence of clinically significant distress." A posttransition specifier was also added to identify individuals who were "living full-time as the desired gender," as well as difference in presentation in children and adolescents. Although the intent behind this decision was to be less stigmatizing and pathologizing, we must still be aware that individuals who identify as a gender that was not their sex assigned at birth can be thought of as having a diagnosable mental disorder. Moreover, this inherently affects the treatment that trans people may receive, specifically from mental health providers. Numerous studies have noted transphobia, the intense dislike of or prejudice against transgender people, as significant barriers within the mental health system (Colton Meier, Fitzgerald, Pardo, & Backcok, 2011; Kidd, Veltman, Gately, Chan, & Cohen, 2011; Lucksted, 2004; Shipherd, Green, & Abramovitz, 2010).

This stigma and prejudice are not limited to mental health providers, and are unfortunately present in larger society. As such, transgender people experience high rates of violence and trauma, which ultimately have consequences on their mental health. Rates of violence vary depending on the study, but many tend to range between 50% and 80% of transgender people experiencing some form of violence in their lifetime (Bockting, Miner, Romine, Hamilton, & Coleman, 2013; Nemoto, Bödeker, & Iwamoto, 2011). Even when looking within the larger LGBTQ community, trans people continue to experience higher rates of violence. The most recent report on hate crimes against LGBTQ people noted that trans women were 1.6 times more likely to experience physical violence, 6.1 times more likely to experience physical police violence, 2.4 times more likely to experience harassment, and 2.9 times more likely to experience discrimination when compared to other survivors of violence (NCAVP, 2015). Additionally, 50% of reported homicides to the NCAVP were trans women of color.

Given the alarming rates of violence against this community, it is not surprising they also struggle with a variety of mental health problems. Hopwood and Dickey (2014) cite a variety of research that indicates lifetime rates of suicidal thoughts in trans people from 48% to 79%, and suicide attempts range between 21% and 41%. This is much higher than the national average, which notes that 1.9% to 8.7% of adults attempt suicide (Nock et al., 2008). Moreover, other research has indicated the incidence of depression of trans women was three times higher than the general population (Nuttbrock et al., 2010).

Given the higher rates of psychiatric conditions, it is also not surprising that trans individuals would develop both negative and positive tools for coping. There is evidence to suggest that trans people have higher rates of self-injurious behavior than their cisgender counterparts (Davey, Arcelus, Meyer, & Bouman, 2016; Walls, Laser, Nickels, & Wisneski, 2010). It has also been found that trans individuals turn to drugs and alcohol to cope more frequently than cisgender individuals (Grant et al., 2011; Lombardi, 2008). Despite some of the negative coping mechanisms that trans people may use, a study done on protective factors against suicide in trans adults identified the themes of social support, gender identity-related factors (e.g., acceptance and comfort with identity), transition-related factors (e.g., coming out/disclosing), individual difference factors (e.g., optimism, coping and problem skills), and reasons for living (e.g., being a positive role model, spiritual or religious reasons) (Moody, Fuks, Pelaez, & Smith, 2015).

Resilience

There has also been a growing amount of research focused on resilience in the trans community. Sanchez and Vilain (2009) explored the role of self-esteem on overall psychological distress in trans women. They found that trans women who felt they were valued members of the trans community, evaluated the community positively, and felt that the trans community incorporated important aspects of their identity had fewer mental health symptoms. Other studies have found self-esteem, sense of personal mastery, hope, activism, and serving as a role model as other factors promoting resiliency in trans-identified individuals (Grossman, D'Augelli, & Frank, 2011; Singh, Hays, & Watson, 2011).

Summary

Research presented in this chapter indicates that sexual- and gender-minority women have specific needs and issues, which need more targeted research. It is a great disservice to these women to group them within larger LGBT research. Furthermore, it has been shown that they all have unique qualities and characteristics, which warrants even further delineation within the research (e.g., studying bisexual women as their own identity). Although sexual- and gender-minority women face much adversity, they still possess resilient qualities, and can continue to thrive in clinical treatment, and in their overall lives.

References

American Psychiatric Association. (1973). Position statement on homosexuality and civil rights. *American Journal of Psychiatry, 131*, 497.

American Psychiatric Association. (2013a). *Diagnostic and statistical manual of mental disorders* (5th ed.). Washington, DC: American Psychiatric Association.

American Psychiatric Association. (2013b). *Gender dysphoria* [fact sheet]. Retrieved from http://www.dsm5.org/documents/gender%20dysphoria%20fact%20sheet.pdf (accessed November 4, 2016).

Anton, B. S. (2010). Proceedings of the American Psychological Association for the legislative year 2009: Minutes of the annual meeting of the Council of Representatives and minutes of the meetings of the Board of Directors. *American Psychologist, 65*, 385–475. doi:10.1037/a0019553.

Austin, S. B., Jun, H. J., Jackson, B., Spiegelman, D., Rich-Edwards, J., Corliss, H. L., & Wright, R. J. (2008). Disparities in child abuse victimization in lesbian, bisexual, and heterosexual women in the Nurses' Health Study II. *Journal of Women's Health, 17*(4), 597–606. doi: 10.1089/jwh.2007.0450.

Balsam, K. F. (2003). Trauma, stress, and resilience among sexual minority women: Rising like the phoenix. *Journal of Lesbian Studies, 7*(4), 1–8. doi: 10.1300/J155v07n04_01.

Bloomfield, K. (1993). A comparison of alcohol consumption between lesbians and heterosexual women in an urban population. *Drug Alcohol Dependence, 33*(3), 257–269.

Bockting, W. O., Miner, M. H., Romine, R. E. S., Hamilton, A., & Coleman, E. (2013). Stigma, mental health, and resilience in an online sample of the U.S. transgender population. *American Journal of Public Health, 103*(5), 943–951.

Bostwick, W. (2012). Assessing bisexual stigma and mental health statues: A brief report. *Journal of Bisexuality, 12*(2), 214–222. doi: 10.1080/15299716.2012.674860.

Bowers, R., Plummer, D., & Minichiello, V. (2005). Homophobia in counseling practice. *International Journal for the Advancement of Counseling, 27*, 471–489. doi:10.1007/s10447-005-8207-7.

Bowleg, L., Huang, J., Brooks, K., Black, A., & Burkholder, G. (2003). Triple jeopardy and beyond: Multiple minority stress and resilience among black lesbians. *Journal of Lesbian Studies, 7*(4), 87–108. doi: 10.1300/J155v07n04_06.

Bradford, J., Ryan, C., Honnold, J., & Rothblum, E. (2001). Expanding the research infrastructure for lesbian health. *American Journal of Public Health, 91*(7), 1029–1032.

Bradford, J., Ryan, C., & Rothblum, E. D. (1994). National lesbian health care survey: Implications for mental health care. *Journal of Consulting and Clinical Psychology, 62*(2), 228–242.

Bradford, J., & White, J. (2000). Lesbian health research. In M. B. Goldman & M. C. Hatch (Eds.), *Women and health* (pp. 64–77). San Diego, CA: Academic Press.

Colton Meier, S. L., Fitzgerald, K. M., Pardo, S. T., & Backcok, J. (2011). The effects of hormonal gender affirmation treatment on mental health in female-to-male transsexuals. *Journal of Gay and Lesbian Mental Health, 15*(3), 281–299. doi: 10.1080/19359705.2011.581195.

Cooper, M. L., Frone, M. R., Russell, M., & Mudar, P. (1995). Drinking to regulate positive and negative emotions: A motivational model of alcohol use. *Journal of Personality and Social Psychology, 69*(5), 990–1005. doi: 10.1037/0022-3514.69.5.990.

Cooperman, N. A., Simoni, J. M., & Lockhart, D. W. (2003). Abuse, social support, and depression among HIV-positive heterosexual, bisexual and lesbian women. *Journal of Lesbian Studies, 7*(4), 49–66. doi: 10.1300/J155v07n04_04.

Corliss, H. L., Cochran, S. D., & Mays, V. M. (2002). Reports of parental maltreatment during childhood in a United States population-based survey of homosexual, bisexual, and heterosexual adults. *Child Abuse and Neglect, 26*, 1165–1178.

D'Augelli, A. R. (2003). Lesbian and bisexual female youths aged 14 to 21: Developmental challenges and victimization experiences. *Journal of Lesbian Studies, 7*(4), 9–29. doi: 10.1300/J155v07n04_02.

Davey, A., Arcelus, J., Meyer, C., & Bouman, W. P. (2016). Self-injury among trans individuals and matched controls: Prevalence and associated factors. *Health and Social Care in the Community, 24*(4), 485–494. doi: 10.1111/hsc.12239.

Ford, J., & Soto-Marquez, J. G. (2016). Sexual assault victimization among straight, gay/lesbian, and bisexual college students. *Violence and Gender, 3*, 1–9. doi: 10.1089/vio.2015.0030.

Grant, J. M., Mottet, L. A., Tanis, J., Harrison, J., Herman, J. L., & Keisling, M. (2011). Injustice at every turn: A report of the national transgender discrimination survey, executive summary. *National Center for Transgender Equality and National Gay and Lesbian Task Force.* Retrieved April 29, 2016 from http://www.thetaskforce.org/static_html/downloads/reports/reports/ntds_summary.pdf (accessed November 4, 2016).

Green, B. (2007). Delivering ethical psychological services to lesbian, gay, and bisexual clients. In K. J. Bieschke, R. M. Perez, & K. A. DeBord (Eds.), *Handbook of counseling and psychotherapy with lesbian, gay, bisexual, and transgender clients* (pp. 181–199). Washington, DC: American Psychological Association.

Green, K. E., & Feinstein, B. A. (2012). Substance use in lesbian, gay, and bisexual populations: An update on empirical research and implications for treatment. *Psychology of Addictive Behaviors, 26*(2), 265–278. doi: 10.1037/a0025424.

Grossman, A. H., D'Augelli, A. R., & Frank, J. A. (2011). Aspects of psychological resilience among transgender youth. *Journal of LGBT Youth, 8*(2), 103–115. doi: 10.1080/19361653.2011.541347.

Hopwood, R., & Dickey, L. M. (2014). Mental health services and support. In L. Erickson-Schroth (Ed.), *Trans bodies, trans selves: A resource for the transgender community* (pp. 291–332). New York: Oxford University Press.

Hughes, T. L., Smith, C., & Dan, A. (Eds.) (2003). *Mental health issues for sexual minority women: Redefining women's mental health.* Binghamton, NY: Harrington Park Press.

Hughes, T. L., Szalacha, L. A., Johnson, T. P., Kinnison, K.E., Wilsnack, S. C., & Cho, Y. (2010). Sexual victimization and hazardous drinking among heterosexual and sexual minority women. *Addictive Behaviors, 35*(12), 1152–1156. doi: 10.1016/j.addbeh.2010.07.004.

Institute of Medicine. (2011). *The health of lesbian, gay, bisexual, and transgender people: Building a foundation for better understanding.* Washington, DC: The National Academies Press.

Israel, T., Gorcheva, R., Walther, W. A., Sulzner, J. M., & Cohen, J. (2008). Therapists' helpful and unhelpful situations with LGBT clients: An exploratory study. *Professional Psychology: Research and Practice, 39*, 361–368. doi:10.1037/0735-7028.39.3.361.

Kerr, D., Ding, K., Burke, A., & Ott-Walter, K. (2015). An alcohol, tobacco, and other drug use comparison of lesbian, bisexual, and heterosexual undergraduate women. *Substance Use and Misuse, 50*(3), 340–349. doi: 10.3109/10826084.2014.980954.

Kerr, D. L., Ding, K., & Chaya, J. (2014). Substance use of lesbian, gay, bisexual and heterosexual college students. *American Journal of Health Behavior, 38*(6), 951–962. doi: 10.5993/AJHB.38.6.17.

Kidd, S. A., Veltman, A., Gately, C., Chan, K. J., & Cohen, J. N. (2011). Lesbian, gay, and transgender persons with severe mental illness: Negotiating wellness in the context of multiple sources of stigma. *American Journal of Psychiatric Rehabilitation, 14*(1), 13–39. doi: 10.1080/15487768.2011.546277.

Kwon, P. (2013). Resilience in lesbian, gay and bisexual individuals. *Personality and Social Psychology Review, 17*(4) 371–383. doi: 10.1177/1088868313490248.

Lehavot, K., & Simpson, T. L. (2014). Trauma, posttraumatic stress disorder, and depression among sexual minority and heterosexual women veterans. *Journal of Counseling Psychology, 61*(3), 392–403. doi: 10.1037/cou0000019.

Lehavot, K., Williams, E. C., Millard, S. P., Bradley, K. A., & Simpson, T. L. (2016). Association of alcohol misuse with sexual identity and sexual behavior in women veterans. *Substance Use and Misuse, 51*(2), 216–229. doi:10.3109/10826084.2015.1092988.

Lewis, R. J., Milletich, R. J., Kelly, M. L., & Woody, A. (2012). Sexual minority stress, substance use, and intimate partner violence among sexual minority women. *Aggression and Violent Behaviors, 17*(3), 247–256. doi: 10.1016/j.avb.2012.02.004.

Lombardi, E. L. (2008). Substance use treatment experiences of transgender/transsexual men and women. *Journal of LGBT Health Research, 3*(2), 37–47.

Lucksted, A. (2004). Lesbian, gay, bisexual, and transgender people receiving services in the public mental health system: Raising issues. *Journal of Gay and Lesbian Psychotherapy, 8*(3–4), 25–42. doi: 10.1300/J236v08n03_03.

Lytle, M. C., Vaughan, M. D., Rodriguez, E. M., & Shmerler, D. L. (2014). Working with LGBT individuals: Incorporating positive psychology into training and practice. *Psychology of Sexual Orientation and Gender Diversity, 1*(4), 335–347. doi: 10.1037/sgd0000064.

McCabe, S. E., Hughes, T. L., Bostwick, W. B., West, B. T., & Boyd, C. J. (2009). Sexual orientation, substance use behaviors and substance dependence in the United States. *Addiction, 104,* 1333–1345.

McCabe, S. E., Hughes, T. L., & Boyd, C. J. (2004). Substance use and misuse: Are bisexual women at greater risk? *Journal of Psychoactive Drugs, 36,* 217–225.

McKirnan, D. J., & Peterson, P. L. (1989). Alcohol and drug use among homosexual men and women: Epidemiology and population characteristics. *Addictive Behaviors, 14,* 545–563.

Mason, T. B., Lewis, R. J., Gargurevich, M., & Kelly, M. L. (2016). Minority stress and intimate partner violence perpetration among lesbians: Negative affect, hazardous drinking, and intrusiveness as mediators. *Psychology of Sexual Orientation and Gender Diversity, 3*(2), 236–246. doi:10.1037/sgd0000165.

Mathy, R. M., & Kerr, S. K. (Eds.) (2003). *Lesbian and bisexual women's mental health.* Binghamton, NY: Haworth Press.

Mattocks, K. M., Sadler, A., Yano, E. M., Krebs E. E., Zephyrin, L., Brandt, C., . . . & Haskell, S. (2013). Sexual victimization among lesbian and bisexual OEF/OIF veterans. *Journal of General Internal Medicine, 28,* 604–608. doi: 10.1007/s11606-013-2357-9.

Meyer, I. H. (2003). Prejudice, social stress, and mental health in lesbian, gay, and bisexual populations: Conceptual issues and research evidence. *Psychological Bulletin, 129*(5), 674–697. doi: 10.1037/0033-2909.129.5.674.

Moody, C., Fuks, N., Pelaez, S., & Smith, N. G. (2015). "Without this, I would for sure already be dead": A qualitative inquiry regarding suicide protective factors among trans adults. *Psychology of Sexual Orientation and Gender Diversity, 2*(3), 266–280. http://dx.doi.org/10.1037/sgd0000130.

National Coalition of Anti-Violence Programs. (2015). *Lesbian, gay, bisexual, transgender, queer, and HIV-affected intimate partner violence in 2014.* New York: Author.

Neisen, J. H. (1993). Healing from cultural victimizations: Recovery from shame due to heterosexism. *Journal of Gay and Lesbian Psychotherapy, 2*(1), 49–63. doi: 10.1300/J236v02n01_04.

Nemoto, T., Bödeker, B., & Iwamoto, M. (2011). Social support, exposure to violence and transphobia, and correlates of depression among male-to-female transgender women with a history of sex work. *American Journal of Public Health, 101*(10), 1980–1988.

Newcomb, M. E., Heinz, A. J., & Mustanski, B. (2012). Examining risk and protective factors for alcohol use in lesbian, gay, bisexual, and transgender youth: A longitudinal multilevel analysis. *Journal of Studies on Alcohol and Drugs, 73*(5), 783–793.

Nock, M. K., Borges, G., Bromet, E. J., Cha, C. B., Kessler, R. C., & Lee, S. (2008). Suicide and suicidal behavior. *Epidemiology Review, 30*(1), 133–154. doi: 10.1093/epirev/mxn002.

Nuttbrock, L., Hwahng, S., Bockting, W., Rosenblum, A., Mason, M., Macri, M., & Becker, J. (2010). Psychiatric impact of gender-related abuse across the life course of male-to-female transgender persons. *Journal of Sex Research, 47*(1), 12–23. doi: 10.1080/00224490903062258.

Razzano, L. A., Cook, J. A., Hamilton, M. M., Hughes, T. L., & Matthews, A. K. (2006). Predictors of mental health service use among lesbian and heterosexual women. *Psychiatric Rehabilitation Journal, 29*(4), 289–298.

Riggle, E. D. B., Whitman, J. S., Olson, A., Rostosky, S. S., & Strong, S. (2008). The positive aspects of being a lesbian or gay man. *Professional Psychology: Research and Practice, 39*(2), 210–217. doi: 10.1037/0735-7028.39.2.210.

Rogers, T. L., Emanuel, K., & Bradford, J. (2002). Sexual minorities seeking services: A retrospective study of the mental health concerns of lesbian and bisexual women. *Journal of Lesbian Studies, 7*(1), 127–146. doi: 10.1300/J155v07n01_09.

Root, M. P. (1992). Reconstructing the impact of trauma on personality. In L. S. Brown & M. Ballou (Eds.), *Personality and psychopathology: Feminist reappraisals* (pp. 229–265). New York: Guilford.

Rostosky, S. S., Riggle, E. D. B., Pascale-Hague, D., & McCants, L. E. (2010). The positive aspect of a bisexual self-identification. *Psychology and Sexuality, 1*(2), 131–144. doi: 10.1080/19419899.2010.484595.

Sanchez, F. J., & Vilain, E. (2009). Collective self esteem as a coping resource for male to-female transsexuals. *Journal of Counseling Psychology, 56*(1), 202–209. http://dx.doi.org/10.1037/a0014573.

Scheer, S., Parks, C. A., McFarland, W., Page-Shafer, K., Delgado, V., Ruiz, J. D., Molitor, F., & Klausner, J. D. (2003). Self-reported sexual identity, sexual behaviors and health risks. *Journal of Lesbian Studies, 7,* 69–83.

Shelton, K., & Delgado-Romero, E. A. (2013). Sexual orientation microaggressions: The experience of lesbian, gay, bisexual, and queer clients in psychotherapy. *Psychology of Sexual Orientation and Gender Diversity, 1*(S), 59–70. doi: 10.1037/2329-0382.1.S.59.

Shipherd, J. C., Green, K., & Abramovitz, S. (2010). Transgender clients: Identifying and minimizing barriers to mental health treatment. *Journal of Gay and Lesbian Mental Health, 14*(2), 94–108. doi: 10.1080/19359701003622875.

Singh, A., Hays, D., & Watson, L. (2011). Strength in the face of adversity: Resilience strategies of transgender individuals. *Journal of Counseling and Development, 89*(1), 20–27. doi: 10.1002/j.1556-6678.2011.tb00057.x.

Skinner, W. F., & Otis, M. D. (1992). Drug use among lesbian and gay people: Findings, research design, and policy issues from the Trilogy project. In R. Kelly (Ed.), *The research symposium on alcohol and other drug problem prevention among lesbians and gay men* (pp. 34–60). Sacramento, CA: EMT Group.

Solarz, A. L. (Ed.) (1999). *Lesbian health: Current assessment and directions for the future.* Washington, DC: National Academy Press.

Stoddard, J. P., Dibble, S. L., & Fineman, N. (2009). Sexual and physical abuse: A comparison between lesbians and their heterosexual sisters. *Journal of Homosexuality, 56*(4), 407–420. doi: 10.1080/00918360902821395.

Stoltenborgh, M., van Ijzendoorn, M. H., Euser, E. M., & Bakermans-Kranenburg, M. J. (2011). A global perspective on child sexual abuse: Meta-analysis of prevalence around the world. *Child Maltreatment, 16*(2), 79–101. doi:10.1177/1077559511403920.

Szymanski, D. M., & Owens, G. P. (2009). Group-level coping as a moderator between heterosexism and sexism and psychological distress in sexual minority women. *Psychology of Women Quarterly, 33*(2), 197–205. doi: 10.1111/j.1471-6402.2009.01489.x.

Walls, N. E., Laser, J., Nickels, S. J., & Wisneski, H. (2010). Correlates of cutting behavior among sexual minority youths and young adults. *Social Work Research, 34*(4), 213–226. doi: 10.1093/swr/34.4.213.

Chapter Seven
Leveraging Integrated Health Services to Promote Behavioral Health Among Women with Disabilities

Colleen Clemency Cordes, Rebecca P. Cameron, Ethan Eisen, Alette Coble-Temple, and Linda R. Mona

According to the Centers for Disease Control and Prevention (CDC, 2016), there are currently 27 million women living with disabilities (WWD) in the United States, which represents approximately 20% of the female population (Center for Research on Women with Disabilities (CROWD), 2016). The prevalence of disability among women rises with age, at least in part as a result of increased prevalence of chronic health conditions that limit functioning (World Health Organization (WHO), 2011). Given that WWD are nearly twice as likely as their non-disabled peers to experience psychiatric concerns, such as depression, anxiety, or substance use disorders (Turner, Lloyd, & Taylor, 2006), it is critical to address the behavioral health needs of WWD across the lifespan.

Definitions of disability have evolved over recent decades, and increasingly recognize the disability experience as a multifaceted interaction of medical, social, environmental, and political factors (WHO, 2011). According to the *International Classification of Functioning, Disability, and Health,* disability is an "umbrella term" for functional limitations that result from the complex relationship between one's physical impairments and their contextual environment (WHO, 2011, p. 4). This biopsychosocial conceptualization of disability encourages a focus on improving quality of life by reducing and removing environmental, institutional, and attitudinal barriers that hinder WWDs' ability to live flourishing lives. WWDs who live with episodic and/or chronic behavioral and behavioral health concerns face the unique challenge of the intersectionality of stigma stemming from physical, cognitive, or sensory differences in addition to that of their mental/behavioral health conditions. Given the multiple layers of societal and body/mind-specific complexities faced by WWDs who live with psychological distress, it is essential that these individuals have access to services that can comprehensively address the intersections of their identity and experiences.

What does all this mean in real life for WWD? Let's consider a WWD wheelchair user who has recently given birth, is a single parent, works as an elementary school teacher with limited family leave, and relies on extended family for childcare. She incurs extensive disability-related medical expenses and high infant care costs, and barely earns enough money to cover her monthly bills. In addition, her parents live in an inaccessible house, limiting her ability to observe the set-up for her child, and this may add to the stress that she experiences adjusting to parenthood combined with work and caring for her own health, each of which is significant in isolation. Thus, the interplay of inadequate parental leave, limited access to quality childcare, financial constraints, parenting pressures, healthcare needs, and an inaccessible environment may result in greater disablement in her role as a mother, and potentially have repercussions for her functioning at work. As noted in this example, multiple specific disability factors can influence overall quality of life, coping abilities, and resilience, and each of these factors must be acknowledged and/or addressed in order to result in positive outcomes.

Integrated Behavioral Healthcare

Given the dynamic nature of the experiences that contribute to WWDs' wellbeing, it is essential that these individuals have access to services that are multifaceted, integrated, and responsive to their lived realities. Integrated behavioral healthcare (IBH) is the provision of mental and behavioral health services within the primary medical environment (most commonly, primary care), wherein interprofessional teams work collaboratively in order to meet the biopsychosocial needs of their patients (Peek, 2013). IBH is delivered on a continuum of collaboration with diverse behavioral health providers (e.g., social workers, counselors, marriage and family therapists, psychologists; Heath, Wise Romero, & Reynolds, 2013). Its roots lie in the Primary Care Medical Home (PCMH) model, originally developed specifically to promote the whole-person healthcare of children with chronic diseases and/or disabling conditions (Auxier, Miller, & Rogers, 2013). Despite its existence since the 1960s, the PCMH has only more recently become commonplace since the passage of the Patient Protection and Affordable Care Act of 2010, with 21 million patients receiving care in 114 PCMH programs in 2013 (Edwards, Bitton, Hong, & Landon, 2014).

At its core, a PCMH embodies five principles that are particularly relevant for the promotion of whole-person health, inclusive of psychological wellbeing, for WWD (Clemency Cordes, Cameron, Mona, Syme, & Coble-Temple, 2016): comprehensive care, patient-centered care, coordinated care, accessible services, and quality and safety (Agency for Healthcare Research and Quality (AHRQ), 2016). The PCMH care delivery system allows for diverse providers to work together, often through a shared medical record and treatment plan, in order to increase access to, and reduce fragmentation of healthcare services, and address the stigmatization and marginalization that have historically been commonplace for WWD (Clemency Cordes et al., 2016).

Such collaborative care has led to improved behavioral health outcomes among patients with arthritis, cancer, diabetes, heart disease, and diabetes when compared to usual primary care (Watson et al., 2013). While PCMH has primarily focused on care delivery within the primary care environment, it is important to note that IBH strategies and approaches have similarly been utilized in specialty healthcare services with positive health outcomes (Blumenthal et al., 2016). This chapter will highlight the knowledge, skills, and abilities necessary for IBH providers to address the psychosocial needs of WWD in primary care and/or the specialty care medical environment in which they are receiving treatment in order to ensure that behavioral health issues can be detected, screened, assessed, and treated at the most accessible point of care.

Addressing Behavioral Health Concerns in Primary Care

As noted above, the PCMH was born out of a need to comprehensively address the physical and behavioral health needs of children with complex physical health conditions. In its current standards surrounding the PCMH, the National Committee for Quality Assurance has expanded its focus on the need to address the behavioral and psychological needs of patients through IBH (SAMHSA-HRSA Center for Integrated Health Solutions, 2014). This shift represents an important recognition of the significant behavioral health needs of patients presenting in the medical environment. Approximately 70% of patient visits in primary care are related to psychosocial concerns (Gatchel & Oordt, 2003), and 85% of patient concerns in primary care are not a direct function of organic etiology (e.g., tension headaches, chronic non-specified pain; Kroenke & Mangelsdorff, 1989). As such, in the United States, primary care has become the *de facto* mental health system, with the majority of psychotropic medications currently being prescribed by primary care providers (Olfson, 2016), and there is an increased need to provide competent IBH services in this arena.

The nature of the behavioral health services provided in the context of IBH is at least, in part, a function of the level of integration within the clinic system (Heath et al., 2013), and can range from co-located specialty mental health services providing traditional mental health services in the context of a 50-minute clinical hour, to fully integrated services with shared cultures and service delivery mechanisms and workflows. Full integration in practice is most commonly delivered in the context of the Primary Care Behavioral Health (PCBH) model of care, where a behavioral health consultant (BHC), typically a psychologist, social worker, or licensed professional counselor, provides mental and behavioral healthcare to patients in 15- to 30-minute visits, with follow-up typically limited to one to four visits, though intermittent treatment across the lifespan is not uncommon, similar to the provision of medical services in primary care (Robinson & Reiter, 2007).

IBH providers working with WWD in this environment provide brief, problem-focused care, with an emphasis on attaining the highest level of functioning and quality of life possible, rather than symptom elimination (Robinson & Reiter, 2007). Issues addressed might include anxiety, depression, self-management of physical or mental health conditions, and coping with stress (herein referred to as "behavioral health"). Furthermore, the degree to which the mind and body interact with each other is often explored to address presenting health circumstances as well as within the context of preventive care. For WWD who require more long-term intervention, such as those related to trauma or untreated severe and persistent mental illness, BHCs assist in the facilitation of, and follow-through with, specialty mental healthcare referrals.

When IBH providers are capable of addressing the biopsychosocial needs of WWD as part of an interprofessional and collaborative team, the focus of care becomes on promoting quality of life and whole-person care, rather than on managing the collection of ailments experienced by a WWD (Clemency Cordes et al., 2016). This chapter will address the intermingling of social, physical, psychological, and environmental factors that influence the behavioral health of WWD, as well as evidence-based approaches to culturally sensitive assessment, and intervention strategies that are relevant for the BHC in the primary medical environment.

Sources of Marginalization for WWD

In order to provide high-quality care to WWD, BHCs in primary care need to be cognizant of the medical and functional aspects of patients' disabilities, as well as a number of contextual factors that affect the behavioral health of WWD across their lifespan. There are myriad ways that gender and disability status can fundamentally affect exposure to, and management of, stigma and/or problematic exclusionary societal attitudes, interpersonal relationships, access to employment, parenting experiences, and sexuality. Providers working with WWD in IBH environments need to avoid colluding with oppressive and limiting circumstances, and instead, both acknowledge these factors and assist WWD in coping with them.

WWD are at risk of negative interactions with others that range from microaggressions to outright abuse that may begin in childhood or adulthood, and that may involve unexpected perpetrators: parents and other close family members, caregivers and healthcare providers, intimate partners, peers, and strangers. We will provide an overview of the risk factors that make WWD more vulnerable to mistreatment, and discuss the prevalence of various types of mistreatment and abuse. Our goals are twofold. First, we hope to encourage IBH providers to examine their own interactions with WWD that may include subtle, but damaging, communications, and to make them more aware of the unique factors that render WWD vulnerable to mistreatment and abuse, as well as those factors that may make it difficult for WWD to challenge mistreatment or disclose abuse. Second, we recognize that these circumstances contribute to overall suffering among WWD, and it is imperative that IBH providers need to become effective partners in addressing these issues.

Microaggressions

Because the provision of healthcare is a social interaction, and often-subtle stigmatizing attitudes toward disability are pervasive in our culture, WWD risk experiencing common and problematic social interactions within healthcare encounters, and at times may encounter frank abuse at the hands of providers. In order to provide optimal care, it is helpful to understand the kinds of inter-actions that may be experienced negatively. One common form of stigmatizing experience has been labeled microaggressions, first identified and defined in relation to racial-minority group members as "the brief, commonplace, daily verbal, behavioral, and environmental indignities, whether intentional or unintentional, that communicate hostile, derogatory, or negative racial slights and insults to the target person or group" (Sue, Bucceri, Lin, Nadal, & Torino, 2007, p. 72.). When considered in relation to WWD, this type of behavior falls within the broader phenomenon of "ableism," generally meaning a worldview that privileges able-bodied perspectives, diminishes and marginalizes disability perspectives, and results in the construction of disabling and demeaning contexts for individuals with disabilities, and according preferential treatment to those without disabilities (Campbell, 2008).

Researchers have noted that, since the passage of Americans with Disabilities Act in 1990 (www.ada.gov), overt acts of discrimination against people with disabilities (PWD), consistent with abuse experiences described below, have declined (Snyder & Mitchell, 2006). Nevertheless, healthcare professionals may still carry subtle stigmatizing attitudes and engage in disability-specific offensive interactions with PWD. According to Keller and Galgay (2010), microaggressions that may be commonplace in medical settings include offer-ing, "let me do that for you" to a WWD, which may be perceived as infantilizing, or communicate the message that a WWD is not capable. Some healthcare providers may avoid eye contact with a WWD, conveying the message that WWD provoke disgust or other negative emotions, and should be avoided. Similarly, while rooming a patient, a care team member may express surprise, either verbally or non-verbally, that a WWD is partnered, and accordingly likely sexually active, thereby potentially conveying that WWD are asexual.

Regardless of whether problematic attitudes are expressed directly to the WWD, they may still impact the quality of care by the integrated team. For example, the assumption by a care team member that "everyone has some disability" reflects a minimization or denial of the disability experience, and may lead to less attention to the specific needs of the WWD. Alternatively, providers may be intrigued by, and discuss openly, aspects of a disability that are irrelevant to the care of a WWD; in this way, the WWD endures a denial of the privacy that is often afforded to non-disabled patients (Keller & Galgay, 2010). Beyond these examples, there are a number of other stigmatizing themes and messages that may be communicated explicitly or implicitly, and awareness of their ubiquity is a critical first step to healthcare providers moving beyond ableism to create safe, therapeutic interactions and relationships for WWD in medical settings.

Although it can initially be uncomfortable for healthcare providers to become more aware of their own ableist assumptions and communications, attention to these issues often leads to heightened empathy and attunement with PWD. Engaging in intentional self-assessment on disability attitudes and beliefs can ultimately translate to activism and advocacy on behalf of, and in partnership with, PWD, resulting in more effective and efficient therapeutic encounters due to enhanced rapport and greater insight into a potential source of patients' stress, anger, or alienation.

Abuse

Abuse is an all too common experience for WWD across the lifespan. In 2012, one study found that 87.2% of PWD experienced emotional abuse, 50.6% reported a history of physical abuse, 41.6% experienced sexual abuse, and 32% reported financial abuse (Baladerian, Coleman, & Stream, 2013). Researchers have identified that children with disabilities are at higher risk for abuse than their non-disabled peers (Jones et al., 2012; Stalker & McArthur, 2012), and a wide range of childhood abuse experiences predict negative behavioral health outcomes later in life (Smith & Harrell, 2013). Because, for example, there are some indications that boys with disabilities may be at greater risk of emotional, physical, and sexual abuse than girls with disabilities, it is important not to generalize from non-disabled experiences to those of PWD (Algood, Hong, Gourdine, & Williams, 2011; Sobsey, Randall, & Parrila, 1997). Factors that contribute to risk for abuse include lower believability, lack of appropriate sex education, social isolation, and failure to ensure that individuals with disabilities have a means to protect themselves from bullying in mainstreamed educational settings (Bowers-Andrews & Veronen, 1993).

Among adult WWD, intimate-partner violence (IPV) is an important concern (Curry, Hassouneh-Phillips, & Johnston-Silverberg, 2001), as research has shown that WWD have 40% greater odds of experiencing IPV than those without disability (Brownridge, 2006). Many aspects of living with a disability amplify the risk of IPV, including dependence upon personal attendants as well as self-defense and mobility limitations that may complicate access to help (Glover-Graf & Reed, 2006). It is critical to note that IPV may take different, difficult-to-recognize forms for WWD than those with which the IBH provider may be familiar, including removing or destroying a person's mobility devices, denying access to and/or taking prescribed medication from someone, forcing someone to take medication against his or her will, forcing someone to remain in soiled undergarments, preventing access to food, inappropriately touching a person while assisting with bathing and/or dressing, and denying access to disability-related resources in the community and/or to healthcare appointments (American Psychological Association, n.d.). Notably, WWD are at risk for abuse by their attendants or healthcare providers in addition to intimate partners, and the duration of the abuse is typically longer when it occurs than for non-disabled women (Young, Nosek, Howland, Champong, & Rintala, 1997). IBH providers should be aware of the increased risk of abuse among WWD, as women experiencing IPV frequently present to their healthcare providers for treatment of secondary injuries related to abuse.

WWD who experience abuse and IPV have higher rates of depression, anxiety, and posttraumatic stress disorder than able-bodied women who experience abuse and IPV, respectively (Holden, McKenzie, Pruitt, Aaron, & Hall, 2012; Swedlund & Nosek, 2000). Among WWD, a number of factors may contribute to reduced recognition of abuse by professionals or insufficient treatment, including societal barriers, physical and attitudinal barriers, isolation, and internalized oppression. Professionals with expertise in abuse may not be well versed in disability, and providers who work with PWD may not have adequate expertise in assessing and treating people dealing with abusive relationships (Williams & Colvin, 2016). Importantly, research shows that PWD who were victims of abuse do not report due to fear of retaliation, futility, and a basic lack of information (Baladerian et al., 2013).

In addition to the abuse experiences noted above, WWD may be uniquely at risk for abuse by healthcare providers, as one study documented 8.7% of WWD reporting any abuse, and 4.8% reporting sexual abuse by their providers (Young et al., 1997), and almost 25% of individuals living in nursing homes experiencing at least one incidence of abuse; for this population, limitations in activities of daily living and previous victimization were predictors of higher rates of abuse (Schiamberg et al., 2012). Despite these findings, there is a paucity of research on the overall topic of abuse by medical providers. However, given the aforementioned factors that contribute to WWDs' increased vulnerability to abuse, IBH providers are encouraged to take the necessary steps to ensure that WWD are safe in integrated care settings.

Employment

One of the important areas in which the complex interplay among disability status, gender, physical and socioemotional wellbeing, and healthcare access and experiences for WWD arises is employment status. WWD face barriers to entering the workforce, obtaining adequate employment, achieving job satisfaction, and balancing job demands with self-care, including accessing healthcare. For decades, researchers have noted that WWD face particularly challenging job prospects (Russo & Jansen, 1988), which may be at least partially attributed to accessibility barriers in educational and employment settings: rates of employment hover around 32% (Kruse, Schur, & Ali, 2010). This is critical, as employment status and job satisfaction play an essential role in an individual's overall physical and psychological health (Jin, Shah, & Svoboda, 1995; McKee-Ryan, Song, Wanberg, & Kinicki, 2005). Researchers have found that rates of unemployment are directly related to poorer health outcomes among women (Rosenthal, Carroll-Scott, Earnshaw, Santilli, & Ickovics 2012). WWD experience higher rates of long-term unemployment compared to women without disabilities, and research demonstrates a twofold increase in likelihood for depression and anxiety for unemployed WWD, as well as higher mortality rates, when compared with employed WWD (Herbig, Dragano, & Angerer, 2013).

Employment concerns may also have direct impact on the provision of IBH for WWD. For WWD who are facing unemployment or underemployment, transportation to appointments may be a significant expense, and may result in not scheduling appointments, cancelling, or no-showing. Due to the stigma surrounding an inability to pay, it is important for IBH providers to be sensitive to this possibility, and help facilitate the identification and obtainment of accessible and affordable transportation services, or to offer a sliding-scale fee structure, in order to decrease the impact of financial barriers. Conversely, for those who are sufficiently employed, there may be a reluctance to miss time at work or to appear to be prioritizing healthcare, because of concerns about appearing to have greater needs than one's co-workers, and of fear of losing one's job. This concern may lead to delaying contact with medical professionals and potentially ignoring critical medical issues. For the WWD receiving IBH services, these barriers may be addressed through the provision of services via telephone or other telehealth technologies, and the brief, focused treatment provided intermittently across the lifespan further reduces the time burden for WWD accessing treatment.

Parenting and Disability

For the IBH provider working with WWD of childbearing age, it is critical to be aware of the challenges associated with the pursuit and attainment of motherhood. WWD often meet resistance, skepticism, and discrimination from people and systems (e.g., medical and legal) regarding their ability to conceive, safely carry a fetus to term, and care for a child physically and emotionally. Historically, pregnancy and motherhood have been viewed as excessive risks for WWD or their children (Hershey, 2003; Krotoski, Nosek, & Turk, 1996; National Council on Disability (NCD), 2012; Thomas, 1997), and 11 states within the United States still have involuntary sterilization laws directed towards WWD, though these laws most commonly focus on WWD with significant psychiatric and/or intellectual disabilities (Lawrence, 2014; NCD, 2012.)

For those who decide to start a family (whether via pregnancy, surrogacy, or adoption), 37 out of 50 states, and the District of Columbia, allow disability to be grounds for termination of parental rights (NCD, 2012), and WWD are at a higher risk of having their children removed from their care solely based on their documented disability (NCD, 2012). As a result, many WWD fear that their children will be taken away from them, and/or feel that they must go to great lengths to appear to be functioning "normally" (Grue & Laerum, 2002). Similarly, a mother with a disability is twice as likely to have at least one interaction with a child welfare agency (Mingus, n.d.), and women with mental health disabilities have an 80% likelihood of having at least one encounter with Child Welfare Services before their child reaches the age of 15 (Marsh, 2009; NCD, 2012). When WWD are forced to prove their parenting ability, they are often evaluated by professionals who have no working knowledge of adaptive parenting strategies (DeVault, 2005). This leads to incorrect evaluations and increased stress for the WWD (NCD, 2012).

Despite a lack of societal support for WWD as mothers, many WWD actively pursue motherhood. A recent epidemiological survey found that 2.0% of women with chronic physical disability between the ages of 18 and 49 are pregnant during any given year, compared to 3.8% without chronic physical disability; though with increased disability severity, there is a decrease in rate of pregnancy (Iezzoni, Yu, Wint, Smeltzer, & Ecker, 2013). This suggests important considerations for those working in IBH. While communicating the additional risks some WWD may face during pregnancy is a critical role of the healthcare team, IBH providers should be cautious to not overstate such risks or unnecessarily dissuade a WWD considering pregnancy, as this reduces the decision-making autonomy of WWD.

IBH providers should be prepared to provide advocacy and education to other members of the care team regarding WWD and parenting issues, and may also benefit from familiarizing themselves with the legal concerns WWD have about parenting in order to provide appropriate guidance. Through the Looking Glass (http://www.lookingglass.org/) and the Disabled Parenting Project (http://www.disabledparenting.com/) are two nationally recognized non-profit organizations providing resources and adaptive parenting strategies for WWD (see Appendix). It is imperative to note that research demonstrates that parents with disabilities exhibit higher levels of resilience and engage in higher levels of creativity compared to parents without disabilities (Prilleltensky, 2004). Furthermore, despite WWD encountering high rates of discrimination and obstacles associated with parenting and disabilities, children being raised by WWD experience typical development and enhanced levels of functioning when compared to children being raised by non-disabled women (NCD, 2012).

Sexuality and Sexual Expression

Though most healthcare providers recognize that sexuality and sexual expression are integral facets of wellbeing, they often overlook sexual functioning among WWD (Esmail, Esmail, & Munro, 2001). Integrated healthcare teams that recognize the importance of sexuality to WWD can address barriers that exist to being able to experience optimal sexual expression.

Overall, WWD report lower levels of satisfaction with dating and relationship opportunities than non-disabled women (Nosek, Howland, Rintala, Young, & Chanpong, 2001). Studies have found that, for PWD, body and sexual esteem are related to general wellbeing (see Lease, Cohen, & Dahlbeck, 2007), as well as to physical pain or physical limitations that impede aspects of sexual expression.

A commonly used model for IBH providers who are not extensively trained in sex therapy is the PLISSIT model (permission, limited information, specific suggestions, intensive therapy; Annon, 1976), which can provide a framework for providing sexual education and counseling for WWD, and is readily adaptable for the primary care setting (see Clemency Cordes, Mona, Syme, Cameron, & Smith, 2013, for more information). IBH providers, like other healthcare providers, may have implicit ableist assumptions about what constitutes satisfying sexual expression, and what disability means for one's sexual life. Yet PWD report views of sexuality that may be more creative, expansive, and affirming than they may have experienced prior to becoming disabled (Leibowitz & Stanton, 2007).

To the extent that IBH providers are willing to consider sexual satisfaction to be an appropriate target of intervention, and to ally themselves with WWD around this, they can actively counter assumptions of asexuality, and the tendency to deny WWD full adult agency in their lives. Resources that cover comprehensive assessment and intervention around sexual concerns among WWD include Clemency Cordes et al. (2013), Mona et al., (2009), and Mona (2003), among others. Integrated care settings are ideal for addressing the interplay of biopsychosocial factors that affect sexual expression as such; IBH providers need to be familiar with these comprehensive sexual healthcare approaches in order to educate WWD about their treatment options and to instill hope.

We have briefly reviewed some of the areas of particular concern to WWD, including whether their interactions with healthcare teams will replicate the kinds of marginalizing social interactions they may experience pervasively; their vulnerability to abuse, as children, in intimate relationships, and even in health-care settings; and some of the ways that full access and participation in important adult roles are compromised for many WWD: employment, parenthood, and sexuality. These issues serve as a partial backdrop to employ a disability culture inclusive examination within initial healthcare meetings with WWD.

Assessment of WWDs' Behavioral Health in Primary Care

For psychologists working in IBH, the assessment process should take into consideration a wide range of factors, including, but not limited to, the unique and intersectional experiences that arise from being disabled and being women in the context of additional cultural identities; environmental barriers; and experiences of marginalization; as well as the assessment of behavioral health concerns (Clemency Cordes, Saxon, & Mona, 2016; Olkin, 1999). First and foremost, WWD are more than a sum of the "problem list" in their medical records, but rather see the world within the context of multiple intersecting identifies, of which disability is just one. Pamela Hays' (1996) ADDRESSING model for cultural identity can help organize one's understanding of facets of identity, and includes Age and generational influences, Developmental and acquired Disability, Religion, Social status, Sexual orientation, Indigenous heritage, National origin, and Gender.

When engaging in an assessment of WWD, IBH providers need to balance the fast-paced nature of primary care with the time-intensiveness of a culturally sensitive assessment, and as such, may choose to utilize the WWD's medical record to identify some relevant demographic information about the patient's identities (e.g., age, gender, ethnicity), while being sensitive to the fact that membership with a particular demographic group does not always ensure iden-tification with the target group (Clemency Cordes et al., 2016), and that there is considerable diversity within groups that share demographic characteristics.

Given that the goal of IBH is to improve quality of life, often in lieu of the resolution of symptoms, assessment is typically focused on a functional analy-sis of the WWD's presenting concerns. Treatment priorities can be identified in light of salient identities and social history information (e.g., quality of social relationships, vocational satisfaction, health status, and behaviors), with attention to identifying strengths and resources, specifying the problem, generating hypotheses, and then targeting new coping strategies and behaviors for WWD (Robinson & Reiter, 2007).

In addition to a focused clinical interview that includes a social history, assessment can be facilitated by the use of brief, validated screening measures appropriate to primary care. Screens such as the Patient-Health Questionnaire (PHQ-9), Generalized Anxiety Disorder-7 (GAD-7), and the Alcohol Use Disorders Identification Test (AUDIT) are frequently used to assess for depression, anxiety, and alcohol use in primary care, respectively. These tools may assist in both identifying concerns and monitoring treatment over time. However, IBH providers must be sensitive to the fact that these screens have not been specifically validated for use with WWD, and should therefore be interpreted with caution (Clemency Cordes et al., 2016). While less commonly used as standard of care in IBH primary care workflows, the Abuse Assessment Screen-Disability (AAS-D) may assist IBH providers in facilitating conversations regarding abuse and violence, which are particularly common experiences for WWD, as noted above. When using such assessments, providers should be attuned to the potential need to modify delivery format (e.g., verbally asking screening questions for the WWD who is not able to respond via paper-and-pencil survey) in order to ensure WWD are included in practice standards for screening as set forth by the IBH system.

The purpose of the assessment in IBH is to understand the WWD and her presenting concerns with attention to the biopsychosocial factors most salient in the present moment. Through brief screens and clinical interview, IBH providers should be prepared to engage both the WWD and her healthcare team in the establishment of a shared treatment plan utilizing evidence-based treatment approaches appropriately adapted to be delivered in a disability-affirmative manner.

Culturally Appropriate Treatment in Integrated Care

An important tool to assist the IBH provider in delivering culturally appropriate treatment to WWD in primary care is disability-affirmative therapy (DAT) (Olkin, 1999). This approach capitalizes on the broad, multifactor conceptualization we have been advocating, is geared toward empowerment of WWD, and is readily adapted for use with evidence-based practices for WWD in IBH environments.

Disability Affirmative Therapy

Given the complex lives of WWD, IBH treatment is likely the most appropriate approach to meet the biopsychosocial health needs of women in this community as it actively promotes collaboration among the multiple providers with whom WWD interface. As such, a starting framework in considering behavioral health treatment for WWD is DAT. DAT is a metatheoretical approach in which clinicians embrace their role as co-advocates with WWD on behalf of reducing barriers, challenging ableist assumptions, and creating enabling environments to replace disabling ones (see Olkin, 1999). Disability is seen from a social lens in which the experience of disablement is only partially a function of biological factors and health status, and largely a result of choices affecting the political, constructed, and cultural realities that privilege able-bodied modes of functioning.

The IBH provider is, therefore, someone who questions the dominant model that is culturally embedded in his or her own ways of thinking, and adopts an affirmative and empowering approach to the therapeutic relationship and to clinically indicated interventions. Thus, providers may need to flex their intervention strategies that may typically focus on individual- and family-level changes to include broader awareness of supportive resources, and bolder advocacy for systems change when needed. In some cases, this may include challenging systems-level issues in the healthcare arena which are predicated on ableist assumptions, such as the standard 15-minute patient appointment in primary care.

Evidence-Based Practices

When evidence-based (e.g., cognitive-behavioral therapy: CBT) techniques are integrated within a disability-affirmative framework, IBH providers are able both to treat the individual's psychological concerns and address social and political factors impacting her functioning (Mona et al., 2009). Culturally competent care for WWD emphasizes a collaborative approach (Clemency Cordes et al., 2016), and research has shown that CBT techniques (e.g., relaxation, mindfulness), motivational interviewing, life-skills training, psychoeducation, and multiple family-focused therapies are effective for individuals with specific disabilities (Perry & Weiss, 2005). For example, CBT has been recommended for individuals with spinal cord injury to address depression, anxiety, and adjustment-related issues (Mehta et al., 2011). Similarly, CBT and mindfulness have been found to be effective for mood and behavioral issues for women with mild to moderate intellectual disabilities (Harper, Webb, & Rayner, 2013; Hassoitis et al., 2013).

While there are proposed models and resources to assist IBH providers in addressing abuse, vocational training, and parenting for WWD, their utilization is limited and requires attention by researchers. A major issue facing IBH providers is unfamiliarity with culturally relevant resources for use in treatment with WWD. Culturally competent resources are necessary to deliver comprehensive care for WWD. For example, the Appendix to this chapter provides a list of resources for IBH providers to consider when addressing the contextual issues of abuse, employment, and parenting for WWD seeking behavioral health treatment. Facilitating healthy living for WWD means addressing multiple areas in their lives. As such, housing, transportation, personal assistance, services, public benefits, healthcare delivery systems, peer support, and competency levels of healthcare service providers are all factors that must be considered in the treatment of WWD in primary care.

Conclusions

IBH is an approach to care that has much to offer to WWD given the complexity of ways in which their identities are marginalized by condescension in the form of pity, distancing, or excessive admiration; their resourcefulness and autonomy are trivialized; and their goals, for safety and freedom from abuse, for meaningful work and financial stability, for relationship and family, for love and sexuality, are often elusive or require a commitment to living a countercultural life in order to achieve. Practically speaking, finances, transportation, and time may be in short supply given underemployment and lack of accessible transportation for WWD. Emotionally, concerns about stigma and its consequences, which include the possibility that interactions with healthcare providers may be unempathic or unsafe, can further complicate access to behavioral healthcare.

Yet WWD have significant needs for behavioral healthcare to address: self-care, stress, coping, and symptoms and syndromes of mental illness. Thus, coordinated services that allow for multiple healthcare needs to be addressed in a way that is geographically and temporally efficient; that allow for providers to work together as a team, promoting better communication about the biopsychosocial factors affecting the patient; and that provide pragmatic and advocacy-informed strategies and solutions for managing wellbeing are highly desirable.

However, IBH providers may need to become both more self-aware of their own attitudes, and better informed about the realities of living with disability, in order to effectively address excess stress and behavioral health disparities that have been documented for WWD. Conducting a culturally sensitive assessment that is adequately comprehensive requires fluency in disability experiences, just as adapting empirically supported treatment strategies to become explicitly disability-affirmative requires commitment to being a clinician, educator, and advocate for WWD.

We recommend that IBH providers continue to read about disability experiences and DAT, and continue to develop self-awareness regarding personal disability attitudes, and how they mirror cultural norms and intersect with attitudes about gender and other identities to perpetuate disablement. Disrupting assumptions by, for example, learning about the creativity and resilience of WWD can promote greater therapeutic range in clinical work with other marginalized groups as well.

References

Agency for Healthcare Research and Quality. (2016). *Defining the PCMH*. Retrieved from: https://pcmh.ahrq.gov/page/defining-pcmh (accessed November 4, 2016).

Algood, C. L., Hong, J. S., Gourdine, R. M., & Williams, A. B. (2011). Maltreatment of children with developmental disabilities: An ecological systems analysis. *Children and Youth Services Review, 33*, 1142–1148.

American Psychological Association (n.d.) *Abuse of women with disabilities: Facts and resources.* Retrieved from: http://www.apa.org/topics/violence/women-disabilities.pdf

Annon, C. J. (1976). The PLISSIT model: A proposed conceptual scheme for the behavioral treatment of sexual problems. *Journal of Sex Education and Therapy, 2*, 1–15.

Auxier, A. M., Miller, B. F., & Rogers, J. (2013). Integrated behavioral health and the patient-centered medical home. In M. R. Talen & A. B. Valeras (Eds.), *Integrated behavioral health in primary care: Evaluating the evidence, identifying the essentials* (pp. 33–52). New York: Springer.

Baladerian, N., Coleman, T. F., & Stream, J. (2013). *Abuse of people with disabilities: Victims and their families speak out: A report on the 2012 National Survey on Abuse of People with Disabilities.* Retrieved from: http://disabilityandabuse.org/survey/index.htm (accessed November 21, 2016).

Blumenthal, J. A., Sherwood, A., Smith, P. J., Watkins, L., Mabe, S., Kraus, W. E., & Hinderliter, A. (2016). Enhancing cardiac rehabilitation with stress management training: A randomized, clinical efficiency trial. *Circulation, 133*, 1341–1350.

Bowers-Andrews, A., & Veronen, L. J. (1993). Sexual assault and people with disabilities. *Journal of Social Work and Human Sexuality, 8*(2), 137–159.

Brownridge, D. A. (2006). Partner violence against women with disabilities: Prevalence, risk, and explanations. *Violence Against Women, 12*, 805–822.

Campbell, F. A. K. (2008). Exploring internalized ableism using critical race theory. *Disability and Society, 23*(2), 151–162. doi: 10.1080/09687590701841190.

Center for Research on Women with Disabilities (2016). *Demographics*. Retrieved from: https://www.bcm.edu/research/centers/research-on-women-with-disabilities/general-info/demographics (accessed November 4, 2016).

Centers for Disease Control and Prevention. (2016). *Women with disabilities*. Retrieved from: http://www.cdc.gov/ncbddd/disabilityandhealth/women.html (accessed November 4, 2016).

Clemency Cordes, C., Cameron, R. P., Mona, L. R., Syme, M. L., & Coble-Temple, A. (2016). Perspectives on disability within integrated healthcare. In L. Suzuki, M. Casas, C. Alexander, & M. Jackson (Eds.), *Handbook of multicultural counseling* (4th ed., pp. 401–410). Thousand Oaks, CA: Sage Publications.

Clemency Cordes, C., Mona, L. R., Syme, M. L., Cameron, R. P., & Smith, K. (2013). Sexuality and sexual health among women with physical disabilities. In D. Castaneda (Ed), *An essential handbook of women's sexuality: Diversity, health, and violence introduction* (Vol. 2, pp. 71–92). Santa Barbara, CA: Praeger.

Clemency Cordes, C., Saxon, L. C., & Mona, L. R. (2016). Women veterans with disabilities: An integrated care perspective. In S. Miles-Cohen & C. Signore (Eds.), *Eliminating inequities for women with disabilities: An agenda for health and wellness.* Washington, DC: American Psychological Association.

Curry, M. A., Hassouneh-Phillips, D., & Johnston-Silverberg, A. (2001). Abuse of women with disabilities: An ecological model and review. *Violence Against Women, 7*(1), 60–79.

DeVault, E. N. (2005). "Reasonable efforts not so reasonable": The termination of the parental rights of a developmentally disabled mother. *Roger Williams University Law Review, 10*, 764.

Edwards, S. T., Bitton, A., Hong, J., & Landon, B. E. (2014). Patient-centered medical home initiatives expanded in 2009–2013: Providers, patients, and payment incentives increased. *Health Affairs, 33*, 1823–1831.

Esmail, S., Esmail, Y., & Munro, B. (2001). Sexuality and disability: The role of health care professionals in providing options and alternatives for couples. *Sexuality and Disability, 19*, 267–282.

134 • C.C. Cordes et al.

Gatchel, R. J., & Oordt, M. S. (2003). *Clinical health psychology and primary care: Practical advice and clinical guidance for successful collaboration.* Washington, DC: American Psychological Association.

Glover-Graf, N. M., & Reed, B. J. (2006). Abuse against women with disabilities. *Rehabilitation Education, 20*(1), 43–56.

Grue, L., & Lærum, K. T. (2002). 'Doing motherhood': Some experiences of mothers with physical disabilities. *Disability and Society, 17,* 671–683.

Harper, S., Webb, T., & Rayner, K. (2013). The effectiveness of mindfulness-based interventions for supporting people with intellectual disabilities: A narrative review. *Behavior Modification, 37,* 431–453.

Hassoitis, A., Serfaty, M., Azam, K., Strydom, A., Blizard, R., Romeo, R., & King, M. (2013). Manualised individual cognitive behavioural therapy for mood disorders in people with mild to moderate intellectual disability: A feasibility randomized controlled trial. *Journal of Affective Disorders, 151,* 186–195.

Hays, P. A. (1996). Addressing the complexities of culture and gender in counseling. *Journal of Counseling and Development, 74,* 332–338.

Heath, B., Wise Romero, P., & Reynolds, K. A. (2013). *A standard framework for levels of integrated healthcare.* Washington, DC: SAMHSA-HRSA Center for Integrated Health Solutions.

Herbig, B., Dragano, N., & Angerer, P., (2013). Health in the long-term unemployed. *Deutsch Arztebl International, 110*(23–24), 413–419.

Hershey, L. (November 26, 2003). *Disabled woman's lawsuit exposes prejudices.* Retrieved December 8, 2014, from http://www.raggededgemagazine.com/extra/hersheychamberstrial. html (accessed November 4, 2016).

Holden, K. B., McKenzie, R., Pruitt, M. V., Aaron, M. K., & Hall, M. S. (2012). Depressive symptoms, substance abuse, and intimate partner violence among pregnant women of diverse ethnicities. *Journal of Health Care for the Poor and Underserved, 23*(1), 226.

Iezzoni, L. I., Yu, J., Wint, A. J., Smeltzer, S. C., & Ecker, J. L. (2013). Prevalence of current pregnancy among US women with and without chronic physical disabilities. *Medical Care, 51,* 555.

Jin, R. L., Shah, C. P., & Svoboda, T. J. (1995). The impact of unemployment on health: A review of the evidence. *Canadian Medical Association Journal, 153*(5), 529–540.

Jones, L., Bellis, M. A., Wood, S., Hughes, K., McCoy, E., Eckley, L., . . . & Officer, A. (2012). Prevalence and risk of violence against children with disabilities: A systematic review and meta-analysis of observational studies. *The Lancet, 380,* 899–907.

Keller, R. M., & Galgay, C. E. (2010). Microaggressive experiences of people with disabilities. In D. W. Sue (Ed.), *Microaggressions and marginality: Manifestation, dynamics, and impact* (pp. 241–268). Hoboken, NJ: John Wiley.

Kroenke, K., & Mangelsdorff, A. (1989). Common symptoms in primary care: Incidence, evaluation, therapy and outcome. *American Journal of Medicine, 86,* 262–266.

Krotoski, D. M., Nosek, M. A., & Turk, M. A. (1996). *Women with physical disabilities: Achieving and maintaining health and well-being.* Baltimore, MD: Paul H. Brookes.

Kruse, D., Schur, L., & Ali, M. (2010). Disability and occupational projections. *Monthly Labor Review,* Retrieved from http://www.jstor.org/stable/monthlylaborrev.2010.10.031 (accessed November 4, 2016).

Lawrence, M. (2014). *Reproductive rights and state institutions: The forced sterilization of minority women in the United States* (Senior Thesis). Retrieved from http://digitalrepository.trincoll. edu/theses/390 (accessed May 18, 2016).

Lease, S. H., Cohen, J. E., & Dahlbeck, D. T. (2007). Body and sexual esteem as mediators of the physical disability–interpersonal competencies relation. *Rehabilitation Psychology, 52,* 399–408.

Leibowitz, R. Q., & Stanton, A. L. (2007). Sexuality after spinal cord injury: A conceptual model based on women's narratives. *Rehabilitation Psychology, 52,* 44–55.

McKee-Ryan, F., Song, Z., Wanberg, C. R., & Kinicki, A. J. (2005). Psychological and physical well-being during unemployment: A meta-analytic study. *Journal of Applied Psychology, 90*(1), 53–76.

Marsh, D. T. (2009). Parental mental illness: Issues in custody determination. *American Journal of Family Law, 23*(1), 29.

Mehta, S., Orenczuk, S., Hansen, K., Aubut, J., Hitzig, S., Legassic M., & Spinal Cord Injury Rehabilitation Evidence Research Team. (2011). An evidence-based review of the effectiveness of cognitive behavioral therapy for psychosocial issues post-spinal cord injury. *Rehabilitation Psychology, 56,* 15–25.

Mingus, M. (n.d.). *Disabled women and reproductive justice*. Retrieved from http://protectchoice.org/article.php?id=140 (accessed February 23, 2014).

Mona, L. R. (2003). Sexual options for people with disabilities: Using personal assistance services for sexual expression. In M. E. Banks and E. Kaschak (Eds.), *Women with visible and invisible disabilities: Multiple intersections, multiple issues, multiple therapies* (pp. 211–222). Gloucestershire, UK: Hawthorn Press.

Mona, L. R., Cameron, R. P., Goldwaser, G., Miller, A. R., Syme, M. L., & Fraley, S. S. (2009). Prescription for pleasure: Exploring sex-positive approaches in women with spinal cord injury. *Topics in Spinal Cord Injury and Rehabilitation, 15*, 15–28.

National Council on Disability (NCD). (September 27, 2012). *Rocking the cradle: Ensuring the rights of parents with disabilities and their children*. Washington, DC: National Council on Disability.

Nosek, M. A., Howland, C., Rintala, D. H., Young, M. E., & Chanpong, G. F. (2001). National study of women with physical disabilities: Final report. *Sexuality and Disability, 19*, 5–39.

Olfson, M. (2016). The rise of primary care physicians in provision of US mental health care. *Journal of Health Politics, Policy, and Law, 28*, epub ahead of print.

Olkin, R. (1999). *What psychotherapists should know about disability*. New York: Guilford Press.

Peek, C. J. (2013). Integrated behavioral health and primary care: A common language. In M. R. Talen & A. B. Valeras (Eds.), *Integrated behavioral health in primary care: Evaluating the evidence, identifying the essentials* (pp. 9–31). New York: Springer.

Perry, A., & Weiss, J. (2005). Evidence-based practice in developmental disabilities: What is it and why does it matter? *Journal of Developmental Disabilities, 13*, 167–171.

Prilleltensky, O. (2004). My child is not my carer: Mothers with physical disabilities and the well-being of children. *Disability and Society 19*(3), 210.

Robinson, P. J., & Reiter, J. T. (2007). *Behavioral consultation and primary care: A guide to integrating services*. New York: Springer.

Rosenthal, L., Carroll-Scott, A., Earnshaw, V. A., Santilli, A., & Ickovics, J. R. (2012). The importance of full-time work for urban adults' mental and physical health. *Social Science Medicine, 75*(9), 1692–1696.

Russo, N., & Jansen, M. (1988). Women, work, and disability: Opportunities and challenges. In M. Fine & A. Asch (Eds.), *Women with disabilities: Essays in psychology, culture, and politics* (pp. 229–244). Philadelphia, PA: Temple University Press.

SAMHSA-HRSA Center for Integrated Health Solutions. (2014). *Advancing behavioral health integration within NCQA recognized patient-centered medical homes*. Washington, DC: National Council for Behavioral Health.

Schiamberg, L. B., Oehmke, J., Zhang, Z., Barboza, G. E., Griffore, R. J., Von Heydrich, L., & Mastin, T. (2012). Physical abuse of older adults in nursing homes: A random survey of adults with an elderly family member in a nursing home. *Journal of Elder Abuse and Neglect, 24*(1), 65–83.

Smith, N., & Harrell, S. (2013). *Sexual abuse of children with disabilities: A national snapshot*. New York: Vera Institute of Justice.

Snyder, S., & Mitchell, D. (2006). Eugenics and the racial genome: Politics at the molecular level. *Patterns of Prejudice, 40(4r-3)*, 399–412.

Sobsey, D., Randall, W., & Parrila, R. K. (1997). Gender differences in abused children with and without disabilities. *Child Abuse and Neglect, 21*, 707–720.

Stalker, K., & McArthur, K. (2012). Child abuse, child protection and disabled children: A review of recent research. *Child Abuse Review, 21*(1), 24–40.

Sue, D. W., Bucceri, J. M., Lin, A., Nadal, K. L., & Torino, G. C. (2007). Racial microaggressions and the Asian American experience. *Cultural Diversity and Ethnic Minority Psychology, 13*(1), 72–81.

Swedlund, N. P., & Nosek, M. A. (2000). An exploratory study on the work of independent living centers to address abuse of women with disabilities. *Journal of Rehabilitation, 66*(4), 57–64.

Thomas, C. (1997). The baby and the bath water: Disabled women and motherhood in social context. *Sociology of Health and Illness, 19*, 622–643.

Turner, R. J., Lloyd, D. A., & Taylor, J. (2006). Physical disability and mental health: An epidemiology of psychiatric and substance disorders. *Rehabilitation Psychology, 51*, 214–223.

Watson, L. C., Amick, H. R., Gaynes, B. N., Brownley, K. A., Thaker, S., Viswanathan, M., & Jonas, D. E. (2013). Practice-based interventions addressing concomitant depression and chronic medical conditions in the primary care setting: A systematic review and meta-analysis. *Journal of Primary Care and Community Health, 4*, 294–306.

Williams, J., & Colvin, L. (2016). Coming together to end violence against women and girls with disabilities. In S. E. Miles-Cohen and C. Signore (Eds.), *Eliminating inequities for women with disabilities: An agenda for health and wellness*. Washington, DC: American Psychological Association.

World Health Organization. (2011). *World report on disability*. Geneva, Switzerland: Author.

Young, M. E., Nosek, M. A., Howland, C., Chanpong, G., & Rintala, D. H. (1997). Prevalence of abuse of women with physical disabilities. *Archives of Physical Medicine and Rehabilitation, 78*(12), S34–S38.

Appendix

Abuse and Treatment for WWD

American Psychological Association

http://apa.org/topics/violence/women-disabilities.aspx
Offers fact sheets and current best practices for clinicians when assessing and providing treatment related to abuse for WWD.

Center for Research on Women with Disabilities (CROWD) at Baylor College of Medicine

https://www.bcm.edu/research/centers/research-on-women-with-disabilities/topics/violence
Current comprehensive research and recommended screening and intervention tools for healthcare providers.

Oak Hill's Center for Relationship and Sexuality Education

http://www.oakhillcrse.org/provider-resources/index.asp
A comprehensive curriculum addressing sexuality, sexual health, healthy relationships, safe boundaries, and breast health for women with intellectual and developmental disabilities across the lifespan.

Vocational Coaching and Treatment

Department of Vocational Rehabilitation (VR)

VR is a nationwide federal–state program for assisting eligible people with disabilities to define a suitable employment goal and become employed. Each state capital has a central VR agency, and there are local offices in most states. VR provides medical, therapeutic, counseling, education, training, and other services needed to prepare people with disabilities for work. VR is an excellent place for a youth or adult with a disability to begin exploring available training and support service options.

To identify the VR office in your vicinity, consult your local telephone directory or visit: http://askjan.org/cgi-win/TypeQuery.exe?902.

JobAccess and ABILITYJobs

http://abilityjobs.com/

The goal of JobAccess and ABILITYJobs is to enable people with disabilities to enhance their professional lives by providing a dedicated system for finding employment. By posting job opportunities, or searching resumes, employers can find qualified persons with disabilities as well as demonstrate their affirmative action and open-door policies.

Job Accommodation Network (JAN)

Tel: +1-800-526-7234 (voice); +1-877-781-9403 (TTY)

Spanish spoken; Spanish materials available http://askjan.org/

JAN is the leading source of free, expert, and confidential guidance on workplace accommodations and disability employment issues. Working toward practical solutions that benefit both employer and employee, JAN helps people with disabilities enhance their employability, and shows employers how to capitalize on the value and talent that people with disabilities add to the workplace.

National Center on Workforce and Disability/Adult (NCWD)

http://www.onestops.info/

NCWD provides training, technical assistance, policy analysis, and information to improve access for all in the workforce development system. Areas of expertise include accommodations and assistive technology, relationships with employers, helping clients with disabilities find jobs, and advising employers as to how to provide job-related supports.

Office of Disability Employment Policy (ODEP)

U.S. Department of Labor

Tel: +1-866-633-7365 (voice); +1-877-889-5627 (TTY) www.dol.gov/odep

ODEP provides national leadership on disability employment policy by developing and influencing the use of evidence-based disability employment policies and practices, building collaborative partnerships, and delivering authoritative and credible data on employment of people with disabilities. Find a wealth of employment-related information on ODEP's website.

WorkSupport

http://worksupport.com/index.cfm

WorkSupport is a web portal that highlights the funded projects of Virginia Commonwealth University on many topics related to the employment of individuals with disabilities. This includes the Rehabilitation Research and Training Center on Employment of People with Physical Disabilities, Autism Center for Excellence, School 2 Work, and the Center on Transition to Employment for Youth with Disabilities.

Parenting with a Disability

Disabled Parenting Project

http://www.disabledparenting.com/
The Disabled Parenting Project launched in 2016 to provide people with disabilities firsthand practical knowledge related to reproductive healthcare, pregnancy, and parenting with a disability. This online community provides parents and prospective parents with disabilities a space to share experiences, advice, and conversations about parenting with a disability. It also serves to disseminate scholarly research, fact sheets, and training resources to both professionals and the public community about successful parenting with a disability.

Know Your Rights Toolkit

http://ncd.gov/sites/default/files/Documents/Final%20508_Parenting%20 Toolkit_Standard_0.pdf
The National Council on Disability and the Christopher and Dana Reeve Foundation published the Know Your Rights Toolkit in April 2016. It provides parents with disabilities a comprehensive review of the barriers and facilitators people with diverse disabilities experience when exercising their fundamental right to create and maintain families. The toolkit analyzes how US disability law and policy apply to parents with disabilities in the child welfare and family law systems.

Rocking the Cradle: Ensuring the Rights of Parents with Disabilities and Their Children

http://ncd.gov/sites/default/files/Documents/NCD_Parenting_508_0.pdf
The National Council on Disability's 2012 publication provides a comprehensive overview of the current state of knowledge, attitudes, and practices towards parents with disabilities and their children. The research includes a legal analysis of disability laws and their implications for parents and prospective parents with disabilities, and a review of federal and state legislation concerning child welfare, family law, and adoption as it relates to parents with disabilities.

Through the Looking Glass (TLG)

http://www.lookingglass.org/

Tel: +1-800-644-2666 (voice); +1-510-848-1005 (TTY)

TLG, in Berkeley, California, is the leading national agency for research, training, and services for families with disabilities. TLG provides comprehensive training for mental health and developmental practitioners regarding parents with all disabilities and their children. TLG's research documents strengths of parents with disabilities and their families, the environmental/ social obstacles faced, and the impact of disability-appropriate parenting resources, such as babycare adaptive equipment for parents with physical disabilities, or adaptations in intervention for parents with cognitive disabilities.

Chapter Eight
Women in the Military

Jackie Hammelman

Being a woman in the military is a unique professional experience. It is difficult to determine the influence of gender in this culture on things such as mental health and well-being as this is an underattended area of research. According to recent surveys, women are a small minority in the military. Depending on their job and unit, a female service member may find herself as the only woman in her environment. Imagine the daily experience of going to work with the absence of contact of another woman. What influence may this have on one's sense of self and sense of belonging in the community?

As you read this chapter, keep this in the forefront of your mind and consider the implications the military culture has on identity and mental health diagnoses we are observing in our servicewomen. My Military Occupational Specialty (MOS) is a 73B (Clinical Psychologist) in the U.S. Army. I help comprise the 2.9% of women who hold the position of a female officer. Part of my job is being responsible for the mental health of a Brigade size element of airborne infantry soldiers (approximately 4,500 paratroopers). There are support MOS positions (i.e., medics, linguistics, military police) that include women, but my entire patient caseload continues to be comprised of men. My day-to-day responsibilities include standard assessment, diagnosis, and treatment of common behavioral health diagnoses as part of a multidisciplinary team. In addition, I conduct evaluations pertaining to medical fitness for continued military service and specialty duties. The different roles are important to highlight because they significantly contribute to the motivation of soldiers seeking behavioral health care and what is or is not openly discussed and thus addressed in treatment.

As a woman in the military, I am often at a disadvantage. I've had Commanders disregard my professional recommendations because I am a female medical officer. Depending on where one practices, the Commander and unit make it known that women are still not accepted. Nor is there movement in the military to accept women as equals. The military is a microcosm of the larger population, but is, perhaps, a more stereotypically male version of it. My gender dictates how I am viewed, my career progression, and so many other facets of my time in the military. This is a shared experience of women in the service, and an important stage to acknowledge and give its due respect when conceptualizing pathology. I am excited for the shift that will transpire when this is not as apparent for my fellow servicewomen. Today, however, this is still a very present force in our professional lives. It impacts how we define ourselves. And I argue that it is an impetus to clinical symptoms that are developed in response to such challenges.

Many of the resources that I utilized for this chapter are specific to women in the Army, as the majority of those I consulted are Army providers and researchers. I am aware of the vast differences across military branches, and between the enlisted and officer ranks. Thus, I want to acknowledge that my experience is even further representative of a minority group. The cultural diversity in the military is immense, and I caution the reader please not to consume my words as overgeneralizations.

You may find the chapter heavy in numbers in the attempt to paint a more accurate picture of the experience of women in the service. For those of you with minimal to no contact with the military culture, it has its own separate language, heavy in acronyms that I will also use and define through the chapter to give the reader some experience that even how we communicate is fundamentally different.

I want to thank you for taking the time to read what I have written, and your interest in the mental health of female service members. More so, I want to thank my fellow servicewomen, my sisters in arms, who walk in a world where we are not yet equal, and where the conversation about us is still an unspoken one.

Women in the Military: A Brief History

A rather progressive male Company Commander of an Infantry Stryker Brigade recently said to me, "Women in the military? We have those?" He meant it as a joke. But his attempt at humor revealed even his unease regarding the place of women in service, and more so for women in combat. My response was, "Yes, in fact, we do." Women have served their country alongside their military husbands dating back to 1775, most commonly as nurses or cooks, with the authorization of a Commander.

It was not until 1901 that women were allowed to join the military, when the Army Nurse Corps was established. Prior to that, women's involvement was restricted to volunteer status. In 1948, Congress passed the Women's Armed Services Integration Act, allowing permanent military status and entitlement to veteran benefits. The most recent act of integration came at the conclusion of 2015 when Defense Secretary, Ashton B. Carter, opened combat-specific jobs to female service members.

Those changes sounded more like a movement towards more equality. But what does this decision mean? For many, it is a challenge to a long-standing order of *brotherhood*. For others, it is concern for the safety of men and women in units that will now have to integrate without clear instruction as to how to carry this out. The impact this will have on mission readiness is not known. Nor is the impact it will have on the mental health of women who are part of this cultural shift.

The Demographics of Women in the Military

The total number of people in the U.S. military (including guard, reserve, retired, and civilians) is just over 3.5 million according to the Department of Defense's (DoD's) demographics report for fiscal year 2014 (Office of the Deputy Assistant Secretary of Defense, 2014). The total active duty strength, however, is 1,326,273. Women comprise 15.1% (200,692) of the total force, and the ratio of female enlisted (161,415) to female officers (39,277) is 4:1. The makeup of the remaining active force is male enlisted (929,524) and male officers (196,057).

These numbers are important, because they shed light on how small the society is—approximately equal to the population of Maine. The society of men is comparable to the state of Delaware, while the female population is near the population of Samoa. Of note, no U.S. state population is low enough to use as comparison group for the female force.

Men and women in the military are young, with nearly half of enlisted members 25 years of age or younger, and a quarter of officers are 41 years or older. There is the absence of higher education, with only 7% of enlisted members having a Bachelor's degree or higher. Over half are married (55.3%), and less than one-third identify themselves as a minority. When one looks closer at the rank structure, individuals who are in positions of the highest authority to facilitate policy change (O7–O10), there are only 65 women compared to 853 men. The discrepancy is not much different on the enlisted side of the house, with opportunities for positions of leadership as senior non-commissioned officers, or NCOs (E7-E9)—females make up only 12.3% of the ranks.

Rates of Mental Health Diagnoses for Women in the Military

General rates of mental health diagnoses specific to women in the service to this date are not well researched or documented. In a 2014 joint study between the U.S. Army and U.S. National Institute of Mental Health (aka the STARRS Report) examining rates of mental health diagnoses in *all* soldiers, the rate of major depression was five times higher, intermittent explosive disorder was six times higher, and posttraumatic stress disorder (PTSD) was nearly 15 times higher when compared to a civilian population (Kessler et al., 2014). Servicewomen had significantly elevated odds of any internalizing disorder (1.5 times higher), and higher rates of major depressive disorder, general anxiety disorder, and PTSD.

Substance Abuse

The STARRS Report also identified that, among those with a reported diagnosis, approximately 85% reported mental health problems *prior* to their time in service. And some diagnoses (i.e., substance-related diagnoses) had an earlier onset when compared to civilians. This is a familiar story I have experienced with many of my patients. It is not uncommon for them to report extensive and complicated histories of childhood trauma, which are further complicated by their experiences while in the service. At any given time approximately half of my patients have a current problem or a history positive for alcohol or substance abuse. Many have also received treatment through the Army Substance Abuse Program (ASAP), or a civilian inpatient dual-diagnosis facility. This is not surprising, given soldiers who make it to the Embedded Behavioral Health (EBH) clinic for treatment tend to be representative of soldiers who are more distressed, and often come by the request of a spouse or their chain of command.

What contributes to this? We anticipate some experimentation with substances with the college-aged population, but this behavior transpires in a context. Social expectations also have a significant impact on soldiers' behaviors. The military culture historically has encouraged the consumption of alcohol. The press to engage in this behavior can still be observed during mandatory events, such as a "dining in," where an open bar is frequently present. Being a non-drinker makes a soldier the statistical anomaly. This culturally expected behavior has implications for the development or exacerbation of pre-existing substance use disorders. Furthermore, multiple places in the environment make purchasing alcohol easy and affordable (i.e., gas stations, Post Exchange (PX), Commissary, and the Class VI). Such storefronts are similar to wholesale markets in the civilian community (i.e., Sam's Club or Costco). The PX and Commissary, for instance, offer reduced-price food items to include alcohol, and each military installation has at least one of these facilities. In particular, there is also a "Class VI" which in military terms represents "personal demand items," specifically to include alcohol; these may essentially be conceptualized as liquor stores on military installations. As a behavioral health provider, the combination is worrisome, as we have service members with intensely stressful jobs who can too easily utilize alcohol and substances to cope with the demands of the profession. This creates an environment where judgment is impaired, and individuals are victimized. Unfortunately, many of those victims are our servicewomen.

Mental Health Disorders

While in the deployed environment the Army Mental Health Advisory Team (MHAT) examines factors that influence the mental health and well-being of our soldiers. The most recent version, MHAT-9, was conducted in 2013 in Afghanistan in support of Operation Enduring Freedom (OEF) (Office of the Surgeon General United States Army Medical Command and Office of the Command Surgeon Headquarters, U.S. Army Central Command (USCENTCOM) and Office of the Command Surgeon U.S. Forces Afghanistan (USFOR-A), 2013). Compared to previous years, rates of soldiers meeting criteria for acute stress, depression, or anxiety, and all diagnoses were significantly lower than observed in 2012, and comparable to rates in 2009. These researchers highlighted that levels of stigma related to seeking behavioral health care remained stable, but perceptions related to barriers to treatment steadily improved compared to 2009. Of note, the sample was composed of maneuver platoons of Army Brigade Combat Teams (BCTs), and statistics related to women were not incorporated into the analysis. The assessment of women in the deployed environment is required to better understand how they respond, if any differently, to the same environment as our male counterparts. If we generalize these findings to female service members who will soon be assigned combat jobs and deploy, stigma is definitely an immensely strong cultural barrier to care.

Stigma in Seeking Care

I have the discussion of impact of stigma with all of my patients. Most soldiers openly admit to not coming to the EBH clinic sooner, when their situation was more manageable, given fear of how they would have been seen by their peers or Commanders. Soldiers freely identify how they do not report symptoms out of fear of being removed from their job, or the negative impact this may have on future career stability or progression. Being viewed as "weak" or "crazy" again discourages both men and women from receiving the care they require for difficulties in a manner that is not comparable to civilian counterparts.

The fear of separation from the unit or social ostracization is very real, and understandably dictates behavior until soldiers can no longer successfully cope on their own. The impact of stigma is constantly discussed in leadership meetings, as we understand that is a significant risk factor for the sustainment and progression of behavioral health symptoms for all service members. Regardless of the attempts of leadership, some of the fear and stigma is founded, and soldiers will be excluded from certain instructor positions or "positions of trust," depending on their pathology, levels of security clearance, or even flight status. The culture of "suck it up" or "rub dirt on it" is not doing clinical justice for our daughters, mothers, sons, or fathers in uniform. I do want to stress that service members are some of the most resilient human beings I have encountered. But that true resilience is observed in those who seek out care, and that bravery lies in the act of asking for guidance as opposed to continued suffering.

Rates of Mental Health Disorders

A study conducted by Wells and colleagues (2010) examined depression in deployed men and women. As anticipated, those exposed to combat had the highest rates when compared to a sample of non-deployed service members. Women had an odds ratio of 2.13, while the men's ratio was 1.32. The difference in rates was not elaborated on, and may reflect a pattern of help-seeking behavior, provider's propensity to diagnose mood disorders, or a variety of other factors. Considering this, clinical providers may need to be prepared to expect more women in aide stations, or the EBH, presenting with possible depression as combat roles are filled by servicewomen in the upcoming years. Civilian providers who treat active duty or veterans off-post should also be informed of such trends to inform which evidence-based treatments they will employ with these patients.

Wojcik and colleagues in 2009 examined psychiatric hospitalization of soldiers when deployed to Iraq and Afghanistan. The most common clinical presentations were related to negative alterations in mood, adjustment difficulties, anxiety, and substance abuse. Their research showed that female enlisted soldiers had significantly greater risk for hospitalization in Operation Iraqi Freedom (OIF) and OEF compared to their male and non-enlisted counterparts. The risk was 1.6 to 3.0 and 2.0 to 6.0 respectively. Younger women also had the highest incident of attempted suicide and self-inflicted injuries.

Suicide

Other research (Rundell, 2006) also identified that OEF/OIF psychiatric evacuees were more likely to be female. Hospitalization and evacuation are costly not only to the individual but also to the mission. If that solider is specialized, she may very well be the only individual in her unit that is able to carry out a specific duty, such as operating an unmanned aircraft (UAV), which has the potential to cripple a mission. Depending on the MOS of the solider, attempted suicide may stop her career, and she is no longer permitted to carry out her duties. This has long-term implications outside of her situational level of distress that contributed to the suicide attempt or self-harm behavior. After such an event, service members find themselves evacuated to an inpatient hospital where they also undergo an evaluation for medical fitness, and may be considered for reclassification, or separation from the service, due to a disqualifying behavioral health condition. These young women now face transition into a civilian world, where they may not have received comprehensive treatment for the difficulties that led up to the attempt or self-injurious behavior.

As a provider, I have witnessed this with very different outcomes where women have, or have not, received care depending on the Command climate. For instance, I encountered a new solider in her 20s who attempted suicide by overdose in response to information that her husband was pursuing a divorce. She was found by a Battle Buddy (trusted peer soldier) when she was not present for morning formation. It was decided that she would remain in the United States as part of the rear detachment of her Company when they deployed, but this was an environment without friends or support. Her clinical presentation decompensated with her attributing symptoms to the new isolation in conjunction with personal relationship problems. The solider not only communicated an immense sense of guilt and shame for her actions related to her attempt, but also to the impact that she had on her fellow soldiers, and failure to carry out the mission.

This response is often heavy with a sense of a burden: the failure to be there for fellow soldiers. The impact that she has "failed" others, and the guilt of leaving others behind to do more work, far supersedes even the guilt related to almost taking her life. Approximately one month later, she was sexually assaulted by another solider and this resulted in a future suicide attempt and second hospitalization. Her care was discontinued, as she was administratively separated under Uniform Code of Military Justice (UCMJ) action related to other behavior. She was provided with services available to her in the community, and therapeutic intervention with me was terminated, as the system does not allow for treatment to continue after separation. What happens to these servicemen and women after separation is not known. If these individuals do not receive services from the Veterans Affairs, information pertaining to aspects of diagnosis, treatment, and outcome is not formally assessed and chronic difficulties related to mental health symptoms remain unknown.

Over the past few years, suicide both in the veteran and active-duty population has received more specific attention along with funding to better assess and increase prevention efforts. We have observed that suicide rates are higher in the active-duty military population compared to civilians. The DoD releases an annual report related to suicide events, called the DoDSER, and includes both attempts that result in hospitalization, and death by suicide declared by the armed forces medical examiner. The most recent report prepared by the National Center for Telehealth and Technology (T2) identified that the suicide rate per 100,000 service members was 18.7, with differential rates across branches (Marine 23.1, Army 23.0, Air Force 14.4, and Navy 13.4) (Smolenski et al., 2013). In comparison, according to the American Foundation for Suicide Prevention (2016), the rate of suicide in the United States is 12.93 per 100,000. For those service members who died by suicide, the most common diagnoses were mood and adjustment disorders. For suicide attempts, the most common diagnoses were mood and anxiety disorders. Regarding gender differences, 15 women and 244 men were included in the report.

Death and Dying

Death and dying are arguably the more difficult existential issues we all face. Culturally, service members are exposed to higher rates of both. The society is unique in that part of the innate job requirement is to place oneself in positions of danger where life may be jeopardized. This has an impact, regardless of how much training they do. To place this into perspective, at any given time, over half of my caseload is related to patients presenting with bereavement-related difficulties, and approximately half of those are death as the result of suicide. Research shows that loss of a close family member or other significant inter-personal relationship to suicide places individuals at increased risk for harm to themselves. This is a culturally magnified risk factor and demands more spe-cific treatment. I use strong language on this issue as currently there are no organizational programs that have been standardized to offer as treatment for these men and women. Where I currently practice, there is not even a single process-oriented group for loss or bereavement. The inability to grieve appro-priately has longstanding implications for development of future mood-related disorders, or more commonly observed complicated bereavement reactions.

PTSD

More statistics are available related to time after military separation, and according to the National Center for PTSD, the increased risk for mental health diagnosis is not a new trend. The National Vietnam Veterans Readjustment Study in 1988 revealed the lifetime prevalence for PTSD among Vietnam veter-ans was 30.9% for men, and 26.9% for women (Kulka et al., 1988). The statistics also noted the chronic nature of the PTSD, because at the time of when the study was conducted, 15.2% of men, and 8.1% of women were still currently diagnosed with PTSD—more than a decade after service.

Moving forward to the first Gulf War, Kang, Natelson, Mahan, Lee, and Murphey (2003) reported a prevalence rate of PTSD across all sampled veterans to be approximately 12.2%. The RAND Corporation and Center for Military Health Policy Research identified that the rate of current PTSD was 13.8% for veterans of OEF and OIF (Taniellan & Jaycox, 2008). These numbers compared to the U.S. population rate of PTSD (about 7% to 8%). The rate for women is approximately 10%. These numbers are not inconceivable given the increased risk of exposure to combat, or other horrific or life-threatening experiences. Others have suggested the impact of exposure is multiplied, and contributes to difficulty and symptom development, when you take into consideration the demands of the living situation: constant noise, absence of privacy, lack of food, limited water supply, and minimal, if any, facilities required for hygiene. Additionally, the triggering events are not always exposure to enemy engagement, but rather having to retrieve body parts or relocate graves, which are all tasks required of soldiers that many are unprepared to carry out.

Military Sexual Trauma

I will conclude the section with discussion related to what has received more attention in the media in the past few years: military sexual trauma (MST). It is a significant contributing factor to mental health diagnoses, and is defined as any sexual harassment or sexual assault that transpires while in the military. The DoD Directive 6495.01 defines sexual assault as:

> Intentional sexual contact characterized by use of force, threats, intimidation, or abuse of authority or when the victim does not or cannot consent. The crime of sexual assault includes a broad category of sexual offenses consisting of the following specific Uniform Code of Military Justice offenses: rape, sexual assault, aggravated sexual contact, abusive contact, forcible sodomy (forced oral or anal sex), or attempts to commit these offenses.
>
> (DoD, 2012a)

According to the National Center for PTSD, in a sampled veteran population, approximately 23% of women said they had been sexually assaulted, and 55% had been sexually harassed. These numbers are higher compared to male counterparts, with 38% of men reporting previous harassment. According to the Defense Women's Health Research Program (DWHRP, 2015), harassment rates were higher in units with fewer women and increased soldier stress levels. Women were not accepted in these communities, and the units had lower scores when examining aspects of mission readiness.

This is the exact situation that women integrating into the combat arms profession are facing now. The Commander that I noted at the beginning of the chapter now has one female assigned to his Company. He expressed frustration and concern over "what to do with her," and having to find another female for "logistical purposes," so that she may have a Battle Buddy as an escort during trainings and while carrying out certain duties. The new solider was already discussed in terms of being a complication for his mission, as opposed to an asset, prior to even meeting her.

The integration of women in specialty combat positions, such as Ranger Regiments and Special Forces, has also received a great deal of attention. I urge interested readers to reference some of the interviews conducted by Szayna and colleagues in conjunction with the RAND Corporation in 2014 with combat troops in these societies (Szayna et al., 2015). It is a comprehensive report, with noted concerns about how not only may women change the operational functioning of these teams, but also how it may impact the women who enter into these worlds.

MST is not a new phenomenon. The 2014 Defense Advisory Committee on Women in the Services (DACOWITS) report identifies a few key points related to MST, including systemic policy issues that may be contributing to the continued problem. The report indicates that the rate of MSTs is most likely underreported. In many cases, there is the absence of transparency in the resulting disciplinary action taken against perpetrators. This may communicate to victims that offenses may be disregarded, and perpetrators will not be held accountable. I have heard victims blatantly identify this as a lack of confidence in the system, and reason for further underreporting of such offenses.

Reporting is a lengthy and difficult process, and a woman's status in her unit is changed forever. In many cases the woman is relocated to a different unit as a *rehabilitative* measure, but clinically I have seen this, time and time again, experienced as a punishment, a sense of social isolation, and rejection from her peers, and chain of command. If punitive action is not a 100% guarantee after an event is reported, then many women struggle with the question of why to report any events.

Furthermore, it is common for soldiers to move to new units, and records of previous sexual offenses are not always transferred to the new Commander. This is a large issue related to the potential reoffense rate. I have been involved in care where perpetrators were relocated to a unit with a *previous* victim (again a "rehabilitative" move) because they had again committed an act of sexual violence in the unit they were first transferred to. Imagine the impact this may have on the emotional well-being of a woman who goes to work for months two doors down from her previous assailant, prior to bringing this up in therapy as a contributing factor to her depressive condition. This woman noted that she felt as if she requested a move again, it would not transpire, would reflect poorly on her career, and would negatively color her new Commander's view of her utility in the unit.

This is not an isolated case. According to the DoD publication in May 2014 on substantiated incidents of sexual harassment in the armed forces, alleged *repeat* offenders comprised 11% of formal sexual harassment cases (U.S. Department of Defense, 2014). To provide a scope of the issue during fiscal year 2013, there were 1,266 formal harassment complaints, which then translates into 139 repeat offenders. That same year, there were also 5,061 reports of sexual assault, which is a 50% increase from the previous fiscal year.

Finally, the DoD published the *Red Book* in 2010, a 350-page report that addressed health promotion, risk reduction, and suicide prevention (United States Army, 2010). A 2012 publication, known as the *Gold Book* (DoD, 2012b), informs leaders about the unique challenges and health of soldiers, families, and veterans that were first addressed by the prior publication. The report is a 210-page document that covers behavioral health diagnoses and treatment, mild traumatic brain injury, PTS/PTSD, depression, substance use, polytrauma, suicide, psychopharmacotherapy, and numerous other topics.

In both publications, there is no discussion of issues specific to women's health in the service. The exception was acknowledgment of one study where rates in female veterans endorsing MST ranged between 20% and 40%, resulting in PTSD, depression, and sleep difficulties. Despite efforts on the part of the DoD, the report includes analysis of data from 2006 to 2011 that identifies that the rate of violent sex crimes is growing at an average of 14.6% per year, which translates into approximately 79 new offenses.

Other Unique Issues for Women

Pregnancy and Postpartum

I will conclude with brief identification of other female-specific issues that arise in the military, which have significant impact on the mental health of service members, but are not commonly discussed. The DWHRP in 1994 examined how social roles impact women's overall health. An area of particular focus was being pregnant while on active duty. One study showed that psychological health of mothers, and the outcome of the birth of their children, were correlated with Command climate and level of support regarding the pregnancy. There are significant issues related to a woman's readiness when she is pregnant, and the months to follow that are not guided by clear policy for how Commanders are to appropriately respond, and thus the experience of women greatly varies.

I have treated women with postpartum depression, who have deployed a few months after the birth of their child, only to return home with worsened depression, and the absence of a mother–child bond. Even field training exercises pose difficulties for women who have no available space or time to utilize a breast pump and increased physical demands commonly result in the cessation of lactation. This is an issue for all women that is magnified in the training environment. The time and space also vary across duty stations, as certain posts such as Ft. Lewis McChord have relaxing lactation stations positioned through the hospital and a variety of outlying places for this exact purpose; this is exceptionally progressive compared to the majority of other duty stations, and there are no such facilities at the Military Training Facility Hospital where

I am currently stationed. The depression and guilt that women like this patient struggle with challenge their concept of being a "good solider" and being a "good mother."

Many women make numerous sacrifices and are loyal patriots to this country, which has an impact on their mental health, but arguably also the health and development of their children. Other women decide to not have children while on active duty, and leave the service to raise their children, and have expressed frustration regarding the impact this has on career progression. Others still, more silently, decide to not have their children at all as the demands of filling both roles is too great, and to make a sacrifice in either role is incongruent with their self identity.

The 2014 DACOWITS annual report also focused on challenges related to pregnancy in the military. Pregnancy is considered to be a "deployment-limiting" medical condition, and access to proper contraceptive care is a large barrier for women, especially in a deployed environment. The choices that are available are limited as well. In addition, large military hospitals are not required to stock long-term birth control options, such as intrauterine devices or the vaginal contraceptive ring. Research available from women deployed in OIF reveals that 22% of women received no gynecological exam in the past year, 58% of contraceptive patches fell off while in theatre, 43% of women had to change their contraception due to unavailability, and 40% of women who required gynecological care had to be removed from their operating base and transported for care via a ground convoy, or even on a bird (aircraft) (Neilsen et al., 2009; Thomson & Nielson, 2006). Furthermore, in the event of an unwanted pregnancy, women are not provided medical care coverage through their military-related insurance and must fully pay for and receive a termination by a private community provider.

The Total Army Injury and Health Outcomes Database (TAIHOD, 2014), created by the U.S. Army Research Institute of Environmental Medicine (USARIEM), has additionally looked into the impact military service may have on women's overall health given approximately 10% of female warfighters are pregnant at any given time. Factors of exposure to hazardous toxic chemicals, prophylactic drugs, sound/vibration, radiation, and electromagnetic fields all clearly have a physical impact on health, but an additional impact on emotional well-being. For a moment, envision being an expectant mother exposed to the sound of a flight line as part of your job in 95-degree weather wearing a service uniform. The added stress is clearly present, yet not comprehensively assessed. Many women will work as long as possible up until the day of the birth of their child to meet mission demands.

A service member's readiness continues to be impacted months postpartum, with approximately half of such women failing to return to pre-pregnancy fitness levels, even six to nine months postpartum. Postpartum soldiers have been shown to be more likely to fail their annual physical fitness test (APFT) compared to non-pregnant soldiers. This may not come across as a significant issue, but a failure of two APFTs allows a Commander to administratively separate a soldier from the Army. Many soldiers experience excessive anxiety related to their physical performance, and one may argue women in this category who are not provided a standardized, graded return-to-exercise program may have an additional stress related to job insecurity, in combination with being a new mother.

Physical Requirements

There are also the physical requirements, and the utilization of gear that is not designed for the structural frame of the female service member. The weight and design of the rucksack, and even some of the moisture wicking and cooling shirts, are not developed for women, and thus not as effective for intended design, resulting in medical problems. TAIHOD has identified that certain MOS positions in the Army place women at a greater risk for certain complications, such as light-wheeled mechanics, who have the highest rate of musculoskeletal hospitalizations, and female parachutists, who have a high rate of injury due to landings. Again, according to the research, women, even in initial training (basic training), have twice as many musculoskeletal injuries, specifically a high rate of stress fractures. I highlight this at the end to point out that, as women, even at the point of induction in our training and integration into the military, the simplest tools are not developed with us in mind. The simple aspects of how a bag is designed and distributes weight carry over into how we are accepted and integrated into the system, as *others* or as the *non-standard*.

This has shaped me as a provider in system. It would be ignorant not to acknowledge this. I exist in a world of men, where the language, dress, and manner of walking and sitting are arguably more masculine in nature. This shapes how I think, my relationships with others, and the relationship I have with myself. As a woman, I take specific countermeasures to achieve balance and acceptance of my womanhood while on active duty. But it has not been my personal or professional experience that any of this is discussed with other women, and definitely not my fellow servicemen, whom I do love and respect. The military culture has demands that, according to some researchers, may be interpreted as mental health "risk factors" to women. This may be true. The society is difficult to navigate, and is isolating, at times.

I do, however, want to highlight the opportunities for personal strength and growth within the organization, and empowering experiences I have had— opportunities that would not be available to me as a civilian. As a minority in society, the deck is stacked against me. But that does not mean that other women and I are forced to succumb to the above-noted behavioral health symptoms and diagnoses. Rather, I would like women to be informed. I hope those in my sisterhood will take smart precautionary and preparatory behaviors to secure their health, and place them in a more advantageous position to care for each other and our brothers, and carry out the larger mission.

Disclaimer

All of the views and opinions expressed in this chapter are those of the author and do not reflect the official policy or position of the U.S. Army, Department of Defense, or the U.S. Government.

References

American Foundation for Suicide Prevention. (2016). *Suicide statistics*. Retrieved from www.afsp. org/about-suicide/suicide-statistics/ (accessed November 4, 2016).

Defense Women's Health Research Program (DWHRP). (2015). Retrieved from htps:momrp. amedd.army.mil/dwhrp_index.html.

Department of Defense. (2012a). *Sexual assault prevention and response (SAPR) program, number 6495.01*. Retrieved from: http://www.vi.ngb.army.mil/html/sapr/docs/DoD%20Directive%20 6495.01.pdf

Department of Defense. (2012b). *Army 2020: Generating health and discipline in the force: Ahead of the strategic resent*. Retrieved from https//www.Army.mil/e2/c/downloads/233874.pdf

Kang, H., Natelson, B., Mahan, C., Lee, K., & Murphey, F. (2003). Post-traumatic stress disorder and chronic fatigue syndrome-like illness among Gulf War veterans: A population-based survey of 30,000 veterans. *American Journal of Epidemiology, 157*(2), 141–148.

Kessler, R., Heeringa, S., Stein, M., Colpe, L., Fullerton, C., Hwang I., Naifeh, J., Nock, M., Petukhova, M., Sampson, N., Schoenbaum, M., Zaslavsky, A., & Ursano, R. (2014). Thirty-day prevalence of DSM-IV mental disorders among non-deployed soldiers in the U.S. Army: results from the Army Study to Assess Risk and Resilience in Servicemembers (ARMY STARRS). *Journal of American Medical Association Psychiatry, March 3*, 504–513.

Kulka, R., Schlenger, W., Fairbank, J., Hough, R., Jordan, K., Marmar, C., & Weis, D. (1988). *Contractual report of findings from the National Vietnam Veterans Readjustment Study, Volume I: Executive summary, description of findings, and technical appendices*. Retrieved from www. ptsd.va.gov/professional/articles/article-pdf/nvvrs_vol1.pdf (accessed November 4, 2016).

Neilsen, P., Murphy, C., Schultz, J., Deering, S., Truong, V., McCartin, T., & Clemons, J. (2009). Female soldiers' gynecologic healthcare in Operation Iraqi Freedom: A survey of camps with echelon three facilities. *Military Medicine, 174*(11), 1171–1176.

Office of the Deputy Assistant Secretary of Defense. (2014). *Department of Defense demographics report for fiscal year 2014*. Retrieved from download.militaryonesource.mil.12038/MOS/ Reports/2014-Demographics-Report.pdf.

Office of the Surgeon General United States Army Medical Command and Office of the Command Surgeon Headquarters, U.S. Army Central Command (USCENTCOM) and Office of the Command Surgeon U.S. Forces Afghanistan (USFOR-A). (2013). *Army Mental Health Advisory Team (MHAT-9) Operation Enduring Freedom (OEF) 2013 Afghanistan*. Retrieved from armymedicine.mil/Documents/MHAT_9_OEF_Report.pdf.

Rundell, J. (2006). Demographics of and diagnosis in Operation Enduring Freedom and Operation Iraqi Freedom personnel who were psychiatrically evacuated form the theater of operations. *General Hospital Psychiatry, 28*(4), 352–356.

Smolenski, D., Reger, M., Bush, N., Skopp, N., Zhang, Y., & Campise, R. (2013). *The National Center for Telehealth and Technology (T2) Department of Defense suicide defense report (DoDSER) 2013*. Retrieved from t2health.dcoe.mil/sites/default/files/DoDSER-2013-Jan-2015-Final.pdf

Szayna, T., Larson, E., O'Mahony, A., Robson, S., Schaefer, A., et al. (2015). *Considerations for integrating women into closed occupations in the U.S. Special Operations Forces, RAND Corporation*. Retrieved from: http://www.defense.gov/Portals/1/Documents/wisr-studies/SOCOM%20-%20

Considerations%20for%20Integrating%20Women%20into%20Closed%20Occupations%20
in%20the%20US%20Special%20Operations%20Forces.pdf (accessed November 21, 2016).

Taniellan, T., & Jaycox, L. (2008). *Invisible wounds of war: Psychological and cognitive injuries, their consequences, and services to assist recovery.* Santa Monica, CA: RAND Cooperation.

Thomson, B., & Nielson, P. (2006). Women's health care in Operational Iraq Freedom: A survey of camps with echelon I or II facilities. *Military Medicine, 171*(3), 216–219.

Total Army Injury and Health Outcomes Database (TAIHOD). (2014). Retrieved from www.usariem. army.mil

United States Army. (2010). *Army health promotion risk reduction suicide prevention report 2010 (red book).* Retrieved from csf2.army.mil/downloads/HP-RR-SReport2010.pdf

U.S. Department of Defense. (2014). *Fiscal year 2013 Department of Defense report on substantiated incidents of sexual harassment in the armed forces.* Washington, DC: U.S. Department of Defense.

Wells, T., LeardMann, C., Smith, B., Smith, T., Ryan, M., Boyko, E., & Blazer, D. (2010). A prospective study of depression following combat deployment in support of the wars in Iraq and Afghanistan. *American Journal of Public Health, 100*(1), 90–99.

Wojcik, B., Akhtar, F., & Hassel, H. (2009). Hospital admissions related to mental disorders in U.S. Army soldiers in Iraq and Afghanistan, *Military Medicine, 174*(10), 1010–1018.

Part III

Specific Disorders Related to Women's Mental Health

Chapter Nine
Mood and Anxiety Disorders in Women

Kimberly D. Thompson

Mood and anxiety disorders are of particular importance when discussing women's mental health. Not only are depression and anxiety the most prominent mental health problems in modern society (e.g., Gibbs, Lee, & Kulkarni, 2012), most manifestations of these problems occur at far higher rates in females (e.g., Patten et al., 2015). Women are at two to three times higher risk than men of developing a depressive disorder, a trend that begins in adolescence and continues through old age (e.g., Chou & Cheung, 2013). Anxiety disorders also occur more frequently in women than men, at a ratio of 2:1 (McLean, Asnaani, Litz, & Hofmann, 2011). This chapter provides an overview of mood and anxiety disorders and their importance to women's mental health.

Defining Disorder

How do normal negative emotional or psychological states differ from disordered ones? There are four distinct qualities of disordered states not shared by normal experiences. These qualities are distress, or disability; danger to self or others; dysfunction in one or more important aspects of life; and deviance, either statistical deviance or in terms of social norms (Davis, 2009). A disordered state exhibits at least one of these qualities, and usually more than one. This framework is important to understand how mood and anxiety disorders differ from adaptive forms of fear and anxiety, and from normal shifts in mood.

Anxiety and Fear

Anxiety is a common response to stress, and can be adaptive to the extent that it prepares people for unpleasant contingencies. However, at times anxiety becomes excessively severe, leading to distorted beliefs about the nature and extent of the anticipated threat. The unusual intensity, duration, or nature of the anxiety becomes painful and may be disabling (McLean et al., 2011; Williams et al., 2010).

Likewise, fear can be a necessary and adaptive response to immediate threat. However, when relatively minor real or imagined threats provoke persistent fight, flight, or freeze responses (Maack, Buchanan, & Young, 2015), fear becomes harmful. This is particularly true for women, with women overall missing more days of work due to anxiety than their male counterparts (McLean et al., 2011).

Phobias

Phobias are undue fears of an object or situation. Phobic individuals avoid what they fear, or go through it with considerable discomfort. Some phobias are quite limited, such as a fear of dogs, thunderstorms, needles, or clowns. These specific phobias can be debilitating despite their limited nature. For example, a needle or medical procedure phobia can interfere with someone getting vital medical care; a choking phobia may lead to avoiding whole food groups, or refusal to take medication in pill form.

Other forms of phobia are more generalized. Social phobia, also known as social anxiety disorder, is an intense fear of being criticized or evaluated by other people, and it also can be debilitating. It often leads to avoiding social situations out of fear of being judged by other people. Agoraphobia is an intense fear of being stuck in a situation where help is not available, especially a public place. People suffering from agoraphobia partially or totally withdraw from normal activities that require going into these feared situations. Every year, between 7% and 9% of the population experiences a specific phobia, about 7% has a social phobia, and around 2% is agoraphobic in any given year. Women experience these disorders at twice the rate of men. The prevalence of both specific phobia and agoraphobia tapers off with age, so that older adults of both sexes are less likely to suffer from them (American Psychiatric Association, 2013).

Panic Disorder

Recurrent, unexpected surges of intense fear are known as panic attacks. Panic attacks immediately result in intense physical symptoms, such as a racing heart, nausea, sweating, and a sense of being cut off from reality. Fearful thoughts quickly follow these physical symptoms. It is common for those in throes of a panic attack to fear that they are dying, that they are going to lose control of themselves, or that they are going insane. These fears lead to avoidance of any situation associated with a panic attack, or situations where they might not be able to get help, which can seriously restrict their activities and lead to agoraphobia. Women are again about twice as likely as men to qualify for a panic disorder diagnosis (Leskin & Sheikh, 2004). About 2% to 3% of the population experience panic disorder in any given year. However, panic disorder prevalence also tends to decrease as the population ages, so that less than 1% of adults over the age of 64 experience a panic attack yearly (American Psychiatric Association, 2013).

Generalized Anxiety Disorder

Generalized anxiety disorder (GAD) is a pervasive pattern of anxiety and worry about many things. Unlike other anxiety disorders in which the individual is distressed about specific concerns, GAD produces significant distress and functional impairments precisely because it is generalized. GAD sufferers tend to see threat lurking in many or most things that they face daily, resulting in a chronic state of anxiety and anticipation of the worst. Per year, almost 3% of the adult population suffers from GAD. As has been discussed with other anxiety disorders, adult females are twice as likely to meet diagnostic criteria for GAD as males (American Psychiatric Association, 2013; Mclean et al., 2011).

Illness Anxiety

A woman experiencing illness anxiety is overly concerned about her health and the possibility of becoming ill. If she is actually suffering from a medical illness, or is truly at risk for becoming ill, then her anxiety is exaggerated considering the objective medical facts (American Psychiatric Association, 2013).

Genito-Pelvic Pain/Penetration Disorder (GPD)

GPD includes vaginismus, or painful contractions of the vagina when penetration is attempted, and dyspareunia, or pain with sexual intercourse. Anxiety may not always be the cause of GPD, since it is a diagnosis of exclusion; medical problems and insufficient sexual stimulation must be ruled out first. However, GPD is relevant to a discussion of anxiety disorders because fear or anxiety about penetration may be the source of the problems. The pain of GPD, and the associated anxiety and fearfulness, can interfere with forming and maintaining sexually intimate relationships. It also may interfere with medical exams and treatment. It is estimated that 15% of North American women experience pain with intercourse, but what the prevalence is for GPD overall is not known (American Psychiatric Association, 2013; Seibell, Hamblin, & Hollander, 2015).

Obsessive-Compulsive Disorder (OCD)

Individuals suffering from OCD experience unwelcome thoughts and urges that feel uncontrollable; they also feel compelled to carry out ritualized behaviors that are pointless except for their usefulness in managing the obsessive thoughts. Evidence is accumulating that OCD is neurologically distinct from the other anxiety disorders, responds to different treatments, and, unlike other types of anxiety, occurs equally in males and females (López-Solà et al., 2014). Therefore, OCD is no longer technically considered to be an anxiety disorder. However, in most people, obsessive thoughts cause anxiety. Compulsions are usually performed to reduce the anxiety associated with the obsessive thoughts. The combination of obsessions and compulsions meets some or all of the criteria for disorders, since both the thoughts and the rituals fall far outside the range of normal experience, are very distressing to the person, and can become severe enough to disrupt job performance or intimate relationships. Compulsions may also pose a danger by leading the sufferer to behavioral excesses that cause physical damage or put the person in harm's way (American Psychiatric Association, 2013).

Mood Disturbance

The term euthymia is used to describe a normal resting mood state. A euthymic mood state is mildly positive, producing psychological energy and motivation to accomplish desired goals and to nurture interpersonal relationships. It is accompanied by a positive sense of self, a sense of a reality shared with other people, and an optimal level of arousal that enables the individual do her best work.

Throughout life, virtually everyone will experience non-euthymic moods. Most of these mood changes are normal and expectable responses to experiences. It is expected that good experiences will induce positive moods, and that bad experiences will induce negative moods. The duration, intensity, and appropriateness of normal mood fluctuations are not disabling, and by themselves are not harmful.

By contrast, mood disorders manifest as abnormally dysphoric or euphoric mood. Episodes of dysphoria, accompanied by debilitating changes in cognition, physiology, and behavior, characterize the depressive disorders. Physiological and cognitive impairments include unexplained exhaustion, difficulty concentrating, impaired motivation and sense of enjoyment in usual activities, fragmented sleep, and either agitation or sluggishness. Some depressed individuals may also struggle with an exaggerated sense of guilt, of being worthless, or thoughts of death or suicide (American Psychiatric Association, 2013).

Episodes of euphoria characterize the bipolar disorders. Euphoria is an elevated mood state, but in the bipolar disorders, the negative consequences of an elevated mood far outweigh any feelings of enjoyment or pleasure. Euphoric mood includes increased irritability, agitation, or anxiety. It is accompanied by an accelerated cognitive tempo, constant physiological arousal, and some form of risky behavior. A severe form, mania, can bring on psychosis.

The cognitive and physiological symptoms are uncomfortable and upsetting, while high-risk behaviors are dysfunctional at best and dangerous at worst. Most women who suffer from a bipolar mood disorder also experience episodes of depression, although this is not a requirement for all forms of bipolar disorder. While bipolar disorders are fairly evenly distributed among women and men, women are overrepresented in the types of bipolar disorders that include prominent depressive episodes (e.g., American Psychiatric Association, 2013; Miquel et al., 2011).

Major Depression

Major depression consists of much more than transient unhappiness in response to a sad or stressful event. This diagnosis specifies that a depressed mood be present for at least two weeks, and must be accompanied by five or more depressive symptoms. The younger the woman is, the greater her risk for major depression, with the rate of depression in women under the age of 30 being three times the rate of women over the age of 60. It has been estimated that almost 5% of women experience a major depressive episode in any given year (American Psychiatric Association, 2013; Patten et al., 2015).

Dysthymia

Dysthymia is a milder form of depression that is nonetheless disabling because it is so long lasting. Dysthymia consists of dysphoria plus at least two other depressive symptoms, and lasts at least two years. About 2% of the population every year meets criteria either for dysthymia or for a major depressive episode that has lasted at least two years (American Psychiatric Association, 2013).

Premenstrual Dysphoric Disorder (PMDD)

PMDD consists of dysphoric mood and other depressive symptoms that fluctuate predictably with the menstrual cycle. These episodes appear premenstrually and resolve once menstruation begins. Approximately 2% to 6% of women who are still menstruating experience PMDD in any given 12-month period (American Psychiatric Association, 2013).

Bipolar I

A lifetime history of at least one manic episode is diagnostic for bipolar I disorder. A manic episode is characterized by an abnormally elevated mood that persists for at least a week and is accompanied by disabling changes in functioning. These include exaggerated self-esteem; the inability to sleep, or lack of interest in sleep, without corresponding fatigue; speaking very rapidly with a sense of underlying urgency; tangential speech and thoughts; easy distractibility; and a problematic increase in purposeful, aimless, or high-risk activity. Symptoms of psychosis may be present; these include hallucinations or delusional beliefs.

Those with bipolar I disorder usually experience both hypomanic and major depressive episodes as well. Hypomanic episodes are characterized by mood elevations that are similar to manic episodes, but are of shorter duration with less impairment than a manic episode. Major depressive episodes in bipolar disorder are similar to those experienced in unipolar depression. Men and women suffer from this disorder at about the same rate (American Psychiatric Association, 2013).

Bipolar II

Bipolar II is diagnosed when true mania is absent, as defined by the persistence and severity of the elevated mood. Women with bipolar II cycle between normal, depressed, and hypomanic episodes. This form of bipolar disorder may be more common in females, and women are more likely to have episodes that combine symptoms of both hypomania and depression. They are also more likely to rotate quickly through abnormal mood episodes. Depression in bipolar II tends to be severe and resistant to treatment (American Psychiatric Association, 2013).

Cyclothymia

Cyclothymia is a persistent alternation between elevated and depressed mood states that do not quite meet the criteria for either hypomania or major depression. The abnormal mood states must be persistent and pervasive for at least two years. Many cases of cyclothymia will evolve over time into a more severe form of bipolar disorder. Cyclothymia is unusual, estimated to be no more than 1% of the general population, with the male and female rates about the same (American Psychiatric Association, 2013).

Related Disorders

Adjustment Disorders

Adjustment disorders develop in response to particular stressors, and can manifest with depression, anxiety, or a combination of the two. A woman with an adjustment disorder experiences discomfort and impairment above and beyond what would usually be expected, given the nature of the stress. These disorders are very common. It is estimated that up to 20% of people seen in psychiatric outpatient settings, and up to 50% of those seen by consulting psychiatrists in hospitals, have an adjustment disorder (American Psychiatric Association, 2013).

Schizoaffective Disorder

Schizoaffective disorder, primarily a schizophrenia spectrum disorder, has an important mood component. Mood disturbance is a prominent part of schizoaffective disorder and the mood and psychotic symptoms occur together to the extent that they are considered to be one disorder rather than a comorbidity. A schizoaffective diagnosis can be difficult to determine, because psychotic symptoms must present when affective symptoms are absent. This is an important distinction, since psychosis can also be a feature of severe mood disturbance, such as psychotic depression and mania. The mood component of schizoaffective disorder can be unipolar depression or a form of bipolar illness (American Psychiatric Association, 2013).

Borderline Personality Disorder (BPD)

Another disorder with a prominent mood component is BPD. BPD is characterized by, among other things, a marked emotional instability. This instability may include brief but intense dysphoria accompanied by suicidal behavior. The impairment associated with BPD varies according to the number of symptoms and their severity, but can be seriously disabling. It is estimated that between 2% and 6% of the total population meet criteria for BPD. In all, 70% to 75% of those diagnosed with BPD are women (e.g., Biskin & Paris, 2012). Similar to the trends observed with major depressive disorder, the severity of BPD tends to peak in early adulthood and taper off with age. It is estimated that, over time, as many as half of those diagnosed with BPD improve to the point that they no longer qualify for the diagnosis (American Psychiatric Association, 2013).

Relationship Between Mood Disorder and Anxiety

It has long been known that the mood and anxiety disorders are highly comorbid (Goldberg & Fawcett, 2012) and share common factors, such as persistent negative cognitions. Both anxiety and depression are characterized by rumination and worry. Rumination is difficult-to-control repetitive negative thoughts, while worry is the anxious expectation of bad things to come (Kalmbach, Pillai, & Ciesla, 2016). Blanco et al. (2014), in analyzing known risk factors for both anxiety and depression, found a single risk factor in which the same genetic and environmental inheritance creates vulnerability to major depression, generalized anxiety, specific phobias, posttraumatic stress, social anxiety, and panic.

Experiencing comorbid anxiety and depression leads to increased disability and dysfunction over and above either problem alone. Hettema, Aggen, Kubarych, Neale, and Kendler (2015) describe a syndrome of mixed anxiety and depression, in which individuals did not meet criteria for either major depression or a specified anxiety disorder but were experiencing significant distress nonetheless. Severe anxiety is highly predictive of severe female depression (Weiss et al., 2015); also, women are particularly disabled by a combination of severe anxiety and bipolar disorder (Saunders, Fitzgerald, Zhang, & McInnis, 2012).

Two-Hit Models

Diathesis–stress, or two-hit, models have robust explanatory power for both anxiety and mood disorders. They effectively incorporate the influence of both nature and nurture, forces that were once thought to be diametrically opposed to one another (Eberhart, Auerbach, Bigda-Peyton, & Abela, 2011; Elwood, Mott, Williams, Lohr, & Schroeder, 2009; Oquendo, McGrath, & Weissman, 2013).

First Hit: Diatheses

Anxiety disorders develop when genetics, physiology, and experience interact to increase a woman's sensitivity to classical fear conditioning. For example, maternal psychosocial stress during pregnancy exposes the developing fetus to higher levels of the stress hormone, cortisol. This early exposure results in alterations to the stress regulation system that primes the infant for anxiety (Davis, Glynn, Waffarn, & Sandman, 2011). Dispositional tendencies such as this are long lasting and often have lifelong consequences. In addition to vulnerabilities acquired prenatally, women who experienced neglect and other adversity in childhood are at increased risk of depression and anxiety in adulthood (Brock, Rowse, & Slade, 2016). Normal socialization processes may be implicated. For example, anxiety is thought to be more prevalent in women because men and women are taught different ways to express anxiety and different ways to cope with it (McLean et al., 2011).

Calkins et al. (2009) report that anxiety sensitivity and neuroticism predict the development of new or recurring episodes of anxiety disorders. Neuroticism is a general tendency toward negative affectivity, while anxiety sensitivity refers to a tendency to fear of having feelings of anxiety. As a group, women tend to score higher on both (Chorri, Marsh, Ubbiali, & Donati, 2016; Norr, Albanese, Allan, & Schmidt, 2015). When stressful life events occur, anxiety sensitivity and neuroticism magnify normal anxiety into a disabling and dysfunctional state.

As for unipolar depression, recent advances in identifying genes that may contribute to depression risk, as well as the physiology of depression, have provided greater understanding of how depression risk is conveyed in families. These advances are also shedding light on why women tend to be at greater risk (Nivard et al., 2015). Polymorphisms in the genes *SERF*, *BDNF*, and *COMT* have been identified as contributors to depression risk, and are thought to have a cumulative effect (Kostic et al., 2016). Additionally, variation in the alleles of estrogen receptor genes is thought to influence the development of female depression specifically (Keyes et al., 2015). Evidence that physiological inflammation is associated with the onset of depressive symptoms is accumulating; women in particular appear vulnerable to mood symptoms when inflammatory markers (C-reactive protein, interleukin-6, and interleukin-1β) and tumor necrosis factor-a are elevated (Derry, Padin, Kuo, Hughes, & Keicolt-Glaser, 2015).

Evidence for a diathesis–stress interaction in bipolar disorder can be found in the observed connections between childhood trauma, the misuse of marijuana, and severe bipolar symptoms. Genetic vulnerabilities interact with perinatal stress to create a predisposition to bipolar disorders. Stressful experience during adolescence or early adulthood, including experimentation with drugs, serves as the "second hit" (Aas et al., 2016).

Second Hit: Stress

Studies of stress exposure in rats suggest that, while early-life stress affects males more profoundly, females become more vulnerable to stress after puberty (Hodes, 2013). This may explain why human females are twice as likely as males to become depressed, starting around puberty and continuing throughout life (e.g., Van de Velde, Bracke, & Levecque, 2010). There are certain stressors that are especially associated with female depression.

Domestic Violence

Intimate-partner violence is a major stressor in the lives of many women. Whether psychological, physical, or sexual, domestic abuse is strongly related to anxiety and anxiety-related disorders (Cougle, Timpano, Sachs-Eriksson, Keough, & Riccardi, 2010), depression, and psychosis (Eshelman & Levendosky, 2012; Watkins et al., 2014). The risk is especially strong for women who were abused as children (Ouellet-Morin et al., 2015).

Reproductive Processes and Events

A variety of processes and events related to reproduction or the reproductive system can also serve as stressors for vulnerable women. Women with severe premenstrual syndrome are more likely to have fearful or anxious personality traits (Sassoon, Colrain, & Baker, 2011), to feel little control over things that cause anxiety (Mahon, Rohan, Nillni, & Zvolenski, 2015), and to develop posttraumatic stress disorder (PTSD) after being exposed to trauma (Nillni, Berenz, Pineles, Coffey, & Zvolensky, 2014). Some women struggle with dramatically increased interpersonal sensitivity around the time of menstruation, which manifests in feelings of being persecuted (Brock et al., 2016). Moods fluctuate with the menstrual cycle for some, but not all, women with bipolar illness. The issue is likely to be sensitivity to hormonal changes rather than absolute hormone levels (Marsh, Gershenson, & Rothschild, 2015).

The perinatal period is also a time of particular vulnerability to both anxiety and disordered mood. New mothers may become depressed when lifelong cognitive patterns interact with the physiological and psychosocial stress of pregnancy, childbirth, and new motherhood (Thompson & Bendell, 2014). Discussed at length elsewhere in this volume, it is nevertheless important to point out that perinatal depression is an important public health issue. Estimates of perinatal depressive disorders range from an estimate of 3% to 6% in the *Diagnostic and Statistical Manual of Mental Disorders, Fifth Edition* (DSM-5: American Psychiatric Association, 2013), which only takes into account episodes of major depressive disorder, to over 50% in adolescent mothers (Kleiber & Dimidjian, 2014). Manic or hypomanic episodes also may be triggered by childbirth (Maina, Rosso, Guglia, & Bogetto, 2014).

Another period of hormonal flux is perimenopause. Besides the vulnerability some women have to hormone changes, many women experience new stressors that can trigger depression. These include psychological factors such as the so-called empty nest, divorce, widowhood, or poverty; physiological features, such as severe hot flashes; and lifestyle factors, such as smoking, obesity, and exercise habits (Gibbs et al., 2012; Post et al., 2013).

As women age, they are exposed to more stress in the form of age-related medical conditions. Because they tend to live longer than men, women are more likely to experience profound losses such as widowhood (Weissman & Levine, 2007). Poor sleep quality may complicate elderly women's recovery from stress and loss. A study that measured sleep disturbance in elderly women found that, even in the absence of a prior episode, fragmented sleep predicted the eventual development of depression (Maglione et al., 2014).

Relationship Stress

Interpersonal relationships serve either as a buffer against depression, or as a stressor that triggers it. Women with low social support are more likely to experience both mood and anxiety disorders (Cyranowski et al., 2012). Social support not only refers to the number of relationships in a woman's life, but also relationship quality. A stable, good-quality relationship with a life partner reduces the risk of depression (Leach, Butterworth, Olesen, & MacKinnon, 2013), while an unstable relationship increases it (Whitton & Whisman, 2010). When it comes to depression, women seem to be better off single than in a low-quality relationship (Leach et al., 2013).

Self-Induced Stress

Depression-prone women tend to behave in ways that increase their own stress. This includes a high sensitivity to negative feedback; a tendency to interpret ambiguous situations negatively, including facial expressions (Bento de Souza, Barbosa, Lacerda, dos Santos, & Torro-Alves, 2014); to report stressful experiences that are at least partly under their own control (Bouchard & Shih, 2013); and, to exhaust loved ones with their need for constant reassurance (Stewart & Harkness, 2015). While unintentional, these behaviors interfere with healthy interpersonal relationships.

Depression and anxiety can erode intimacy through a negative impact on sexuality. Depressed women often complain of diminished sexual functioning, which has been traced to anhedonia (Kalmbach, Pillai, Kingsberg, & Ciesla, 2015). Anxiety about one's own appearance also interferes with sexual functioning and a sense of sexual well-being (Vencill, Tebbe, & Garos, 2015).

Symptoms of mania or hypomania can damage interpersonal relationships, since they tend to increase relationship friction (Morriss et al., 2013). There is a high rate of divorce among those with bipolar disorders, thought to be due in large part to burnout among spouses (Granek, Danan, Bersudsky, & Osher, 2016).

Psychosocial Treatments

Psychosocial treatments that have been shown to be effective for mood and anxiety disorders include cognitive-behavioral therapies (CBT), interpersonal therapy, acceptance and mindfulness therapies, such as acceptance and commitment therapy, and dialectical behavior therapy, and metacognitive therapy (e.g., Cort et al., 2014; Koszycki, Bisserbe, Blier, Bradwejn, & Markowitz, 2012).

Cognitive-Behavioral Therapy

CBT is a hybrid type of therapy that combines strategic behavioral modifications with awareness and evaluation of underlying belief systems. In addition to effectiveness with depressive disorders (e.g., Dobson & Dobson, 2009), a meta-analytic review found that CBT is effective in reducing anxiety symptoms and in boosting quality of life for individuals with PTSD, OCD, panic disorder, social anxiety disorder, and GAD (Hofmann, Wu, & Boettcher, 2014).

Mindfulness and Acceptance Therapies

Mindfulness is inversely related to both anxiety sensitivity and symptoms of depression (Waszczuk et al., 2015). Mindfulness and acceptance-based therapies are designed to increase awareness of the present moment, decrease attention given to negative repetitive thoughts, create phenomenological distance from painful experiences, and encourage the acceptance of reality. They have been found to provide significant benefits for the treatment of both anxiety (Vollestad, Nielsen, & Nielsen, 2012) and depression (Hofmann, Sawyer, Witt, & Oh, 2010).

Metacognitive Therapy

Metacognitive therapy differs from traditional cognitive therapies in that it is aimed at altering distorted beliefs about thought processes themselves. This therapy treats what is called the "cognitive attentional syndrome," or repetitive negative thinking patterns that resist distraction or redirection. Some examples of distorted beliefs about thought processes include believing that worry is necessary in order to solve problems, or that depressive rumination is uncontrollable. A meta-analytic review has indicated that metacognitive therapy shows promise for even greater levels of effectiveness than traditional CBT (Norman, Van Emmerik, & Morina, 2014).

Interpersonal Therapy

Interpersonal therapy consists of techniques aimed at improving the way the individual relates to others, in terms of relationship choice, ways to behave in relationships, and ways to respond to others' behaviors. It has been shown to be effective in treating depressive disorders (de Mallo, de Jesus, Bacaltchuk, Verdeli, & Neugebauer, 2005).

Gender and Treatment Response

Do depressed or anxious women respond differently to treatment than their male counterparts? The answer to that question appears to depend upon the treatment. In a meta-analytic study of treatment response to both cognitive-behavioral psychotherapy and antidepressant medications, Cuipers et al. (2014) report no significant gender differences. Conversely, Grubbs et al. (2015) report in a study of the effectiveness of collaborative care that anxious women responded significantly better than treatment as usual. Collaborative care, a model in which psychosocial interventions are provided in primary care settings, performed about as well as treatment as usual for men. Treatment as usual in this case was medication and referral to outside mental health services.

Summary

Anxiety and mood disorders occur across a spectrum of severity and can take many forms. Depressive disorders and most forms of anxiety are more common in women than men across the lifespan. This is likely the result of the interaction of genes, physiological vulnerabilities, gender-specific socialization processes, and adverse life experiences that are unique to, or are more common in, women. These experiences include menstruation, pregnancy, menopause, and being more likely to be a victim of domestic violence or to outlive a spouse. Fortunately, there are now many effective treatments for both anxiety and depression, including antidepressant and anxiolytic medications and a variety of psychosocial modalities.

References

Aas, M., Henry, C., Andreassen, O., Bellivier, F., Melle, I., & Etain, B. (2016). The role of childhood trauma in bipolar disorders. *International Journal of Bipolar Disorders, 4*(2).

American Psychiatric Association. (2013). *Diagnostic and statistical manual of mental disorders, fifth edition.* Arlington, VA: American Psychological Association.

Bento de Souza, I., Barbosa, F., Lacerda, A., dos Santos, N., & Torro-Alves, N. (2014). Evaluation of facial expressions in women with major depression: Is there a negative bias? *Psychology and Neuroscience, 7*(4), 513–519.

Biskin, R., & Paris, J. (2012). Diagnosing borderline personality disorder. *Canadian Medical Association Journal, 184*(16), 1789–1794.

Blanco, C., Rubio, J., Wall, M., Wang, S., Jiu, C., & Kendler, K. (2014). Risk factors for anxiety disorders: Common and specific effects in a national sample. *Depression and Anxiety, 31,* 756–764.

Bouchard, L., & Shih, J. (2013). Gender differences in stress generation: Examination of interpersonal predictors. *Journal of Social and Clinical Psychology, 32*(4), 442–445.

Brock, R., Rowse, G., & Slade, P. (2016). Relationships between paranoid thinking, self-esteem and the menstrual cycle. *Archives of Women's Mental Health, 19,* 271–279.

Calkins, A., Otto, M., Cohen, L., Soares, C., Vitonis, A., Hearon, B., & Harlow, B. (2009). Psychosocial predictors of the onset of anxiety disorders in women: Results from a prospective 3-year longitudinal study. *Journal of Anxiety Disorders, 23,* 1165–1169.

Chorri, C., Marsh, H., Ubbiali, A., & Donati, D. (2016). Testing the factor structure and measurement invariance across gender of the big five inventory through exploratory structural equation modeling. *Journal of Personality Assessment, 98*(1), 88–99.

Chou, K., & Cheung, K. (2013). Major depressive disorder in vulnerable groups of older adults, their course and treatment, and psychiatric comorbidity. *Depression and Anxiety, 30,* 528–537.

Cort, N., Cerulli, C., Poleshuck, E., Bellinger, K., Xia, Y., Tu, X., Mazzotta, C., & Talbot, N. (2014). Interpersonal psychotherapy for depressed women with histories of intimate partner violence. *Psychological Trauma: Theory, Research, Practice and Policy, 6*(6), 700–707.

Cougle, J., Timpano, K., Sachs-Eriksson, N., Keough, M., & Riccardi, C. (2010). Examining the unique relationships between anxiety disorders and childhood physical and sexual abuse in the National Comorbidity Survey-Replication. *Psychiatry Research, 177,* 150–155.

Cuijpers, P., Weitz, E., Twisk, J., Kuehner, C., Cristea, I., David, D., DeRubeis, R., Dimidjian, S., Dunlop, B. W., Faramarzi, M., Hegerl, U., Jarrett, R. B., Kennedy, S. H., Kheirkhah, F., Mergl, R., Miranda, J., Mohr, D., Segal, Z., Siddique, J., Simons, A., Vittengl, J., & Hollon, S. (2014). Gender as predictor and moderator of outcome in cognitive behavior therapy and pharmacotherapy for adult depression: An "individual patient data" meta-analysis. *Depression and Anxiety, 31,* 941–951.

Cyranowski, J., Schott, L., Kravitz, H., Brown, C., Thurston, R., Joffe, H., Matthews, K., & Bromberger, J. (2012). Psychosocial features associated with lifetime comorbidity of major depression and anxiety disorders among a community sample of mid-life women: The SWAN mental health study. *Depression and Anxiety, 29,* 1050–1057.

Davis, E., Glynn, L., Waffarn, F., & Sandman, C. (2011). Prenatal maternal stress programs infant stress regulation. *Journal of Child Psychology and Psychiatry, 52*(2), 119–129.

Davis, T. (2009). Conceptualizing psychiatric disorders using "four d's" of diagnoses. *The Internet Journal of Psychiatry, 1* (1).

de Mallo, M., de Jesus, M., Bacaltchuk, J., Verdeli, H., & Neugebauer, R. (2005). A systematic review of research findings on the efficacy of interpersonal therapy for depressive disorders. *European Archives of Psychiatry and Clinical Neuroscience, 255*(2), 75–82.

Derry, H., Padin, A., Kuo, J., Hughes, S., & Keicolt-Glaser, J. (2015). Sex differences in depression: Does inflammation play a role? *Current Psychiatry Reports, 17*, 78.

Dobson, D., & Dobson, K. (2009). *Evidence-based practice of cognitive-behavioral therapy.* New York: Guilford.

Eberhart, N., Auerbach, R., Bigda-Peyton, J., & Abela, J. (2011). Maladaptive schemas and depression: Tests of stress generation and diathesis-stress models. *Journal of Social and Clinical Psychology, 30*(1), 75–104.

Elwood, L., Mott, J., Williams, N., Lohr, J., & Schroeder, D. (2009). Attributional style and anxiety sensitivity as maintenance factors of posttraumatic stress symptoms: A prospective examination of a diathesis-stress model. *Journal of Behavior Therapy and Experimental Psychiatry, 40*, 544–557.

Eshelman, L. & Levendosky, A. (2012). Dating violence: Mental health consequences based on type of abuse. *Violence and Victims, 27*(2), 215–228.

Gibbs, Z., Lee, S., & Kulkarni, J. (2012). What factors determine whether a woman becomes depressed during the perimenopause? *Archives of Women's Mental Health, 15*, 323–332.

Goldberg, D., & Fawcett, J. (2012). The importance of anxiety in both major depression and bipolar disorder. *Depression and Anxiety, 29*, 471–478.

Granek, L., Danan, D., Bersudsky, Y., & Osher, Y. (2016). Living with bipolar disorder: The impact on patients, spouses, and their marital relationship. *Bipolar Disorders, 18*, 192–199.

Grubbs, K., Cheney, A., Fortney, J., Edlund, C., Han, X., Dubbert, P., Sherbourne, C., Craske, M., Stein, M., Roy-Byrne, P., & Sullivan, J. (2015). The role of gender in moderating treatment outcome in collaborative care for anxiety. *Psychiatric Services, 66*, 265–271.

Hettema, J., Aggen, S., Kubarych, T., Neale, M., & Kendler, K. (2015). Identification and validation of mixed anxiety–depression. *Psychological Medicine, 45*, 3075–3084.

Hodes, G. (2013). Sex, stress, and epigenetics: Regulation of behavior in animal models of mood disorders. *Biology of Sex Differences, 4*(1).

Hofmann, S., Sawyer, A., Witt, A., & Oh, D. (2010). The effect of mindfulness-based therapy on anxiety and depression: A meta-analytic review. *Journal of Consulting and Clinical Psychology, 78*(2), 169–183.

Hofmann, S., Wu, J., & Boettcher, H. (2014). Effect of cognitive-behavioral therapy for anxiety disorders on quality of life: A meta-analysis. *Journal of Consulting and Clinical Psychology, 82*(3), 375–391.

Kalmbach, D., Pillai, V., & Ciesla, J. (2016). The correspondence of changes in depressive rumination and worry to weekly variations in affective symptoms: A test of the tripartite model of anxiety and depression in women. *Australian Journal of Psychology, 68*, 52–60.

Kalmbach, D., Pillai, V., Kingsberg, S., & Ciesla, J. (2015). The transaction between depression and anxiety symptoms and sexual functioning: A prospective study of premenopausal, healthy women. *Archives of Sexual Behavior, 44*, 1535–1549.

Keyes, K., Agnew-Blais, J., Roberts, A., Hamilton, A., De Vivo, I., Ranu, H., & Koenen, K. (2015). The role of allelic variation in estrogen receptor genes and major depression in the Nurses Health Study. *Social Psychiatry and Psychiatric Epidemiology, 50*(12), 1893–1904.

Kleiber, B., & Dimidjian, S. (2014). Postpartum depression among adolescent mothers: A comprehensive review of prevalence, course, correlates, consequences, and interventions. *Clinical Psychology: Science and Practice, 21*(1), 48–66.

Kostic, M., Canu, E., Agosta, F., Munjiza, A., Novakovic, I., Dobricic, V., Maria Ferraro, P., Miler Jerkovic, V., Pekmezovic, T., Lecic Tosevski, D., & Filippi, M. (2016). The cumulative effect of genetic polymorphisms on depression and brain structural integrity. *Human Brain Mapping, 37*, 2173–2184.

Koszycki, D., Bisserbe, J., Blier, P., Bradwejn, J., & Markowitz, J. (2012). Interpersonal psychotherapy versus brief supportive therapy for depressed infertile women: First pilot randomized controlled trial. *Archives of Women's Mental Health, 15*, 193–201.

Leach, L., Butterworth, P., Olesen, S., & MacKinnon, A. (2013). Relationship quality and levels of depression and anxiety in a large population-based survey. *Social Psychiatry and Psychiatric Epidemiology, 48*, 417–425.

Leskin, G., & Sheikh, J. (2004). Gender differences in panic disorder. *Psychiatric Times, 21*(1), 65–66.

López-Solà, C., Fontenelle, L., Alonso, P., Cuadras, D., Foley D., Pantelis, C., Pujol, J., Yücel, M., Cardoner, N., Soriano-Mas, C., Menchón, J., & Harrison, B. (2014). Prevalence and heritability of obsessive-compulsive spectrum and anxiety disorder symptoms: A survey of the Australian twin registry. *American Journal of Medical Genetics, Part B 165*(B), 314–325.

Maack, D., Buchanan, E., & Young, J. (2015). Development and psychometric investigation of an inventory to assess fight, flight, and freeze tendencies: The fight, flight, freeze questionnaire. *Cognitive Behavioral Therapy, 44*(2), 117–127.

McLean, C., Asnaani, A., Litz, B., & Hofmann, S. (2011). Gender differences in anxiety disorders: Prevalence, course of illness, comorbidity and burden of illness. *Journal of Psychiatric Research, 45*, 1027–1035.

Maglione, J., Ancoli-Israel, S., Peters, K., Paudel, M., Yafe, K., Ensrud, K., Stone, K., and the Study of Osteoporotic Fractures Research Group. (2014). Subjective and objective sleep disturbance and longitudinal risk of depression in a cohort of older women. *Sleep, 37*(7), 1179–1187.

Mahon, J., Rohan, K., Nillni, Y., & Zvolenski, M. (2015). The role of perceived control over anxiety in prospective symptom reports across the menstrual cycle. *Archives of Women's Mental Health, 15*, 239–246.

Maina, G., Rosso, G., Guglia, A., & Bogetto, F. (2014). Recurrence rates of bipolar disorder during the postpartum period: A study on 276 medication-free Italian women. *Archives of Women's Mental Health, 17*, 367–372.

Marsh, W., Gershenson, B., & Rothschild, A. (2015). Sympton severity of bipolar disorder during the menopausal transition. *International Journal of Bipolar Disorders, 3*(17).

Miquel, L., Usall, J., Reed, C., Betsch, J., Vieta, E., Gonzalez-Pinto, A., Angst, J., Nolen, W., van Rossum, I., & Haro, J. (2011). Gender differences in outcomes of acute mania: A 12-month follow-up study. *Archives of Women's Mental Health, 14*, 107–113.

Morriss, R., Yang, M., Chopra, A., Bentall, R., Paykel, E., & Scott, J. (2013). Differential effects of depression and mania symptoms on social adjustment: Prospective study in bipolar disorder. *Bipolar Disorders, 15*(1), 80–91.

Nillni, Y., Berenz, E., Pineles, S., Coffey, S., & Zvolensky, M. (2014). Anxiety sensitivity as a moderator of the association between premenstrual symptoms and posttraumatic stress disorder symptom severity. *Psychological Trauma: Theory, Research, Practice, and Policy, 6*(2), 167–175.

Nivard, M., Dolan, C., Kendler, K., Kan, K., Willemsen, G., van Beijsterveldt, C., Lindauer, R., van Beek, J., Geels, L., Bartels, M., Middeldorp, C., & Boomsma, D. (2015). Stability in symptoms of anxiety and depression as a function of genotype and environment: A longitudinal twin study from ages 3 to 63 years. *Psychological Medicine, 45*(5), 1039–1049.

Norman, N., Van Emmerik, A., & Morina, N. (2014). The efficacy of metacognitive therapy for anxiety and depression: A meta-analytic review. *Depression and Anxiety, 31*, 402–411.

Norr, A., Albanese, B., Allan, N., & Schmidt, N. (2015). Anxiety sensitivity as a mechanism for gender discrepancies in anxiety and mood symptoms. *Journal of Psychiatric Research, 62*, 101–107.

Ouellet-Morin, I., Fisher, H., York-Smith, M., Fincham-Campbell, S., Moffitt, T., & Arsenaeault, L. (2015). Intimate partner violence and new-onset depression: A longitudinal study of women's childhood and adult histories of abuse. *Depression and Anxiety, 32*, 316–324.

Oquendo, M., McGrath, P., & Weissman, M. (2013). Biomarker studies and the future of personalized treatment for depression. *Depression and Anxiety, 31*, 902–905.

Patten, S., Williams, J., Lavorato, D., Wang, J., McDonald, K., & Bulloch, A. (2015). Descriptive epidemiology of major depressive disorder in Canada in 2012. *Canadian Journal of Psychiatry, 60*(1), 23–30.

Post, D., Gehlert, S., Hade, E., Reiter, P., Ruffin, M., & Paskett, E. (2013). Depression and SES in women from Appalachia. *Journal of Rural Mental Health, 37*(1), 2–15.

Sassoon, S., Colrain, I., & Baker, F. (2011). Personality disorders in women with severe premenstrual syndrome. *Archives of Women's Mental Health, 14*, 257–264.

Saunders, E., Fitzgerald, K., Zhang, P., & McInnis, M. (2012). Clinical features of bipolar disorder comorbid with anxiety disorders differ between men and women. *Depression and Anxiety, 29*, 739–746.

Seibell, P. J., Hamblin, R. J., & Hollander, E. (2015). Obsessive-compulsive disorder: Overview and standard treatment strategies. *Psychiatric Annals, 45*(6), 297–302.

Stewart, J., & Harkness, K. (2015). The interpersonal toxicity of excessive reassurance-seeking: Evidence from a longitudinal study of romantic relationships. *Journal of Social and Clinical Psychology, 34*(5), 392–410.

Thompson, K., & Bendell, D. (2014). Depressive cognitions, maternal attitudes, and postnatal depression. *Journal of Infant and Reproductive Psychology, 32*(1), 70–82.

Van de Velde, S., Bracke, P., & Levecque, K. (2010). Gender differences in depression in 23 European countries: Cross-national variation in the gender gap in depression. *Social Science in Medicine, 71*(2), 305–313.

Vencill, J., Tebbe, E., & Garos, S. (2015). It's not the size of the boat or the motion of the ocean: The role of self-objectification, appearance anxiety, and depression in female sexual functioning. *Psychology of Women Quarterly, 39*(4), 471–483.

Vollestad, J., Nielsen, M., & Nielsen, G. (2012). Mindfulness- and acceptance-based interventions for anxiety disorders: A systematic review and meta-analysis. *British Journal of Clinical Psychology, 51*(3), 239–260.

Waszczuk, M., Zavos, H., Antonova, E., Haworth, C., Plomin, R., & Eley, T. (2015). A multivariate twin study of trait mindfulness, depressive symptoms, and anxiety sensitivity. *Depression and Anxiety, 32*, 254–261.

Watkins, L., Jaffe, A., Hoffman, L., Gratz, K., Messman-Moore, T., & DiLillo, D. (2014). The longitudinal impact of intimate partner aggression and relationship status on women's physical health and depression symptoms. *Journal of Family Psychology, 28*(5), 655–665.

Weiss, S., Simeonova, D., Kimmel, M., Battle, C., Maki, P., & Flynn, H. (2015). Anxiety and physical health problems increase the odds of women having more severe symptoms of depression. *Archives of Women's Mental Health, 19*(3), 491–499.

Weissman, J., & Levine, S. (2007). Anxiety disorders and older women. *Journal of Women and Aging, 19*(1–2), 79–101.

Whitton, S., & Whisman, M. (2010). Relationship satisfaction instability and depression. *Journal of Family Psychology, 24*(6), 791–794.

Williams, L., Jacka, F., Pasco, J., Henry, M., Dodd, S., Nicholson, G., Kotowicz, M., & Berg, M. (2010). The prevalence of mood and anxiety disorders in Australian women. *Australasian Psychiatry, 18*(3).

Chapter Ten
Women, Trauma, and PTSD

Teresa López-Castro, Tanya Saraiya,
and Denise A. Hien

Beginning in the 1960s, activism and increasing public awareness heralded a new era of research chronicling the pervasiveness and consequences of violence against women. A product of this attention has been a body of epidemiological findings that suggest women are twice as likely as men to develop posttraumatic stress disorder (PTSD) in response to a traumatic event (Tolin & Foa, 2006). With this disparity in mind, this chapter will consider the kinds of traumatic experiences women confront across the lifespan, how responses to traumatic stress are transformed into posttraumatic difficulties, and why certain thera-peutic approaches may hold unique value for women survivors of violence.

Women and Trauma

We begin by charting women's lifetime risk for traumatic exposure, noting the critical developmental periods when trauma may leave its most indelible mark, and concluding with the phenomenon of revictimization as a means of under-standing the liability embedded within traumatic experiences.

Traumatic Exposure

Across a woman's lifespan, the risk for traumatic exposure increases from childhood to young adulthood, peaks at young or middle adulthood, and decreases in older adulthood (Breslau, 2009; Bright & Bowland, 2008). Men report more lifetime traumatic exposure, but women encounter more severe traumatic events, specifically interpersonal violence, that lead to greater detri-ment to their psychological and physical well-being (Tolin & Foa, 2006). These gender disparities begin in childhood when girls show a higher prevalence of child sexual abuse (19.7%) in comparison to boys (7.9%), and are associated with multiple types of victimization (Mccutcheon et al., 2010; Scher, Forde, McQuaid, & Stein, 2004). These rates suggest that, starting from childhood, being female is associated with greater exposure to sexual assault throughout the lifespan (Pratchett, Pelcovitz, & Yehuda, 2010).

Childhood Trauma

Previous research has suggested childhood trauma leads to the most severe outcomes in women, but recent findings point to adolescence as the most vulnerable time period for traumatic exposure with the most distressing long-term symptoms (Kaltman, Krupnick, Stockton, Hooper, & Green, 2005; Krupnick et al., 2004). Epidemiological data have corroborated these findings: across all female age groups; girls from the ages of 16 to 20 have the highest risk of traumatic exposure (Breslau, 2009). Traumatic exposure may not only be frequent in adolescence, but also particularly damaging given that adolescence is a developmental stage marked by change (Krupnick et al., 2004). Indeed, by the time a woman is in her early 20s, she has experienced multiple exposures to trauma: 80% to 85% of sophomore-aged female participants reported more than one traumatic experience (Green et al., 2000). As a woman progresses through late adolescence to early adulthood, the risk for non-assaultive violence decreases, but the risk for assaultive trauma rises after the age of 20 (Breslau, 2009).

Intimate Partner Violence

Intimate partner violence may be the main contributor to the peak in traumatic exposure from early adulthood to late adulthood. Women are three times more likely to experience intimate partner violence, in comparison to men, and experience severe intimate partner violence that can lead to debilitating physical injury and risk for homicide. Further, women suffering from intimate-partner violence are 22.5 times more likely to experience rape (Pratchett et al., 2010). Yet, beyond the high risk for intimate partner violence, women from their late 20s to early 30s are more likely to report multiple traumatic events rather than one (Mezey, Bacchus, Bewley, & White, 2005). Given that exposure to one trauma can increase the risk for being exposed to another trauma, the additive effects of multiple exposure in adult women are an ongoing area of investigation (Cortina & Kubiak, 2006; Pratchett et al., 2010).

Among older women, less research has focused on the prevalence or impact of traumatic exposure. Some studies report older women have a reduced risk for traumatic exposure (Cortina & Kubiak, 2006; Creamer & Parslow, 2008), while other studies, such as that by Wilke and Vinton (2005), have found women from the ages of 45 to 70 to experience higher rates of traumatic violence than younger women, and endure traumatic symptoms from cumulative trauma exposures (as cited by Bright & Bowland, 2008). Epidemiological data support the latter finding; the Minnesota Coalition for Battered Women (2006) found a quarter of women murdered by their partners to be over the age of 55 (as cited by Bright & Bowland, 2008). These numbers suggest that, although researchers have presumed traumatic exposure decreases after middle adulthood in women, it may, in fact, increase across the lifespan.

Revictimization

Research has repeatedly found that female survivors of childhood sexual abuse have a greater probability of experiencing another traumatic occurrence, particularly adulthood sexual abuse or intimate partner violence, in comparison to non-traumatized women; this is known as revictimization (Messman & Long, 1996; Roodman & Clum, 2001). Messman and Long's (1996) seminal review found that 16% to 72% of child sexual abuse survivors, in a primarily White sample, experienced sexual victimization as adults. Put another way, child sexual abuse survivors are 1.5 to 2 times more likely to be assaulted as adolescents or adults than women without a history of child sexual abuse (Arata, 2002). While the influence of childhood sexual abuse on adulthood intimate partner violence, sexual assault, and self-harm behaviors has been well researched, the impact of childhood physical abuse has been less studied (Arata, 2002; Noll, Horowitz, Bonanno, Trickett, & Putnam, 2003). Some research has found childhood physical abuse does not predict physical violence (Arata, 2002), while other research found childhood physical abuse predicts intimate partner violence (Kuijpers, van der Knaap, & Lodewijks, 2011).

Interestingly, despite their co-occurrence, childhood sexual abuse is not a direct predictor of revictimization (Messman-Moore & Brown, 2006; Noll et al., 2003). Instead, substance use, risky behaviors, poor risk recognition, and posttraumatic symptoms from childhood trauma are better direct predictors of revictimization (Breslau, Chilcoat, Kessler, & Davis, 1999; Noll et al., 2003). For example, one study found that revictimized women present more difficulty leaving a hypothetical rape scenario in comparison to non-traumatized women (Messman-Moore & Brown, 2006).

Another line of research has found that adolescent trauma, adolescent risky behaviors, and risky sexual behaviors are all potential mediators between childhood sexual abuse and revictimization (Arata, 2002; Fargo, 2009). However, beyond all of these variables, posttraumatic avoidance, hypervigilance, and re-experiencing symptoms present the strongest predictors of revictimization (Arata, 2002; Messman-Moore, Ward, & Brown, 2009). In fact, posttraumatic symptoms not only increase the risk for revictimization, but also are a result of revictimization. Thus, the cycle between repeated trauma exposure and trauma-related distress suggests that understanding the course of traumatic stress along a woman's lifespan could have widespread effects on reducing chronic pathology as well as subsequent exposure (Bright & Bowland, 2008; Kuijpers et al., 2011).

Women and Trauma-Related Disorders

The majority of women, like men, survive horrific experiences without developing psychological problems. Following a normative distress reaction to the fear/helplessness/horror of a traumatic event, women's posttraumatic course can range widely from growth to pathology (Bonanno et al., 2012; Norris, Tracy, & Galea, 2009). Of critical concern to trauma disorder researchers are the pathways from *distress to disorder*. Other courses, such as posttraumatic resilience and growth trajectories, have traditionally received far less attention, although this is rapidly changing (Vishnevsky, Cann, Calhoun, Tedeschi, & Demakis, 2010). Research has converged to understand the risk for posttraumatic problems as an outcome of complex biopsychosocial processes. Indeed, some have described PTSD as a "biopsychosocial trap" wherein dysfunctions in one domain prohibit the initiation of recovery processes in another (van der Kolk, McFarlane, & Weisaeth, 1996).

The following section will discuss some of the particularities of the biopsychosocial transformation from posttraumatic distress to disorder that are especially relevant to women. We begin with a brief definition of the most recognized posttrauma pathology, PTSD, and its prevalence amongst women. A natural rejoinder is the role of trauma exposure, and the pernicious impact of interpersonal violence in predicting PTSD and other common trauma-related difficulties.

Another extensive area of study has yielded valuable insights on the relationship of peri- and posttraumatic cognitions and affect to PTSD development. To further explore women's risk for trauma-related problems, we turn first to the interaction of biological sex differences and the neurobiological disruptions of traumatic stress, and then to the influence of gender socialization on posttrauma coping styles. Looking beyond the diagnosis of PTSD, we conclude by discussing other frequently experienced psychiatric problems and the complex adaptations in self-regulation and identity that may occur in trauma's wake.

Definition of PTSD

Of the wide range of psychological and biological adaptations that may take place after experiencing a traumatic event, the diagnosis of PTSD represents the most systematically investigated of these consequences. PTSD is an alarmingly common, yet heterogeneous, disorder associated with a substantial degree of life dysfunction, disability, and morbidity (Schnurr, Friedman, Sengupta, Jankowski, & Holmes, 2000). In broad terms, PTSD can be considered an information-processing disorder wherein trauma-related information derails how an individual organizes, integrates, and responds to current experience (van der Kolk et al., 1996). PTSD's most recent *Diagnostic and Statistical*

Manual of Mental Disorders (DSM-5: American Psychiatric Association, 2013) definition is comprised of four symptom clusters: (1) the intrusion of trauma-related memory and/or sensations; (2) avoidance of trauma reminders; (3) negative cognitions and mood; and (4) alterations in arousal and reactivity.

PTSD Prevalence

Repeated findings from large-scale epidemiological surveys point to a troubling gender difference in trauma exposure and PTSD. In the National Comorbidity Survey, a nationally representative sample of Americans, 61% of men and 51% of women reported being exposed to traumatic events during their lifetime, yet 10% of women developed PTSD compared to 5% of men (Kessler, 1995; Kessler et al., 2005), reflecting a twofold greater vulnerability for PTSD among women. Similarly, the Detroit Area Survey of Trauma found 92.2% of men to be exposed to trauma in comparison to 87.1% of women, but women to show a twofold risk of lifetime PTSD in comparison to men (13.0% vs. 6.2%, respectively) (Breslau et al., 1999; Breslau, 2009). Internationally, a survey of 1,784 individuals in Sweden found a greater percentage of men exposed to trauma than women (84% vs. 77%), with women having a greater lifetime conditional risk for PTSD than men (7.4% vs. 3.6%), while, contrastingly, research in Australia found no gender difference in current PTSD prevalence rates (Creamer, Burgess, & McFarlane, 2001).

This discrepancy in international epidemiological data is due to the prevalence of specific traumatic events, and differences in current PTSD versus lifetime PTSD. Both assaultive and sexual trauma have a tenfold greater risk of leading to PTSD in comparison to losing a loved one, and assaultive and sexual experiences are more common in females than in males (Aiim et al., 2006; Perkonigg, Kessler, Storz, & Wittchen, 2000). Australia's lower rates of sexual violence could account for the absence of gender differences in PTSD (Creamer et al., 2001). Furthermore, Perkonigg et al. (2000) found no gender differences in current PTSD, suggesting that gender differences present in lifetime PTSD rates because the course of PTSD across a woman's lifespan may be more chronic.

Trauma Type and PTSD Risk

Various theories have been put forth to explain women's greater odds of developing PTSD. The "situational-vulnerability hypothesis" (Pimlott-Kubiak & Cortina, 2003) attributes the increased likelihood of PTSD in women to the type or severity of trauma women are exposed to. As aforementioned, women are more likely to be exposed to chronic high-impact traumas, such as childhood sexual abuse and rape. Men, in contrast, are more likely to be exposed to non-sexual physical assaults, combat traumas, or accidents (Tolin & Breslau, 2007). This difference in type of trauma exposure is critical since it is known that sexual violence is one of the highest risk factors for the development of PTSD. Studies show that, compared to other types of traumas (e.g., physical assault or combat), rape exposure is most strongly associated with PTSD (Norris, Foster, & Weisshaar, 2002).

Others, however, point to research that controlled for type of trauma exposure and found that women's risk for developing PTSD remained twofold (Olff, Langeland, Draijer, & Gersons, 2007). An often-cited meta-analysis by Tolin and Foa (2006) determined that women and girls were still more likely to develop PTSD after controlling for histories of childhood sexual abuse, as well as following exposure to non-sexual assault. Certain methodological limitations have since been noted, but perhaps the most salient critique against Tolin and Foa (2006) has argued that non-sexual assault experiences cannot be considered equivalent across gender since women must contend with disproportionately more threat of non-sexual assaults becoming sexual (Pratchett et al., 2010). Indeed, assigning accurate weight to the trauma type and frequency has proved challenging, leaving the etiological contribution of trauma type to PTSD gender differences currently unresolved.

Peritraumatic and Posttraumatic Responses

Despite the uncertainty around the severity of non-equivalent trauma exposures in men and women, it is known that reactions to a traumatic event directly influence the risk of PTSD onset (Irish et al., 2011). For women, research has debated what posttraumatic reactions could lead to the twofold risk for PTSD development. Three specific factors—affective reactions, dissociation, and cognitive appraisals of a traumatic event—are common peritraumatic and posttraumatic reactions in women and known contributors to PTSD development in females (Olff et al., 2007). Women in particular appear to experience emotional reactions of intense fear, helplessness, and horror after a traumatic event—acute stress responses, which men are less likely to present (Brewin et al., 2002). Women also experience higher levels of peritraumatic dissociation—the loss of time, place, and inability to experience one's bodily emotions during a traumatic event. Peritraumatic dissociation encourages avoidant coping styles, which then predict the development of PTSD (Irish et al., 2011). Further, women are more likely to appraise traumatic events negatively, partially because of their enhanced threat perception and awareness of threat cues (Irish et al., 2011; Norris et al., 2002). Yet, this enhanced threat perception also makes women more susceptible to fear conditioning after a traumatic event, making the likelihood of developing PTSD in women even more probable (Inslicht et al., 2013). Given that avoidance of stimuli related to a traumatic event, and negative cognitions of oneself and the world are part of the DSM-5 diagnosis for PTSD, it is somewhat unsurprising that these two reactions after a traumatic event lead to increased susceptibility to PTSD development.

In addition to dissociation and cognitive appraisals of trauma, the literature has suggested the prevalence of shame, guilt, isolation, and low self-worth in women's reactions to trauma (Bright & Bowland, 2008). Shame and guilt have been associated with posttraumatic stress symptoms, depression, and avoidance behavior, while isolation has been associated with greater dissociation, depression, and posttraumatic symptoms (Shin et al., 2015; Srinivas, DePrince, & Chu, 2015). A repetitive cycle seems to happen in women's reactions to trauma, where women experience emotional reactions to traumatic events that they are unable to regulate, often utilizing avoidant and suppressive emotion regulation strategies. As a result of this, women may experience dissociation, negative appraisals, or somatization of symptoms, which in turn lead to PTSD (Lilly, Pole, Best, Metzler, & Marmar, 2009). Consequently, the continual experience of these emotional reactions, and the inability to regulate them effectively, can yield chronic PTSD.

A final factor that may influence posttraumatic symptoms in a woman is disclosure of the traumatic event. In contrast to men, the timing of disclosure can influence the onset of PTSD and posttraumatic distress levels in women. Ullman and Filipas (2005) found that negative reactions to a woman's experience of victimization can lead to more psychological harm. More specifically, disclosure of severe forms of abuse, stranger attacks, and longer episodes of abuse elicited negative reactions by others (Ullman & Filipas, 2005). This suggests that, for women with severe abuse, the inability to disclose and receive a positive reaction will contribute to increased self-blame, greater dissociation, and eventually greater risk for PTSD onset.

Neurobiological Factors

Another line of research has explored the impact of the female stress regulatory system on resilience and pathology related to traumatic stress (Peirce, Newton, Buckley, & Keane, 2002; Rasmusson & Friedman, 2002). It is known that women have a more sensitive stress response system after adolescence than men do normatively (e.g., Desantis et al., 2011; Romeo & McEwen, 2006). Following exposure to threats or trauma, hyperactivation of fear-processing networks in women can lead to ongoing stress dysregulation and PTSD (Olff et al., 2007). If fear-processing networks are more readily activated in women during trauma, sustained arousal may follow the trauma and increase the risk for developing PTSD (Bryant, Creamer, O'Donnell, Silove, & McFarlane, 2008). Compared to men, women have been also observed to normatively possess a sharper neuroendocrine response to both acute and chronic stress, evident in alterations in the hypothalamic–pituitary–adrenal (HPA) axis (Bale & Epperson, 2015; Rasmusson & Friedman, 2002). Notwithstanding a diagnosis of PTSD, there is clear evidence that trauma exposure, especially early-childhood trauma, is linked to HPA axis dysregulation in women. In addition to sex hormones, women's oxytocin-mediated responses to trauma have been shown to provide resiliency (Heim & Nemeroff, 2001; Heim et al., 2009).

Importantly, developmental studies of animal (e.g., Cohen & Yehuda, 2011) and human subjects (Bale & Epperson, 2015) reveal that biological sex differences in stress-related dysregulation pathways appear sensitive to critical periods in maturation throughout the lifespan. The pathways are impacted independently by gonadal hormones in early childhood, adolescence, perimenopause (e.g., Freeman et al., 2004; Romeo & McEwen, 2006), and by genes on the sex chromosomes, where both sex hormones and gene interactions shape neural plasticity (e.g., Andersen & Teicher, 2008; Andersen et al., 2008). Studies identify that the regions of neurocircuitry involved in regulation of stress and mood, which include the prefrontal cortex, amygdala, hypothalamus, and hippocampus, mature throughout the pubertal period in human and animal models. These neurobiological processes may explain why for women the developmental period of adolescence has been consistently documented as a such a vulnerable window for stress dysregulation caused by external trauma (Desantis et al., 2011; Kajantie & Phillips, 2006; Ladd, Huot, Thrivikraman, Nemeroff, & Plotsky, 2004; Teicher, Andersen, Polcari, Anderson, & Navalta, 2002).

Gender Socialization and Coping Styles

Social processes, such as gender role socialization, have been heavily implicated in shaping how women respond and cope in the aftermath of trauma (Christiansen & Elklit, 2011; Olff et al., 2007). In particular, certain gendered coping styles often attributed to women are known to carry unique sets of protective and risk factors, forming multiple pathways to posttraumatic health and posttraumatic distress.

The arena of social support offers a compelling example of the interaction between gendered coping responses and posttraumatic risk and resilience. The engagement of social support has long been understood as a powerful buffer against PTSD development (Ozer, Best, Lipsey, & Weiss, 2003). Gender socialization literature has suggested that women are more likely than men to employ *emotion-focused coping*, exemplified by seeking out social support, as well as expressing emotion, i.e., "tend and befriend" strategies (Taylor et al., 2000). Thus, it is likely that women's suite of relationally oriented efforts—from pursuing social contact to interpersonally processing stressful events—enhances the likelihood of posttraumatic resilience. In turn, the reliance on socioemotional resources has also been shown to impart a differential risk for women. Compared to men, women are not only subject to more negative social interactions (i.e., criticism, rejected requests for assistance); they are more impacted by these relational ruptures in the wake of trauma, evidenced by higher posttraumatic symptom severity than men with equivalent social support disruptions (Andrews, Brewin, & Rose, 2003).

It is noteworthy that, following trauma exposure, women have also been found to utilize avoidance coping approaches, such as drinking. Some have theorized that these avoidance efforts may serve as a form of continued dissociation employed specifically when "tend and befriend" attempts prove ineffective (Christiansen & Elklit, 2011). As mentioned earlier, peri- and posttraumatic dissociative responses increase risk for PTSD and slow down the rate of recovery from posttraumatic stress. In turn, research has suggested that women are less prone than men to rely on what some consider "fight or flight" responses (Christiansen & Elklit, 2011)—displaying aggressive behaviors and using problem-focused coping, such as seeking practical or material support. In sum, the manner in which women implement certain combinations of coping responses may considerably influence the development or maintenance of PTSD symptoms.

Beyond PTSD: Other Trauma-Related Issues

PTSD is frequently comorbid with at least one additional psychiatric diagnosis. Based upon findings from the National Comorbidity Study (Kessler, 1995), approximately 80% of women with PTSD meet criteria for at least one other psychiatric diagnosis, with 17% having one other diagnosis, 18% having two other diagnoses, and 44% having three or more additional diagnoses. The most common comorbid conditions with PTSD are substance use disorders (28% alcohol use disorders, 27% substance use disorders), affective disorders (49% major depression, 23% dysthymia, and 6% mania), and other anxiety disorders (ranging from 15% generalized anxiety to 28% with social and 29% with simple phobias). Clients with chronic trauma beginning in childhood are also likely to have a variety of additional psychiatric problems, including dissociation, poor impulse control, and personality-related disturbances. Consistent findings (although lower overall rates of PTSD and posttraumatic stress exposures) in a German sample (Perkonigg et al., 2000) reveal that, following traumatic events, disorders that occur along with PTSD included single or recurrent depressive disorders (62.4%), drug abuse and dependence (65.9%), nicotine dependence (60.0%), and agoraphobia with or without panic disorder, and over 60% of these occurred post trauma exposure.

Recent latent class analysis on a sample of 409 individuals with PTSD (Galatzer-Levy, Nickerson, Litz, & Marmar, 2013) has revealed that there were three patterns of lifetime comorbidity associated with PTSD in this sample. One was characterized by comorbid mood and anxiety disorders; one by comorbid mood, anxiety, and substance use disorders; and the third was a low-comorbidity "pure" PTSD class. Each of the two high-comorbidity patterns had significantly greater severity in terms of PTSD symptoms, suicidal ideation, and domestic violence compared with the pure PTSD group.

Although overall comorbidity rates do not appear different for men and women with PTSD, the *types* of associated disorders do. For example, in contrast to national epidemiology findings among those *without* PTSD, women are two times more likely than men to meet criteria for a depressive disorder, whereas for those *with* PTSD, women have concurrent depressive disorders at equal rates to men (Brady, 1997; Kessler, 1995). Women with comorbid conditions are more likely than men to have PTSD as their primary diagnosis and the typical drinking pattern is more likely to be episodic binge drinking than heavy drinking (Peirce et al., 2002). In line with national epidemiology estimates, women with PTSD are less likely to be diagnosed with antisocial personality disorder and more likely to be diagnosed with borderline personality and panic disorders (Keane & Kaloupek, 1997; Kessler, 1995). When patterns of comorbidity were examined, among three classes (two high comorbidity and one low), women were less likely to fall into the substance dependence comorbidity pattern than men (Galatzer-Levy et al., 2013). On the other hand, despite the findings that men show higher levels of comorbid alcohol use, more women start drinking excessively after trauma (Back, Brady, Sonne, & Verduin, 2006; Deykin & Buka, 1997).

Thus, it bears noting that the relationship between PTSD and other associated disorders is often quite complex. The extent to which associated disorders typically follow the onset of PTSD remains unclear. There appear to be multiple pathways resulting in several different subtypes of PTSD, rather than generalizable patterns of cause and effect. For example, whereas some individuals presenting with PTSD had pre-existing psychological problems prior to exposure to trauma, others developed additional disorders secondary to the onset of PTSD and its often-debilitating symptoms. There are also those for whom PTSD and related psychiatric conditions developed simultaneously at the time of trauma exposure.

The substantial degree of overlap between PTSD and many other psychiatric disorders, most notably depression (i.e., sleep disturbance and social withdrawal), and other anxiety disorders (i.e., panic attacks and avoidance), has led some experts to believe that the PTSD diagnosis is inherently limited in that it fails to take into account the complexity of adaptation to trauma. This argument has led to the proposal that many conditions classified as comorbid disorders should instead be recognized as part of a complex range of trauma-related problems, rather than conceptualized as separate and discrete disorders (van der Kolk et al., 1996). Although future investigation is needed to clarify these issues, at present we do know that exposure to early, severe, and chronic trauma is associated with multifaceted adaptations to trauma, often characterized by impulse control deficits, unstable emotions and relationships, and disruptions in consciousness, memory, identity, and/or perception of the environment. Referred to as complex PTSD (CPTSD) (Courtois & Ford, 2014), or disorders of extreme stress not otherwise specified (DESNOS) (Pelcovitz et al., 1997), the diagnostic formulation of these alterations in self, affect, and relationships has been widely accepted by the clinical field, despite formal exclusion from the DSM-5.

In conclusion, a growing body of neurobiological findings on early trauma exposure and later disruptions in HPA axis functioning suggest gender-specific pathways to development of PTSD and other psychiatric comorbidities. Regardless of etiology, the presence of other psychiatric disorders typically worsens and prolongs the course of PTSD and also complicates clinical assessment and diagnosis. In addition, the presence of additional psychiatric disorders often exacerbates PTSD symptoms and can prolong the course of the disorder.

Women and Trauma Recovery: Therapeutic Considerations

Facilitating Treatment Entry

Research has found that emotional, physical, and sexual abuse female survivors have high health care utilization rates (Lang et al., 2003; Rayburn et al., 2005; Sansone, Wiederman, & Sansone, 1997). However, health care utilization revolves around women addressing secondary symptoms, such as anxiety, sadness, and sleeping issues, with their primary care physicians (Mezey, Bacchus, & Bewley, 2005). Treatment for trauma victimization itself is less common (Acierno, 1997; Mezey et al., 2005). Most physicians fail to screen for traumatization in women, in fear of asking invasive questions and being unable to assist if women are being traumatized (Acierno, 1997). This is unfortunate, given that over 75% of both traumatized and non-traumatized women want regular trauma screenings by their primary care physicians (Friedman et al., 1992, as cited by Acierno, 1997).

Yet, the way trauma is screened is essential in encouraging treatment entry. Secondary traumatization, feeling traumatized by how one is examined or questioned in a medical or mental health care facility, is a common occurrence that prevents women from seeking treatment. Campbell and Raja (2005) found female veterans to be hesitant to enter mental health treatment because staff and procedures could elicit feelings of guilt and symptoms of depression. Similarly, female civilians may re-experience posttraumatic symptoms when physically examined by male practitioners, suggesting that, while primary care physicians should screen for trauma, skill, sensitivity, and compassion in screening are imperative to encourage treatment entrance (Mezey et al., 2005).

Validated PTSD Treatments

Fortunately, a number of well-validated psychotherapies are available to address PTSD-related problems across the lifespan (Foa, Keane, Friedman, & Cohen, 2009). Advances in the field of child and adolescent trauma treatment have produced a wealth of interventions targeting PTSD symptoms in multiply traumatized children across school, home, and clinic settings (Cohen, 2010). To date, cognitive-behavioral approaches for adult PTSD remain the most empirically studied of interventions and have garnered substantial evidence for their efficacy (Foa et al., 2009). Of these, exposure-based therapies, such as prolonged exposure and cognitive processing therapy, are regarded as *the* first-line treatments for adult PTSD (Institute of Medicine, 2008). Manualized and widely disseminated, they involve the cognitive and affective processing of traumatic memories in conjunction with the extinction of trauma-related fear responses through systematic confrontation of safe, yet avoided, situations and activities.

Additionally, in light of the known alterations in critical neurobiological processes associated with traumatic stress, research on PTSD pharmacotherapy has surged in the past decade, with evidence mounting for the value of antidepressants, specifically selective serotonin reuptake inhibitors (SSRIs) and serotonin-norepinephrine reuptake inhibitors (SNRIs). Proponents of psychopharmacological agents point to the collateral benefit of their use in ameliorating frequently comorbid conditions such as major depression and anxiety disorders (Foa et al., 2009). The remission rates after SSRI/SNRI treatments, however, lag significantly behind that of cognitive-behavioral therapy-based interventions (Ipser & Stein, 2012). Thus, their use is presently understood to be limited to the reduction of, rather than recovery from, PTSD symptomatology (Hoskins et al., 2015). Moreover, like most pharmacotherapies for anxiety and mood disorders, associated gains are only maintained with the indefinite continuation of medication. With evidence suggesting that adjunctive pharmacotherapy can boost psychotherapy gains, clinical researchers have lately turned to the study of combined approaches, wherein psychological and pharmacological interventions are optimally integrated (Hien et al., 2015).

Tailoring Treatment to Women's Needs

Few PTSD interventions are formally considered women-specific. However, most empirically supported treatments to date have been studied in largely women-only samples (Foa et al., 1999), and, from the limited data available, women have been shown to respond equally to—if not better than—men to the traditional suite of PTSD treatments (Blain, Galovski, & Robinson, 2010). Nevertheless, attention to particular proximal, pragmatic considerations— such as home environment, childcare, level of social support and practical resources—may not only support a woman's entry into treatment, but raise the likelihood of retention and positive response to therapeutic intervention. Moreover, certain conceptual approaches are relevant to women's recovery given the nature of traumas predominantly experienced by girls and women.

As previously mentioned, individuals with histories of repeated victimization may contend with significant psychological disruptions that fall outside the exclusive domain of PTSD, frequently emerging as psychiatric comorbidities (i.e., major depression, substance use disorders), and/or the profound alterations in self-regulation and identity associated with CPTSD and DESNOS. For survivors of prolonged and repeated interpersonal trauma, clinical consensus and empirical evidence have increasingly coalesced in support of multimodal, comprehensive care (Courtois & Ford, 2014). In sum, therapies must speak to overarching problems related to somatization, dissociation, and emotion dysregulation that reach beyond disorder-specific difficulties, and are aptly described as the legacy of an "interrupted life" (Cloitre, Cohen, & Koenen, 2006).

In her seminal work on trauma-related disorders, Judith Herman (1992) proposed the idea that recovery from prolonged and repeated exposure to traumatic stress occurs in progression through recognizable stages, beginning with the establishment of safety, moving through the processing of traumatic memories, and culminating with the reconnection of social ties. The tripartite model of recovery stages has been widely adopted as a framework for treating prolonged, repeated trauma exposure with approaches falling into the three broad categories of stabilization, processing, and reintegration.

An important outgrowth of these conceptual stages is an appreciation of the value of sequencing interventions to the needs of the client. In order to not only be effective but avoid iatrogenic harm, therapeutic techniques should be matched to clients' specific stage of recovery. From a stage model perspective, therapies such as prolonged exposure or cognitive processing therapy are most beneficial when they are implemented after the early recovery work of establishing personal safety. Designed originally for women survivors of childhood abuse, Skills Training in Affect and Interpersonal Regulation (STAIR: Cloitre et al., 2006) is emblematic of a phase-based approach wherein social and emotional competencies are developed and strengthened prior to commencing trauma-processing work.

In addition to a staged recovery conceptualization, several considerations and modalities are especially salient for the treatment of chronic interpersonal trauma. Always a fundamental backdrop of psychotherapy, the quality of the therapeutic relationship has emerged as a critical factor in recovery in cases of prolonged and repeated trauma (Courtois, 1999). To cultivate and maintain a working alliance, therapists must effectively manage the unique challenges posed by the client's attachment history, including the likelihood of relational re-enactments of trauma and transference/countertransference dilemmas (Dalenberg, 2000). Paramount to working with prolonged and repeated trauma survivors is the establishment of safety through a variety of efforts, collaborative in nature, and focused on provision of clear goals, expectations, and boundaries for therapist and client alike (Cloitre et al., 2006).

Given the social and interpersonal ramifications of trauma-related disorders, systemic treatment modalities such as family, couple, and group psychotherapy have been noted as natural allies in women's recovery from trauma (Courtois & Ford, 2014). Group psychotherapy, for instance, provides a variety of therapeutic benefits across stages of recovery. During the stabilization stage, the homogeneity of a women's group may scaffold the work of self-care and safety building; later in recovery, the group becomes a living representation of each member's effort to reconnect with a greater social world (Herman, 1992).

Overall, as with psychotherapies for other disorders, stronger therapeutic alliance between client and clinician has been shown to be associated with greater retention in trauma-related treatments (e.g., Barber et al., 2001; Ruglass et al., 2012). In support of multimodal care, attendance of 12-step meetings has been associated with retention in treatment programs (Laudet, Magura, Cleland, Vogel, & Knight, 2003; Pinto, Campbell, Hien, Yu, & Gorroochurn, 2011). Interestingly, our knowledge of how women's PTSD treatment outcomes compare to that of men's remains limited. A comprehensive review of empirical studies examining gender differences in PTSD treatment response found that, while a majority of the studies reviewed did not detect differential treatment responses by gender, some significant differences did emerge (Blain et al., 2010). Women were more likely to benefit from trauma-focused treatment and less likely than men to drop out of treatment. Future directions in clinical research have prioritized the identifying optimal treatment pathways for traumatized women.

Summary

Across the lifespan, women inevitably confront the possibility of being exposed to high-impact traumas—most often sexual and physical violence, likely perpetuated by an attachment figure. In the wake of these experiences, most women will demonstrate astonishing resilience. However, for a subset of women, these traumatic experiences lay the groundwork for a vicious cycle of revictimization and a chronic course of trauma-related psychopathology. Research into the biopsychosocial processes activated during and after trauma exposure has deepened our understanding of women's relative risk for trauma-related disorders and underscored the complex adaptations to cognition, affect, and neurobiology which occur in trauma's wake. When treatment is warranted, an assortment of empirically supported interventions is currently available to help women address the psychological disturbances caused by traumatic experiences. Although traditional PTSD-directed therapies, centered on cognitive and affective processing, have proven efficacious for chronic PTSD, a stage recovery model may be especially suited to the unique needs of women survivors of prolonged and repeated violence.

References

Acierno, R. (1997). Health impact of interpersonal violence 1. *Behavioral Medicine, 23*(2), 53.

Aiim, T. N., Graves, E., Meilman, T. A., Aigbogun, N., Gray, E., Lawson, W., & Charney, D. S. (2006). Trauma exposure, posttraumatic stress disorder and depression in an African-American primary care population. *Journal of the National Medical Association, 98*(10), 1630–1636.

American Psychiatric Association. (2013). *Diagnostic and statistical manual of mental disorders: DSM-5.* Washington, D.C.: American Psychiatric Association.

Andersen, S. L., & Teicher, M. H. (2008). Stress, sensitive periods and maturational events in adolescent depression. *Trends in Neurosciences, 31,* 183–191.

Andersen, S. L., Tomada, A., Vincow, E. S., Valente, E., Polcari, A., & Teicher, M. H. (2008). Preliminary evidence for sensitive periods in the effect of childhood sexual abuse on regional brain development. *Journal of Neuropsychiatry and Clinical Neurosciences, 20*(3), 292–301. http://doi.org/10.1176/appi.neuropsych.20.3.292.

Andrews, B., Brewin, C. R., & Rose, S. (2003). Gender, social support, and PTSD in victims of violent crime. *Journal of Traumatic Stress, 16*(4), 421–427. http://doi.org/10.1023/A:1024478305142.

Arata, C. M. (2002). Child sexual abuse and sexual revictimization. *Clinical Psychology: Science and Practice, 9*(2), 135–164.

Back, S. E., Brady, K. T., Sonne, S. C., & Verduin, M. L. (2006). Symptom improvement in co-occurring PTSD and alcohol dependence. *Journal of Nervous and Mental Disease, 194*(9), 690–696. http://doi.org/10.1097/01.nmd.0000235794.12794.8a.

Bale, T. L., & Epperson, C. N. (2015). Sex differences and stress across the lifespan. *Nature Neuroscience, 18*(10), 1413–1420.

Barber, J. P., Luborsky, L., Gallop, R., Crits-Christoph, P., Frank, A., Hospital, B., . . . & Siqueland, L. (2001). Therapeutic alliance as a predictor of outcome and retention in the National Institute on Drug Abuse Collaborative Cocaine Treatment Study. *Journal of Consulting and Clinical Psychology, 69*(1), 119–124. http://doi.org/10.1037//0022-006X.69.U19.

Blain, L. M., Galovski, T. E., & Robinson, T. (2010). Gender differences in recovery from post-traumatic stress disorder: A critical review. *Aggression and Violent Behavior, 15*(6), 463–474. http://doi.org/10.1016/j.avb.2010.09.001.

Bonanno, G. A., Mancini, A. D., Horton, J. L., Powell, T. M., LeardMann, C. A., Boyko, E. J., . . . & Smith, T. C. (2012). Trajectories of trauma symptoms and resilience in deployed US military service members: Prospective cohort study. *British Journal of Psychiatry, 200*(4), 317–323. http://doi.org/10.1192/bjp.bp.111.096552.

Brady, K. T. (1997). Posttraumatic stress disorder and comorbidity: Recognizing the many faces of PTSD. *Journal of Clinical Psychiatry, 58,* 12–15.

Breslau, N. (2009). The epidemiology of trauma, PTSD, and other posttrauma disorders. *Trauma, Violence, and Abuse, 10*(3), 198–210. http://doi.org/10.1177/1524838009334448.

Breslau, N., Chilcoat, H. D., Kessler, R. C., & Davis, G. C. (1999). Previous exposure to trauma and PTSD effects of subsequent trauma: Results from the Detroit area survey of trauma. *American Journal of Psychiatry, 156*(6), 902–907.

Brewin, C. R., Rose, S., Andrews, B., Green, J., Tata, P., McEvedy, C., . . . & Foa, E. B. (2002). Brief screening instrument for post-traumatic stress disorder. *British Journal of Psychiatry, 181,* 158–162. http://doi.org/10.1192/bjp.181.2.158.

Bright, C. L. Y. N., & Bowland, S. E. (2008). Assessing interpersonal trauma in older adult women. *Journal of Loss and Trauma, 13*(4), 373–393. http://doi.org/10.1080/15325020701771523.

Bryant, R. A., Creamer, M., O'Donnell, M. L., Silove, D., & McFarlane, A. C. (2008). A multisite study of the capacity of acute stress disorder diagnosis to predict posttraumatic stress disorder. *Journal of Clinical Psychiatry, 69*(6), 923–929.

Campbell, R., & Raja, S. (2005). The sexual assault and secondary victimization of female veterans: Help-seeking experiences with military and civilian social systems. *Psychology of Women Quarterly, 29*(1), 97–106. http://doi.org/10.1111/j.1471-6402.2005.00171.x.

Christiansen, D. M., & Elklit, A. (2011). Sex differences in PTSD. In A. Lazinica & E. Ovuga (Eds.), *Post traumatic stress disorders in a global context* (pp. 113–142). Rijeka: Open Access Publisher.

Cloitre, M., Cohen, L. R., & Koenen, K. C. (2006). *Treating survivors of childhood abuse: Psychotherapy for the interrupted life.* New York: Guilford Press.

Cohen, H., & Yehuda, R. (2011). Gender differences in animal models of posttraumatic stress disorder. *Disease Markers, 30*(2–3), 141–150.

Cohen, J. A. (2010). Practice parameter for the assessment and treatment of children and adolescents with posttraumatic stress disorder. *Journal of the American Academy of Child and Adolescent Psychiatry, 49*(4), 414–430. http://doi.org/10.1016/j.jaac.2009.12.020.

Cortina, L. M., & Kubiak, S. P. (2006). Gender and posttraumatic stress: Sexual violence as an explanation for women's increased risk. *Journal of Abnormal Psychology, 115*(4), 753–759. http://doi.org/10.1037/0021-843X.115.4.753.

Courtois, C. A. (1999). *Recollections of sexual abuse: Treatment principles and guidelines.* New York: W.W. Norton.

Courtois, C. A., & Ford, J. D. (2014). *Treating complex traumatic stress disorders: Scientific foundations and therapeutic models.* New York: Guilford Press.

Creamer, M., Burgess, P., & McFarlane, A. C. (2001). Post-traumatic stress disorder: Findings from the Australian National Survey of Mental Health and Well-being. *Psychological Medicine, 31*(7), 1237–1247. http://doi.org/10.1017/S0033291701004287.

Creamer, M., & Parslow, R. (2008). Posttraumatic stress disorder in the elderly. *American Journal of Geriatric Psychiatry, 16*(10), 853–856. http://doi.org/10.1097/01.JGP.0000310785.36837.85.

Dalenberg, C. (2000). *Countertransference and the treatment of trauma.* Washington, DC: American Psychological Association.

Desantis, S. M., Baker, N. L., Back, S. E., Spratt, E., Ciolino, J. D., Moran-Santa Maria, M., . . . & Brady, K. T. (2011). Gender differences in the effect of early life trauma on hypothalamic–pituitary–adrenal axis functioning. *Depression and Anxiety, 28*(5), 383–392.

Deykin, E. Y., & Buka, S. L. (1997). Prevalence and risk factors for posttraumatic stress disorder among chemically dependent adolescents. *American Journal of Psychiatry, 154*(6), 752–757.

Fargo, J. D. (2009). Pathways to adult sexual revictimization: Direct and indirect behavioral risk factors across the lifespan. *Journal of Interpersonal Violence, 24*(11), 1771–1791.

Foa, E. B., Dancu, C. V., Hembree, E. A., Jaycox, L. H., Meadows, E. A., & Street, G. P. (1999). A comparison of exposure therapy, stress inoculation training, and their combination for reducing posttraumatic stress disorder in female assault victims. *Journal of Consulting and Clinical Psychology, 67*(2), 194–200.

Foa, E. B., Keane, T. M., Friedman, M. J., & Cohen, J. A. (Eds.). (2009). *Effective treatments for PTSD: Practice guidelines from the International Society for Traumatic Stress Studies* (2nd ed.). New York: The Guilford Press.

Freeman, E. W., Sammel, M. D., Liu, L., Gracia, C. R., Nelson, D. B., & Hollander, L. (2004). Hormones and menopausal status as predictors of depression in women in transition to menopause. *Archives of General Psychiatry, 61*(1), 62–70.

Galatzer-Levy, I. R., Nickerson, A., Litz, B. T., & Marmar, C. R. (2013). Patterns of lifetime PTSD comorbidity: A latent class analysis. *Depression and Anxiety, 30*(5), 489–496.

Green, B. L., Goodman, L. A., Krupnick, J. L., Corcoran, C. B., Petty, R. M., Stockton, P., & Stern, N. M. (2000). Outcomes of single versus multiple trauma exposure in a screening sample. *Journal of Traumatic Stress, 13*(2), 271–286.

Heim, C., & Nemeroff, C. B. (2001). The role of childhood trauma in the neurobiology of mood and anxiety disorders: preclinical and clinical studies. *Biological Psychiatry, 49*(12), 1023–1039. http://doi.org/10.1016/S0006-3223(01)01157-X.

Heim, C., Young, L. J., Newport, D. J., Mletzko, T., Miller, A. H., & Nemeroff, C. B. (2009). Lower CSF oxytocin concentrations in women with a history of childhood abuse. *Molecular Psychiatry, 14*(10), 954–958.

Herman, J. L. (1992). *Trauma and recovery.* New York: Basic Books.

Hien, D. A., Rudnick Levin, F., Ruglass, L. M., López-Castro, T., Papini, S., Hu, M.-C., . . . & Herron, A. (2015). Combining seeking safety with sertraline for PTSD and alcohol use disorders: A randomized controlled trial. *Journal of Consulting and Clinical Psychology, 83*(2). http://doi.org/10.1037/a0038719.

Hoskins, M., Pearce, J., Bethell, A., Dankova, L., Barbui, C., Tol, W. A., . . . & Payne, V. (2015). Pharmacotherapy for post-traumatic stress disorder: Systematic review and meta-analysis. *British Journal of Psychiatry, 206*(2), 93–100. http://doi.org/10.1192/bjp.bp.114.148551.

Inslicht, S. S., Metzler, T. J., Garcia, N. M., Pineles, S. L., Milad, M. R., Orr, S. P., . . . & Neylan, T. C. (2013). Sex differences in fear conditioning in posttraumatic stress disorder. *Journal of Psychiatric Research, 47*(1), 64–71. http://doi.org/10.1016/j.jpsychires.2012.08.027.

Institute of Medicine. (2008). *Treatment of posttraumatic stress disorder: An assessment of the evidence.* Washington, DC: National Academies Press.

Ipser, J. C., & Stein, D. J. (2012). Evidence-based pharmacotherapy of post-traumatic stress disorder (PTSD). *International Journal of Neuropsychopharmacology, 15*, 825–840. http://doi.org/10.1017/S1461145711001209.

Irish, L. A., Fischer, B., Fallon, W., Spoonster, E., Sledjeski, E. M., & Delahanty, D. L. (2011). Gender differences in PTSD symptoms: An exploration of peritraumatic mechanisms. *Journal of Anxiety Disorders, 25*, 209–216. http://doi.org/10.1016/j.janxdis.2010.09.004.

Kajantie, E., & Phillips, D. I. W. (2006). The effects of sex and hormonal status on the physiological response to acute psychosocial stress. *Psychoneuroendocrinology, 31*(2),151–178.

Kaltman, S., Krupnick, J., Stockton, P., Hooper, L., & Green, B. L. (2005). Psychological impact of types of sexual trauma among college women. *Journal of Traumatic Stress, 18*(5), 547–555. http://doi.org/10.1002/jts.20063.

Keane, T. M., & Kaloupek, D. G. (1997). Comorbid psychiatric disorders in PTSD. Implications for research. *Annals of the New York Academy of Sciences, 821*, 24–34.

Kessler, R. C. (1995). Posttraumatic stress disorder in the National Comorbidity Survey. *Archives of General Psychiatry, 52*(12), 1048. http://doi.org/10.1001/archpsyc.1995.03950240066012.

Kessler, R. C., Berglund, P., Demler, O., Jin, R., Merikangas, K. R., & Walters, E. E. (2005). Lifetime prevalence and age-of-onset distributions of DSM-IV disorders in the National Comorbidity Survey replication. *Archives of General Psychiatry, 62*(6), 593. http://doi.org/10.1001/archpsyc. 62.6.593.

Krupnick, J. L., Green, B. L., Stockton, P., Goodman, L., Corcoran, C., & Petty, R. (2004). Mental health effects of adolescent trauma exposure in a female college sample: Exploring differential outcomes based on experiences of unique trauma types and dimensions. *Psychiatry, 67*(3), 264–279.

Kuijpers, K. F., van der Knaap, L. M., & Lodewijks, I. A. J. (2011). Victims' influence on intimate partner violence revictimization: A systematic review of prospective evidence. *Trauma, Violence, and Abuse, 12*(4), 198–219. http://doi.org/10.1177/1524838011416378.

Ladd, C. O., Huot, R. L., Thrivikraman, K. V., Nemeroff, C. B., & Plotsky, P. M. (2004). Long-term adaptations in glucocorticoid receptor and mineralocorticoid receptor mRNA and negative feedback on the hypothalamo-pituitary-adrenal axis following neonatal maternal separation. *Biological Psychiatry, 55*(4), 367–375.

Lang, A. J., Rodgers, C. S., Laffaye, C., Satz, L. E., Dresselhaus, T. S., & Stein, M. B. (2003). Sexual trauma, posttraumatic stress disorder, and health behavior. *Behavioral Medicine, 28*(4), 150–158.

Laudet, A. B., Magura, S., Cleland, C. M., Vogel, H. S., & Knight, E. L. (2003). Predictors of retention in dual-focus self-help groups. *Community Mental Health Journal, 39*(4), 281–297. http:// doi.org/10.1023/A:1024085423488.

Lilly, M. M., Pole, N., Best, S. R., Metzler, T., & Marmar, C. R. (2009). Gender and PTSD: What can we learn from female police officers? *Journal of Anxiety Disorders, 23*, 767–774. http://doi. org/10.1016/j.janxdis.2009.02.015.

McCutcheon, V. V., Sartor, C. E., Pommer, N. E., Bucholz, K. K., Nelson, E. C., Madden, P. A. F., & Heath, A. C. (2010). Age at trauma exposure and PTSD risk in young adult women. *Journal of Traumatic Stress, 23*(6), 811–814. http://doi.org/10.1002/jts.

Messman, T. L., & Long, P. J. (1996). Child sexual abuse and its relationship to revictimization in adult women: A review. *Clinical Psychology Review, 16*(5), 397–420.

Messman-Moore, T. L., & Brown, A. L. (2006). Risk perception, rape, and sexual revictimization: A prospective study of college women. *Psychology of Women Quarterly, 30*, 159–172.

Messman-Moore, T. L., Ward, R. M., & Brown, A. L. (2009). Substance use and PTSD symptoms impact the likelihood of rape and revictimization in college women. *Journal of Interpersonal Violence, 24*(3), 499–521.

Mezey, G., Bacchus, L., & Bewley, S. (2005). Domestic violence, lifetime trauma and psychological health of childbearing women. *British Journal of Obstetrics and Gynaecology, 112*(February), 197–204.

Mezey, G., Bacchus, L., Bewley, S., & White, S. (2005). Domestic violence, lifetime trauma and psychological health of childbearing women. *International Journal of Obstetrics and Gynaecology*, 112(2), 197–204.

Noll, J. G., Horowitz, L. A., Bonanno, G. A., Trickett, P. K., & Putnam, F. W. (2003). Revictimization and self-harm in females who experienced childhood sexual abuse: Results from a prospective study. *Journal of Interpersonal Violence*, 18(12), 1452–1471. http://doi.org/10.1177/0886260503258035.

Norris, F. H., Foster, J. D., & Weisshaar, D. L. (2002). The epidemiology of gender differences in PTSD across developmental, societal, and research contexts. In R. Kimerling, P. Ouimette, J. Wolfe, R. Kimerling, P. Ouimette, & J. Wolfe (Eds.), *Gender and PTSD* (pp. 3–42). New York: Guilford Press.

Norris, F. H., Tracy, M., & Galea, S. (2009). Looking for resilience: Understanding the longitudinal trajectories of responses to stress. *Social Science and Medicine*, 68(12), 2190–2198. http://doi.org/10.1016/j.socscimed.2009.03.043.

Olff, M., Langeland, W., Draijer, N., & Gersons, B. P. R. (2007). Gender differences in posttraumatic stress disorder. *Psychological Bulletin*, 133(2), 183–204. http://doi.org/10.1037/0033-2909.133.2.183.

Ozer, E. J., Best, S. R., Lipsey, T. L., & Weiss, D. S. (2003). Predictors of posttraumatic stress disorder and symptoms in adults: A meta-analysis. *Psychological Bulletin*, 129(1), 52–73.

Peirce, J. M., Newton, T. L., Buckley, T. C., & Keane, T. M. (2002). Gender and psychophysiology of PTSD. In R. Kimerling & P. Ouimette (Eds.), *Gender and PTSD* (pp. 177–204). New York: Guilford Press.

Pelcovitz, D., Van der Kolk, B. D., Roth, S., Mandel, F., Kaplan, S., & Resick, P. (1997). Development of a criteria set and a structured interview for disorders of extreme stress (SIDES). *Journal of Traumatic Stress*, 10(1), 3–16. http://doi.org/10.1023/A:1024800212070.

Perkonigg, A., Kessler, R. C., Storz, S., & Wittchen, H.-U. (2000). Traumatic events and posttraumatic stress disorder in the community: Prevalence, risk factors and comorbidity. *Acta Psychiatrica Scandinavica*, 101(1), 46–59. http://doi.org/10.1034/j.1600-0447.2000.101001046.x.

Pimlott-Kubiak, S., & Cortina, L. M. (2003). Gender, victimization, and outcomes: Reconceptualizing risk. *Journal of Consulting and Clinical Psychology*, 71(3), 528–539. http://doi.org/10.1037/0022-006X.71.3.528.

Pinto, R. M., Campbell, A. N. C., Hien, D. A., Yu, G., & Gorroochurn, P. (2011). Retention in the National Institute on Drug Abuse Clinical Trials Network Women and Trauma Study: Implications for posttrial implementation. *American Journal of Orthopsychiatry*, 81(2), 211–217. http://doi.org/10.1111/j.1939-0025.2011.01090.x.

Pratchett, L. C., Pelcovitz, M. R., & Yehuda, R. (2010). Trauma and violence: Are women the weaker sex? *Psychiatric Clinics of North America*. http://doi.org/10.1016/j.psc.2010.01.010.

Rasmusson, A. M., & Friedman, M. J. (2002). Gender issues in the neurobiology of PTSD. In R. Kimerling & P. Ouimette (Eds.), *Gender and PTSD* (pp. 43–75). New York: Guilford Press.

Rayburn, N. R., Wenzel, S. L., Elliott, M. N., Hambarsoomians, K., Marshall, G. N., & Tucker, J. S. (2005). Trauma, depression, coping, and mental health service seeking among impoverished women. *Journal of Consulting and Clinical Psychology*, 73(4), 667–677. http://doi.org/10.1037/0022-006X.73.4.667.

Romeo, R. D., & McEwen, B. S. (2006). Stress and the adolescent brain. *Annals of the New York Academy of Sciences*, 1094, 202–214.

Roodman, A. A., & Clum, G. A. (2001). Revictimization rates and method variance: A meta-analysis. *Clinical Psychology Review*, 21(2), 183–204. http://doi.org/10.1016/S0272-7358(99)00045-8.

Ruglass, L. M., Miele, G. M., Hien, D. A., Campbell, A. N. C., Hu, M.-C., Caldeira, N., ... & Nunes, E. V. (2012). Helping alliance, retention, and treatment outcomes: A secondary analysis from the NIDA clinical trials network women and trauma study. *Substance Use and Misuse*, 47, 695–707. http://doi.org/10.3109/10826084.2012.659789.

Sansone, R. A., Wiederman, M. W., & Sansone, L. A. (1997). Health care utilization and history of trauma among women in a primary care setting. *Violence and Victims*, 12(2), 165–172.

Scher, C. D., Forde, D. R., McQuaid, J. R., & Stein, M. B. (2004). Prevalence and demographic correlates of childhood maltreatment in an adult community sample. *Child Abuse and Neglect*, 28(2), 167–180. http://doi.org/10.1016/j.chiabu.2003.09.012.

Schnurr, P. P., Friedman, M. J., Sengupta, A., Jankowski, M. K., & Holmes, T. (2000). PTSD and utilization of medical treatment services among male Vietnam veterans. *Journal of Nervous and Mental Disease*, 188(8), 496–504.

Shin, K. M., Chang, H. Y., Cho, S. M., Kim, N. H., Kim, K. A., & Chung, Y. K. (2015). Avoidance symptoms and delayed verbal memory are associated with post-traumatic stress symptoms in female victims of sexual violence. *Journal of Affective Disorders, 184*, 145–148. http://doi. org/10.1016/j.jad.2015.05.051.

Srinivas, T., DePrince, A. P., & Chu, A. T. (2015). Links between posttrauma appraisals and trauma-related distress in adolescent females from the child welfare system. *Child Abuse and Neglect, 47*(2009), 14–23. http://doi.org/10.1016/j.chiabu.2015.05.011.

Taylor, S. E., Klein, L. C., Lewis, B. P., Gruenewald, T. L., Gurung, R. A., & Updegraff, J. A. (2000). Biobehavioral responses to stress in females: Tend-and-befriend, not fight-or-flight. *Psychological Review, 107*(3), 411–429. http://doi.org/10.1037/0033-295X.107.3.411.

Teicher, M. H., Andersen, S. L., Polcari, A., Anderson, C. M., & Navalta, C. P. (2002). Developmental neurobiology of childhood stress and trauma. *Psychiatric Clinics of North America, 25*(2), 397–426.

Tolin, D. F., & Breslau, N. (2007). Sex differences in risk of PTSD. *PTSD Research Quarterly, 18*(2), 1–8.

Tolin, D. F., & Foa, E. B. (2006). Sex differences in trauma and posttraumatic stress disorder: A quantitative review of 25 years of research. *Psychological Bulletin, 132*(6), 959–992. http://doi. org/10.1037/0033-2909.132.6.959.

Ullman, S. E., & Filipas, H. H. (2005). Gender differences in social reactions to abuse disclosures, post-abuse coping, and PTSD of child sexual abuse survivors. *Child Abuse and Neglect, 29*, 767–782. http://doi.org/10.1016/j.chiabu.2005.01.005.

van der Kolk, B. A., McFarlane, A. C., & Weisaeth, L. (1996). *Traumatic stress: The effects of overwhelming experience on mind, body, and society.* New York: Guilford Press. http://doi. org/10.1111/j.2044-8260.1994.tb01095.x.

Vishnevsky, T., Cann, A., Calhoun, L. G., Tedeschi, R. G., & Demakis, G. J. (2010). Gender differences in self-reported posttraumatic growth: A meta-analysis. *Psychology of Women Quarterly, 34*, 110–120.

Wilke, D. J., & Vinton, L. (2005). The nature and impact of domestic violence across age cohorts. *Affilia, 20*(3), 316–328.

Chapter Eleven
Women and Substance Use Disorders

Aimee N. C. Campbell and Margaret Wolff

Up until the last decade of the 20th century, women were effectively excluded from most research on substance use disorders (SUDs) (Lal, Deb, & Kedia, 2015). To address the major gap in scientific knowledge on women with SUDs, in 1994, the National Institutes of Health (NIH) enacted a requirement that federally financed investigations include a larger proportion of women (NIH, 1994). Twenty years later, NIH extended its initial requirement by calling for an explicit examination of biological sex within all research (NIH, 2014), followed by a 2016 strategic plan to enhance health research on sexual orientation and gender identity (NIH, 2016).

Although research on women and addiction has increased since the 1994 NIH research guidelines, it has often focused on women's alcohol use without considering the unique needs of women who use drugs (Lal et al., 2015). Men continue to demonstrate disproportionate rates of drug (Kay, Taylor, Barthwell, Wichelecki, & Leopold, 2010) and alcohol use (Grucza, Norberg, Bucholz, & Bierut, 2008; Khan et al., 2013), but gendered disparities in substance use have dissipated as younger women increasingly report levels of use comparable to male counterparts (Kuhn, 2015; Substance Abuse and Mental Health Services Administration (SAMHSA), 2015a).

Epidemiology of Substance Use Disorders

Alcohol Use

In 2013, over half of all U.S. women age 15 to 44 reported current alcohol use (SAMHSA, 2015a). Among adults, men's current alcohol use surpasses that of women by 10%; among adolescents, however, prevalence rates are similar for males and females (11.2% and 11.9% respectively) (SAMHSA, 2015a). As stigma around women's alcohol use has diminished (Harvard Medical School,

2010), disparities between men's and women's overall alcohol use prevalence have also declined. For example, past-month alcohol use among women increased from 44% in 1996 (Brittingham, 1998) to 48% in 2013 (SAMHSA, 2015a); among men, use decreased from 60% in 1996 (SAMHSA, 2007) to 57% in 2013. Even as women consume alcohol in a lower quantity and frequency than men, they experience more adverse physical health outcomes like liver cirrhosis (Graziani, Nencini, & Nisticò, 2014), as well as comorbid mental health problems and other SUDs (Khan et al., 2013).

About one-third of emerging adult women (age 18 to 25) have engaged in binge drinking (defined as four or more drinks in a sitting) within the past year (SAMHSA, 2015a) and close to 20% of adult women have done so within the past month (Tan, Denny, Cheal, Sniezek, & Kanny, 2015). These rates have prompted the Centers for Disease Control (CDC) to acknowledge binge drinking as a critical health issue, often overlooked in women's health care (CDC, 2013). Still, men continue to binge drink at levels that are disproportionately higher than those among women, with a roughly 12% gap among the ages of 18 to 25, increasing to 50% for those age 26 and older (SAMHSA, 2015a).

Alcohol Use Across the Life Course

Women's alcohol use and dependence fluctuate across the lifespan: prevalence of current alcohol use was about 12% among women aged 12 to 17, compared to 57% among 18- to 25-year-olds, 50% among women over 26, and 42% for those over 65. Binge-drinking rates also sharply drop as women age, from about 33% among women aged 18 to 25 (SAMHSA, 2015a), 9% among 50- to 64-year-olds, and 3% among women 65 and older (Blazer & Wu, 2009). According to the 2001–2002 National Epidemiologic Survey on Alcohol and Related Conditions (NESARC), alcohol use dependence (AUD) follows a similar pattern, with 6% of women aged 30 to 44 meeting AUD criteria, 3% for those 45 to 64, and 0.5% among those 65 and older (Grant et al., 2004). Despite low levels of disordered alcohol use among older women, future generations may deviate from this pattern, as female teens and young adults report increasingly higher levels of heavy drinking and potentially greater risk for drinking problems later in life (Epstein, Fischer-Elber, & Al-Otaiba, 2007). Underage drinking poses specific risks for later alcohol problems. Young people who initiate alcohol use before age 15 have a sixfold risk of developing an AUD compared to those who initiate use after age 21 (SAMHSA, 2015a). Trends in alcohol use among older adults are also shifting as the baby boomers age—a generation with greater alcohol use prevalence compared to previous cohorts (Wang & Andrade, 2013).

Drug Use

In 2013, more than 9% of Americans reported illicit drug use in the past month (SAMHSA, 2014a). Historically, drug use has been perceived as a male phenomenon: men's overall substance use prevalence remains 4% higher than women's, as does men's use of specific substances such as marijuana (9.7% vs. 5.6%), cocaine (0.8% vs. 0.4%), and hallucinogens (0.7% vs. 0.3%) (SAMHSA, 2015a). In recent years, however, rates of drug use are rising among women, who now comprise nearly 60% of the 2.8 million Americans who initiated drug use in 2013 (SAMHSA, 2015a), and over 40% of the 41.5 million individuals who were actively using drugs in 2012 (SAMHSA, 2014b).

Women are also more likely than men to abuse prescription drugs like opioids and tranquilizers (SAMHSA, 2015a). Prevalence of recreational opioid use has been increasing over the past 15 years across the United States, and men and women currently have comparable rates of SUDs involving prescription opioids (about 13%) (SAMHSA, 2015a). The narrowing of the gender gap in drug use is particularly pronounced among adolescents, with overall prevalence at 9.6% and 8.0% for male and female adolescents respectively (Kuhn, 2015; SAMHSA, 2015a). In 1993, 37% of male versus 29% of female high school students reported marijuana use; by 2013, those rates had increased to 42% for males and 39% for females (Executive Office of the President of the United States, 2014).

Drug Use Across the Life Course

Like alcohol use, drug use patterns among women shift over the life course. As observed in the 2013 National Survey on Drug Use and Health (NSDUH), about 7% of women over the age of 12 reported current recreational drug use, and 1.4% reported a current diagnosis of an illicit drug use disorder (DUD). When broken down by age group, rates of current drug use were 8% among women aged 12 to 17, 19% among those 18 to 22 (SAMHSA, 2015a), and about 10% for those 26 and older (SAMHSA, 2015b). Levels of current recreational drug use have risen among older adults (50 to 64), as well, with rates doubling from 2002 to 2013 (3% to 6%) (Wang & Andrade, 2013). Out of all women who engage in drug use, 7% have reported a history of DUD (Compton, Thomas, Stinson, & Grant, 2007).

As with drug use in general, women's rates of DUD decline with age. About 5% of women aged 18 to 25 report illicit drug dependence compared to 1.3% of women over age 25 (SAMHSA, 2015b). Men are more vulnerable to SUDs later in life than their female counterparts (Wu & Blazer, 2011); however, according to the Treatment Episode Data Set—which documents yearly substance abuse treatment admissions across the United States—admissions among those aged 55 and over are disproportionately comprised of women. Further, older women have a higher incidence of substance use compared to older men (Arndt, Gunter, & Acion, 2005). Older women are particularly susceptible to misuse of prescription medications (Voyer, Préville, Roussel, Berbiche, & Béland, 2009) and vulnerable to telescoping, the phenomenon of rapidly progressing from initial substance use to disordered use (Harvard Medical School, 2010; Khan et al., 2013). Telescoping among older women may be the result of higher levels of social seclusion and financial vulnerabilities than those of men in the same age range (Keyes, Martins, Blanco, & Hasin, 2010). The telescoping phenomenon has also been observed among adolescent females (Buccelli, Della Casa, Paternoster, Niola, & Pieri, 2016; Harvard Medical School, 2010).

Lesbian, Gay, Bisexual, and Transgender Women

Sexual-minority women (those who identify as lesbian, gay, or bisexual, who have sex with other women and/or who express sexual attraction to other women regardless of their identity label) are particularly vulnerable to substance use and SUDs compared with their heterosexually identified counterparts (Institute of Medicine, 2011). Lesbian/bisexually identified women's lifetime levels of illicit drug use (Parsons, Kelly, & Wells, 2006) and drinking (Hyde, Comfort, McManus, Brown, & Howat, 2009) are significantly greater than those of heterosexual women. Lesbian/bisexual women's drug prevalence may be up to 49% (compared to 40% among heterosexual women) (Parsons et al., 2006), and they may have 3.5 times the odds of having a current SUD compared to heterosexually identified women (Meyer, 2003).

Sexual-minority women also experience alcohol-associated adverse outcomes more frequently than non-sexual minorities, including driving while intoxicated, engaging in unanticipated sex, suicidal ideation, and perpetrating sexual harrassment when drunk (McCabe, Boyd, Hughes, & d'Arcy, 2003). When examined as a unique group, bisexually identified women are at greater risk for elevated substance abuse (e.g., Kerr, Ding, Burke, & Ott-Walter, 2015), adverse consequences of alcohol use, and higher levels of alcohol dependence (Wilsnack et al., 2008) when compared to both lesbian and heterosexually identified women, even when they report lower levels of use (Bostwick et al., 2007).

Although the literature base is limited, studies have shown that transgender women have higher levels of substance use compared to non-transgender (i.e., cisgender) individuals (e.g., Reisner, White, Bradford, & Mimiaga, 2014). Prevalence of use among transgender women has been documented at 88% for alcohol, 63% marijuana, 30% cocaine, and 9% stimulants and injection drugs in one study (Reisner et al., 2014), prevalence that dwarfs rates among the cisgender population (SAMHSA, 2015a).

Sexual- and gender-minority women's substance use and abuse should not be considered as functions of sexual orientation or gender identity in isolation, but rather in relation to structural factors that adversely affect individuals with stigmatized identities (Hughes, 2011; MacCarthy, Reisner, Nunn, Perez-Brumer, & Operario, 2015; Reisner et al., 2014). Such factors and mechanisms will be discussed in more detail below.

Risk Factors for Addiction and Psychiatric Comorbidities

Adverse Childhood Experiences

SUDs among women are not without pretext and numerous risk factors are associated with addiction. Women diagnosed with SUDs in adulthood often have a history of adverse childhood experiences, including physical and sexual abuse, parental neglect (e.g., Afifi, Henriksen, Asmundson, & Sareen, 2012; Tripodi & Pettus-Davis, 2013), and parental substance use in the home (Douglas et al., 2010). For example, in a study that drew upon NESARC data from over 34,000 U.S. adults, both men and women with childhood neglect or sexual abuse were at significantly greater risk for adult SUDs; however, after adjusting for mental health disorders, childhood sexual abuse continued to be a significant predictor of all SUDs for women but only opioid, cannabis, and cocaine use disorders among men (Afifi et al., 2012).

Theories of SUD

Psychiatric disorders commonly appear along the mediational pathway between adverse childhood events and SUDs (Douglas et al., 2010). The self-medication hypothesis of SUDs—which continues to be the primary mechanistic theory (Lembke, 2012)—posits that people with mental health disorders use drugs and alcohol to treat the associated symptoms, such as anxiety or depression, leading to a cycle of addiction (Khantzian, 1985). Two additional theories of addiction include the stress-coping model (Wills & Hirky, 1996; Wills & Shiffman, 1985) and the tension reduction theory (Conger, 1956). The stress-coping model suggests that substance use is a means of handling stress and that it serves to suppress undesirable feelings while enhancing positive emotions (Wills & Hirky, 1996; Wills & Shiffman, 1985).

Similarly, the tension reduction theory purports that alcohol consumption occurs in order to ease tension. This theory also recognizes the cycle of addiction by noting that the reduction in tension achieved through drinking alcohol perpetuates ongoing alcohol use (Conger, 1956). Both the stress-coping model and the tension reduction theory regard substance use as a form of self-medicating against stress and tension, but unlike the self-medication hypothesis (Khantzian, 1985), these models do not necessarily place mental health disorders as factors that contribute to or are byproducts of such stress and tension.

Depression

Several studies that have examined the relationship between psychiatric disorders and substance abuse outcomes reflect the aforementioned SUD theories. Anxiety and mood problems, such as depression, often exist concurrently with substance use, a situation more prevalent among women than men (Greenfield, Back, Lawson, & Brady, 2010). A recent study using the NSDUH (2005–2010) focused on men and women with SUD, some of whom also had concurrent major depression. Women comprised 30% of the SUD-only group, but 48% of the SUD with depression group (Chen, Strain, Crum, & Mojtabai, 2013). Both men and women with SUD and co-occurring depression were more likely to report unmet SUD treatment needs, but rates of major depression among women with AUD is much more common than among men (48.5% vs. 24.3% in the 2001–2002 National Comorbidity Survey) (Conner, Pinquart, & Gamble, 2009).

Trauma and Posttraumatic Stress Disorder (PTSD)

Similarly, the self-medication model, stress-coping model, and tension reduction theory may also explain high levels of substance abuse among women who have traumatic histories and subsequent symptoms of PTSD (Lazareck et al., 2012; McCauley, Killeen, Gros, Brady, & Back, 2012). Women with PTSD may consume alcohol and drugs in order to temper symptoms associated with PTSD, such as difficulty sleeping, hypervigilance, and hyperarousal (e.g., Ruglass, Hien, Hu, & Campbell, 2014). For example, in a study using the NESARC, 46% of people with PTSD had a co-occurring SUD (Pietrzak, Goldstein, Southwick, & Grant, 2011); rates increase up to 60% among treatment-seeking populations (McCauley et al., 2012). Co-occurring PTSD + SUDs creates a more complex and costly clinical course due to greater health problems, lower social functioning, increased risk of violence, and worse treatment outcomes (McCauley et al., 2012). The interplay between PTSD and SUD symptoms has been examined in several studies demonstrating that reductions in PTSD can in turn reduce substance use (Back, Payne, Simpson, & Brady, 2010; Hien et al., 2009).

Eating Disorders

Eating disorders also occur more frequently in populations with SUDs, with the highest reported rates among individuals with bulimia nervosa and alcohol use disorders (Hudson, Hiripi, Pope, & Kessler, 2007; National Center on Addiction and Substance Abuse at Columbia University (CASA), 2003). Women are more likely than men to develop eating disorders, thus also placing them at greater risk for SUDs (CASA, 2003). As with other comorbidities, eating disorders and SUDs can create a complex and interwoven presentation of symptoms. Drugs and alcohol can be used to facilitate disordered eating through appetite suppression, increasing metabolism, or inducing vomiting (Killeen, Brewerton, Campbell, Cohen, & Hien, 2015). For example, initial motivation for drug use among women in treatment for methamphetamine abuse was for weight loss (Brecht, O'Brien, Von Mayrhauser, & Anglin, 2004) and a significant proportion of women (45%) were concerned that weight gain could trigger relapse (Warren, Lindsay, White, Claudat, & Velasquez, 2013). Further, adverse childhood experiences increase the risk of developing an eating disorder, as well as developing PTSD or SUDs (Baker, Mazzeo, & Kendler, 2007). Thus, these three disorders often co-occur, with substance use and binge eating used as coping strategies to manage negative emotions (Killeen et al., 2015).

Risk Factors for Addiction Among Sexual-Minority Women and Psychiatric Comorbidities

A host of both similar and unique adverse experiences contribute to the disproportionately high rates of substance use among sexual-minority women, which are explored primarily in two theories: minority stress theory (Meyer, 2003) and the psychological mediation framework (Hatzenbuehler, 2009). According to minority stress theory, experiences of stigma and discrimination engender stress for individuals who hold a sexual-minority status, thus leading to adverse health outcomes, such as substance use and resultant SUDs (Meyer, 2003). The psychological mediation framework extends the minority stress theory by examining the causal pathways that link stress-generating stigma and discrimination with mental health problems among sexual minorities. The framework specifically acknowledges how stress impairs emotional and cognitive functioning, which ultimately mediates the association between stress and negative health outcomes, such as SUDs (Hatzenbuehler, 2009).

Sexual-minority women face stigma, discrimination, and victimization across the life course which in turn is associated with SUDs (e.g., Gilmore et al., 2014; Herek, Norton, Allen, & Sims, 2010; Hughes, 2011). Adverse childhood experiences include a lack of family acceptance around sexuality, antigay bullying at school, and childhood physical abuse and sexual assault (Friedman et al., 2011). Moreover, sexual-minority women who are targets of anti-LGBT hate violence and/or discrimination often suffer negative mental health outcomes, such as depression, anxiety, and anger, and subsequently use drugs and alcohol to self-medicate challenging emotion states (Condit, Kitaji, Drabble, & Trocki, 2011; Institute of Medicine, 2011).

Research has shown that, compared to sexual-minority women, exclusively heterosexual women report significantly lower levels of stress and a more positive mental health status, while depression, anxiety, and stress are significantly related to binge drinking and illicit substance use for all sexual-minority women (Hughes, Szalacha, & McNair, 2010). Bisexual women may be at particular risk for stigma and discrimination, both at the hands of mainstream heterosexual society, and among lesbian-identified communities, causing further isolation and resultant psychological distress (Herek, 2002).

Sexual-minority women's substance abuse may also be related to attempts to mask embarrassment, remorse, and internalized homophobia associated with being a sexual minority (Amadio, 2006; Matthews, Lorah, & Fenton, 2005). Furthermore, demographic and social factors, such as presenting with a masculine gender identity or one that does not conform to traditional representations of femininity (Lehavot & Simoni, 2011; Rosario, Schrimshaw, & Hunter, 2008), or holding a racial/ethnic-minority identity (Bowleg, Huang, Brooks, Black, & Burkholder, 2003; Kim & Fredriksen-Goldsen, 2012) are further associated with increased rates of substance use among women who have sex with women as a function of minority stress (Hughes et al., 2006; Meyer, 2003). One study ($n = 577$) found that sexual-minority adults who experienced discrimination related to sexuality, race, and gender had more than four times the odds of having a SUD compared to those who did not experience discrimination (McCabe, Bostwick, Hughes, West, & Boyd, 2010).

Transgender individuals are at especially high risk for adverse health and mental health outcomes. A recent study of 292 transgender female adolescents and young adults found that 61% screened positive for PTSD, and 80% had confronted stigmatization as a result of their gender presentation (Rowe, Santos, McFarland, & Wilson, 2015). Further, youth who had a positive PTSD screen demonstrated almost two times the odds of illicit drug use compared to those who did not report PTSD symptoms. Thus, sexual- and gender-minority women's experiences with stress, stigma, and discrimination across the life course appear to be key drivers of disproportionately higher rates of SUDs and concurrent mental health problems.

Biological Effects of Alcohol and Drugs

Biological differences in the onset and progression of SUD among men and women are arguably of increasing importance as the gap between female and male adolescent substance use becomes smaller, and as social norms around women's substance use become less restrictive. The following section briefly overviews biological differences between males and females specifically for alcohol and stimulant use, the two categories of substances for which the most evidence is available.

Alcohol

The negative effects of alcohol are more pronounced in women for several reasons. First, there is a higher susceptibility to the physiological consequences of alcohol among women, partly based on alcohol being more soluble in water than fat, and women having more fatty tissue and lower percentage of body water compared to men (Buccelli et al., 2016). Further, as compared to men, women produce less alcohol dehydrogenase, the enzyme in the stomach which breaks down alcohol, resulting in more alcohol passing from the digestive system into the blood (Buccelli et al., 2016; Van Der Walde, Urgenson, Weltz, & Hanna, 2002). Women also reach higher blood alcohol levels, have a higher risk for developing cirrhosis of the liver, and sustain greater cognitive damage than men, all while consuming equivalent amounts of alcohol (Graziani et al., 2014; Lynch, Roth, & Carroll, 2002).

Alcohol consumption also influences female reproduction, including menstrual cycle irregularities, infertility, miscarriage, and fetal abnormalities (Emanuele, Wezeman, & Emanuele, 2002; Van Der Walde et al., 2002). Moderate alcohol consumption can lead to hormonal imbalances in women, with binge alcohol use associated with increased estradiol levels (Schliep et al., 2015). Although more research is needed, increasing circulating estrogen may heighten risk of breast cancer among menopausal women. Animal studies reveal that mild to moderate alcohol use can suppress estrogen in females, disrupting puberty and affecting growth and bone health (Emanuele et al., 2002).

Stimulants

Some of the most consistent biologically based findings on sex differences in SUDs are apparent in men's and women's response to the use of stimulant drugs. Women have an overall pharmacological sensitivity to cocaine, whereby subjective mental and physical well-being (i.e., euphoria, energy, and intellectual efficiency) is enhanced (Graziani et al., 2014; Terner & De Wit, 2006). Hormonal levels, especially those related to the menstrual cycle, appear to influence this subjective effect. Women report greater sensitivity to the subjective effects of cocaine when estrogen levels are higher (e.g., during the follicular phase of the menstrual cycle), while progesterone appears to attenuate the subjective effects of cocaine (Buccelli et al., 2016; Graziani et al., 2014; Lynch et al., 2002; Terner & De Wit, 2006). These findings have been borne out in both animal and human lab studies (Buccelli et al., 2016). Despite these consistent findings with regard to stimulants, there has been virtually no research on drugs for treating SUDs during the menstrual cycle (Terner & De Wit, 2006).

Gender differences in the stress system may also help to explain women's greater vulnerability to the negative consequences of substance use, greater prevalence of comorbidities compared to men, and increased risk for relapse to drug and alcohol use (Fox & Sinha, 2009). Women, in general, experience greater emotional sensitivity to biophysiological stress system changes (Fox & Sinha, 2009). Although this is especially acute following cocaine administration, it has also been shown among healthy females who engage in social drinking. Cocaine- and alcohol-dependent women report enhanced emotional response following stress and drug cues, and have a higher likelihood of a dysregulated hypothalamic–pituitary–adrenal axis; both are associated with greater craving and relapse to substance use (Fox & Sinha, 2009). Thus, substance use and fluctuation of sex hormones can influence stress system adaptations that may in turn influence SUD development and recovery outcomes.

Addiction Treatment

Access, Engagement, and Retention

Women and men differ in access to and engagement in SUD treatment. Women with SUDs may be reluctant to disclose problematic use due to perceived stigma and judgment from health care providers (Hecksher & Hesse, 2009). Because women are much more likely to have custody, and take on primary childcare responsibilities compared to men, they are also more likely to be stigmatized for their substance use and to encounter legal issues related to substance use and child protection clauses (Child Welfare Information Gateway, 2014). In order to avoid scrutiny from health care workers, potential jail time, and loss of child custody, pregnant women may forgo prenatal care and women with children may withhold disclosing their substance use to their health care providers (Albright & Rayburn, 2009; Hecksher & Hesse, 2009). As a result, they may be less likely to be referred to or receive appropriate substance abuse treatment (Lal et al., 2015).

Further barriers to women seeking treatment include lack of childcare, costs associated with treatment, family opposition, inadequate diagnostic testing for SUDs, intimate-partner violence, and partner substance use (Grella, 2008; Lynch et al., 2002; Van Der Walde et al., 2002). When women do enter treatment, they arrive with a more severe clinical profile than men, marked by greater psychological distress and co-occurring psychiatric disorders, trauma histories, medical issues, interpersonal conflicts and family-related needs, less social support and stability, and fewer vocational skills (DeVito, Babuscio, Nich, Ball, & Carroll, 2014; Greenfield et al., 2007; Grella, 2008). Thus, although gender is not directly associated with treatment retention and outcomes, treatment barriers, and other common co-occurring problems can greatly influence women's treatment trajectory.

Following traditional social and family responsibilities, women with a SUD treatment history are more likely to have been referred by a social worker, and to have been involved in other social service systems like child welfare (Grella & Joshi, 1999). Eighteen states' child welfare laws continue to classify substance use during pregnancy as a form of child abuse. In 18 additional states, health care workers are legally obligated to report women believed to be using drugs while pregnant; in four states, health care workers must test all pregnant women for prenatal drug use (Guttmacher Institute, 2016). As such, although women may be reluctant to disclose substance use to their health care providers, requisite drug testing of pregnant women may force some women to enter treatment or risk jail time. By comparison, men are more likely to have been referred to substance abuse treatment by family members, an employer, or the criminal justice system (Grella & Joshi, 1999; Lynch et al., 2002). Thus, women's treatment histories are associated with becoming known to outside social systems like child welfare, whereas men are more likely to seek treatment based on family- or job-related consequences or interactions with the police.

SUD Treatment Programming

Although women and men experience similar treatment outcomes, the dynamics of achieving that recovery differ (Grella, 2008). In general, women benefit from programs that are longer or of greater intensity, have women-specific ancillary services (e.g., childcare or child beds in residential care, vocational or income support, housing services, prenatal care, and mental health services, case management, family therapy), and supportive staff with non-judgmental attitudes and positive client–staff interactions (SAMHSA, 2009; Grella, 2008; Hines, 2012).

Single-sex, or women-only, programs are not necessarily more effective than mixed-gender programs; however, they may produce better outcomes for specific subgroups of women, such as with women who have dependent children, lesbian-identified women, or women with histories of childhood sexual abuse (Grella, 2008). According to a meta-analysis of 34 treatment outcome studies of women participating in women-only compared to mixed-gender SUD treatment programs, better drug use outcomes were found in women-only programs; however, women-only programs with specialized programming (i.e., psychiatric services, trauma-informed treatment) produced better outcomes on psychological well-being and HIV risk reduction (Orwin, Francisco, & Bernichon, 2001). Despite this knowledge, a recent national study found that the proportion of SUD treatment programs offering women-centered services decreased from 2002 to 2009, from 43%

to 40% (Terplan, Longinaker, & Appel, 2015). Even in programs that offered some women-centered services, they were often not the resources that women needed most, such as childcare and onsite accommodations for the children of women in residential programming, counseling for intimate-partner violence, and transportation support (Terplan et al., 2015).

A number of factors are thought to be associated with long-term treatment outcomes for women. In particular, ongoing participation in self-help groups may be a protective factor for women in recovery, while mandating treatment appears beneficial to men's recovery (Grella, 2008; Morgan-Lopez et al., 2013). Other protective factors for women are treatment engagement, social support, and life satisfaction, while risk factors include daily stressors, intimate-partner violence, partner substance use, co-occurring mental health issues, low self-esteem, and chronic medical conditions (Comfort, Sockloff, Loverro, & Kaltenbach, 2003; Lynch et al., 2002).

SUD Treatment for Sexual-Minority Women

Research regarding substance abuse treatment engagement, retention, and outcomes for LGBT individuals is severely limited, particularly concerning sexual-minority women. A 2012 literature review found that, since 1996, only six studies have examined drug and alcohol interventions for LGBT populations, and that none were comprised of sexual-minority women participants. Moreover, the majority of the studies in the review focused on illicit drug use while neglecting alcohol abuse, and only a single study contained a comparison condition (Green & Feinstein, 2012).

Sexual-minority women may seek treatment at even lower rates then their heterosexually identified counterparts, partially due to the perception that health care providers may not hold a positive attitude toward sexual minorities (Cochran, Peavy, & Cauce, 2007; Eliason & Schope, 2001). A study examining availability of LGBT-specific substance abuse treatment found that 70% of the services that were advertised as tailored to LGBT needs were no different than mainstream substance abuse services (Cochran, Peavy, & Robohm, 2007). Further, research often doesn't explore or specify where treatment services are designed to meet the needs of LGBT individuals (Institute of Medicine, 2011). Thus, sexual-minority women's risk for persistent substance abuse may be influenced by a lack of access to treatment that is truly affirming of their sexual identity and sexual behavior.

SUD Treatment for Incarcerated Women

Despite decreases in substance use stigma over time, women continue to be uniquely targeted for their substance use. Criminal drug-related activity—together with drug use and possession—accounts for over 60% of all women's arrests (Guerino, Harrison, & Sabol, 2011). Women who abuse substances may also be more vulnerable to interactions with law enforcement since they may turn to sex work to obtain income to purchase drugs, or to exchange sex for drugs, food, shelter, or other essential resources (Gjersing & Bretteville-Jensen, 2014). Despite a growing population of incarcerated women and their unique psychosocial needs, the majority of existing mental health services for prisoners have been grounded in research involving male samples (Drapalski, Youman, Stuewig, & Tangney, 2009). Incarcerated women's mental health and substance use are characterized by critical differences from that of men. Compared to male inmates, women have a higher prevalence of poor physical health, trauma histories, limited economic means, and mental health issues (Lewis, 2006). Without adequate services to address these comorbidities, women are at greater risk for recidivism and ongoing substance use upon release from prison (Bergseth, Jens, Bergeron-Vigesaa, & McDonald, 2011; Tripodi & Pettus-Davis, 2013).

Behavioral SUD Treatments

With few exceptions, evidence-based SUD treatments have been developed generically, and not systematically examined for gender differences (Grella, 2008) . A systematic review of substance abuse treatment literature from 1975 to 2005 found only 252 investigations that explored variations in treatment outcomes by gender; of those, almost half (110) were conducted between 2000 and 2005, and only 12% were empirical studies (Greenfield et al., 2007). Further, women are often recruited to mixed-gender studies at lower rates than men, often due to exclusion criteria (e.g., psychiatric comorbidities) that may disproportionately impact women (as well as ethnic and racial minorities) (Susukida, Crum, Stuart, Ebnesajjad, & Mojtabai, 2016). In randomized controlled trials testing evidence-based SUD treatments among women and men, gender analyses are often relegated to secondary outcomes where findings are complicated by a lack of a priori power calculations.

The following sections highlight the major science-based behavioral and pharmacological treatments available, as well as available evidence on differential responses among women.

Cognitive-Behavioral Therapy (CBT)

CBT encompasses various treatment techniques to promote abstinence and reduce relapse, including identifying and addressing triggers for use, developing coping skills, and using homework assignments to practice and integrate these new techniques into daily living (Emmelkamp & Vedel, 2012; Marlatt & Donovan, 2005). A recent review that included five randomized controlled trials of CBT for cocaine use disorder found no differences in behavioral outcomes by gender even when controlling for baseline gender differences. The lack of differences could mean that behavioral therapies are more broadly applicable and have inherent flexibility to adapt to each individual's unique set of drug use patterns and motivations to use (DeVito et al., 2014); that is, CBT could become gender-specific without having been developed specifically for women. CBT-related clinical trials involving exclusively female samples have often been limited to pregnant women, further limiting generalizability (Grella, 2008).

Contingency Management (CM)

CM is a behavioral approach using a schedule of rewards (e.g., money, program incentives, prizes) to reinforce positive behaviors like abstinence or treatment participation (van Dam, Vedel, Ehring, & Emmelkamp, 2012). There is substantial evidence for the efficacy of CM approaches as a standalone intervention and in combination with other treatments across substances of abuse (Petry, 2010). The available evidence on gender differences in the effect of CM interventions suggests that women and men experience similar benefits (Burch, Rash, & Petry, 2015).

Community Reinforcement Approach (CRA)

CRA is based on the premise that interpersonal interactions and environmental components can serve as critical facilitators or deterrents to substance use. As such, CRA aims to restructure contextual factors such that greater rewards are obtained by refraining from than engaging in substance use (Smith, Meyers, & Miller, 2001).

A recent multisite randomized controlled trial of a technology-based version of CRA (plus CM) did not find gender differences on multiple behavioral outcomes (Campbell et al., 2015), although acceptability of the intervention was associated with abstinence outcomes and only among women. Another randomized controlled trial involved CRA treatment among adolescents with a focus on variations in treatment responsiveness and outcomes by gender. Male and female adolescents were equally as likely to link to and remain in treatment. Males were significantly more likely to report satisfaction with treatment, while females reported higher levels of abstinence and a greater likelihood of being in recovery by the six-month follow-up (Godley, Hedges, & Hunter, 2011). These studies demonstrate that, even when there are no detectable gender differences on major outcomes, there could be subgroups of women for whom the intervention is more or less effective.

Motivational Interviewing (MI) and Motivational Enhancement Treatments

MI employs a client-centered, partially directive communication style aimed at decreasing ambivalence for changing substance use through non-judgmental, individually focused discussion, increasing (or highlighting) commitment to change talk, and bolstering individual motivation (Rollnick & Miller, 1995). The client-centered focus of MI also demands that the therapist "meet the clients where they are," ensuring that the conversation remains relevant to particular motivations and needs of the client.

Like CBT, MI has a formidable evidence base for effectively addressing substance abuse (Smedslund et al., 2011). Specific research with MI has been completed with pregnant women (Grella, 2008; Ondersma et al., 2015), taking advantage of pregnancy as a critical time to leverage motivation to change behavior. A recent systematic review examined the effectiveness of brief MI-based intervention outcomes for women across 36 studies, with those who received the intervention generally reducing their alcohol use. Although about a third of the studies reported comparable findings by gender, others noted that women and men differed in terms of both reductions and increases in alcohol use (de Paula Gebara, de Castro Bhona, Ronzani, Lourenço, & Noto, 2013).

Self-Help/12-Step Models

Finally, 12-step programs (e.g., Alcoholics Anonymous (AA), Narcotics Anonymous) are a mutual-aid, self-help model of SUD treatment with empirical evidence for their immediate and long-standing benefits that match those of specialized treatment approaches (Kelly, Hoeppner, Stout, & Pagano, 2012). Women *may not* benefit from 12-step programs in the same way as men, for reasons such as the fact that 12-step was designed by and for men (Kaskutas, 1994), and women may struggle with ideas of powerlessness (Matheson & McCollum, 2008; Sered & Norton-Hawk, 2011). Others have noted that 12-step programs can be tailored to be more gender-responsive through women-only meetings and adaptation of 12-step tenets and practices (Sanders, 2006). In general, however, women and men do not appear to differ in 12-step attendance (Delucchi & Kaskutas, 2010), and attending AA seems to influence men's and women's alcohol use outcomes equally (Kelly & Hoeppner, 2013). Women may experience a stronger relationship between 12-step participation and abstinence compared to men (Witbrodt et al., 2014), and women who use self-help treatments, especially during aftercare, may have better outcomes (Morgan-Lopez et al., 2013).

Pharmacotherapy Treatments for SUD

Efficacious medications approved by the Food and Drug Administration (FDA) are available for alcohol and opioid use disorders. For alcohol use disorders, medications include: disulfiram (Antabuse), which inhibits the liver metabolism of alcohol and causes an aversive physical reaction that deters alcohol use; naltrexone, an opioid receptor antagonist available as a daily pill or monthly injection (Vivitrol); and acamprosate, which reduces alcohol craving and promotes abstinence. For opioid use disorder, medications include: methadone maintenance, an agonist medication that reduces craving, withdrawal and use; buprenorphine or buprenorphine/naloxone (Suboxone), a high-affinity partial opioid receptor agonist with similar effectiveness to methadone; and naltrexone (or the monthly injectable Vivitrol), an antagonist that fully blocks the effects of opioids.

Although there is still limited exploration of gender differences in response to pharmacological treatment, evidence to date suggests that there may be gender differences in dose–response and dosing schedules to medications for SUD, with poorer outcomes for women (DeVito et al., 2014; Grella, 2008). However, other research has found similar outcomes by gender for acamprosate (Mason & Lehert, 2012) and naltrexone, except among women dependent on both alcohol and cocaine (Greenfield et al., 2010). The effectiveness of methadone maintenance for opioid-dependent women has been demonstrated (Unger, Metz, & Fischer, 2012). Buprenorphine is indicated for women, although studies with women have shown mixed results (Unger, Jung, Winklbaur, & Fischer, 2010), and the majority of early buprenorphine trials were with men (Jones, 2004).

Methadone and Buprenorphine During Pregnancy

The FDA considers both methadone and buprenorphine as category C medications that should be used during pregnancy only if the potential benefit justifies the potential risk to the fetus. The benefits of methadone during pregnancy, compared to detoxification, have been established, although not without side effects, such as altering fetal activity and heart rate and spurring neonatal abstinence syndrome (Unger et al., 2012). There is emerging evidence of the safety of buprenorphine during pregnancy (Fischer et al., 1998; Schindler et al., 2003) and, more recently, findings that buprenorphine may be safer than methadone (Jones et al., 2010; Soyka, 2013).

Summary

There is great unmet need for research on women-centered addiction services. This is compounded by gaps in the research literature on gender-specific needs.

At a particular disadvantage are subgroups of women typically not included in research studies, or not included in large enough numbers for separate analyses (e.g., women who are sexual minorities, racial and ethnic minorities, elderly women, and incarcerated women). The need for women-focused addiction research becomes even more important as substance use becomes increasingly normalized among women and men.

While research and treatment must consider women's substance use in the context of their lived experiences—including women's challenges and resilience (SAMHSA, 2009)—future research endeavors should seek to shift the prevailing perception of women as a "special population" with "unique treatment needs" (Martin & Aston, 2014). Relegating women's addiction issues to a special-interest topic rather than a leading public health concern undermines a full integration of women's treatment needs into a wide array of treatment options. Women must be able to expect services that are responsive to their needs, build on their strengths, and are grounded in scientific research that has adequately tested and examined how to effectively deliver appropriate services.

References

Afifi, T. O., Henriksen, C. A., Asmundson, G. J., & Sareen, J. (2012). Childhood maltreatment and substance use disorders among men and women in a nationally representative sample. *Canadian Journal of Psychiatry, 57*(11), 677–686.

Albright, B. B., & Rayburn, W. F. (2009). Substance abuse among reproductive age women. *Obstetrics and Gynecology Clinics of North America, 36*(4), 891–906.

Amadio, D. M. (2006). Internalized heterosexism, alcohol use, and alcohol-related problems among lesbians and gay men. *Addictive Behaviors, 31*(7), 1153–1162.

Arndt, S., Gunter, T. D., & Acion, L. (2005). Older admissions to substance abuse treatment in 2001. *American Journal of Geriatric Psychiatry, 13*(5), 385–392.

Back, S. E., Payne, R. L., Simpson, A. N., & Brady, K. T. (2010). Gender and prescription opioids: Findings from the National Survey on Drug Use and Health. *Addictive Behaviors, 35*(11), 1001–1007.

Baker, J. H., Mazzeo, S. E., & Kendler, K. S. (2007). Association between broadly defined bulimia nervosa and drug use disorders: Common genetic and environmental influences. *International Journal of Eating Disorders, 40*(8), 673–678.

Bergseth, K. J., Jens, K. R., Bergeron-Vigesaa, L., & McDonald, T. D. (2011). Assessing the needs of women recently released from prison. *Women and Criminal Justice, 21*(2), 100–122.

Blazer, D. G., & Wu, L.-T. (2009). The epidemiology of at-risk and binge drinking among middle-aged and elderly community adults: National Survey on Drug Use and Health. *American Journal of Psychiatry, 166*(10), 1162–1169.

Bostwick, W. B., McCabe, S. E., Horn, S., Hughes, T. L., Johnson, T., & Valles, J. R. (2007). Drinking patterns, problems, and motivations among collegiate bisexual women. *Journal of American College Health, 56*(3), 285–292.

Bowleg, L., Huang, J., Brooks, K., Black, A., & Burkholder, G. (2003). Triple jeopardy and beyond: Multiple minority stress and resilience among Black lesbians. *Journal of Lesbian Studies, 7*(4), 87–108.

Brecht, M.-L., O'Brien, A., Von Mayrhauser, C., & Anglin, M. D. (2004). Methamphetamine use behaviors and gender differences. *Addictive Behaviors, 29*(1), 89–106.

Brittingham, A. (1998). *National household survey on drug abuse: Main findings, 1996.* Darby, PA: DIANE Publishing.

Buccelli, C., Della Casa, E., Paternoster, M., Niola, M., & Pieri, M. (2016). Gender differences in drug abuse in the forensic toxicological approach. *Forensic Science International, 265*, 89–95.

Burch, A. E., Rash, C. J., & Petry, N. M. (2015). Sex effects in cocaine-using methadone patients randomized to contingency management interventions. *Experimental and Clinical Psychopharmacology, 23*(4), 284–290.

Campbell, A. N., Nunes, E. V., Pavlicova, M., Hatch-Maillette, M., Hu, M.-C., Bailey, G. L., . . . & Shores-Wilson, K. (2015). Gender-based outcomes and acceptability of a computer-assisted psychosocial intervention for substance use disorders. *Journal of Substance Abuse Treatment, 53*, 9–15.

CDC. (2013, October 11). *Binge drinking: A serious, under-recognized problem among women and girls.* Retrieved from http://www.cdc.gov/vitalsigns/bingedrinkingfemale/ (accessed March 3, 2015).

Chen, L. Y., Strain, E. C., Crum, R. M., & Mojtabai, R. (2013). Gender differences in substance abuse treatment and barriers to care among persons with substance use disorders with and without comorbid major depression. *Journal of Addiction Medicine, 7*(5), 325–334.

Child Welfare Information Gateway. (2014, October). *Parental substance use and the child welfare system.* Retrieved from https://www.childwelfare.gov/pubs/factsheets/parentalsubabuse.cfm (accessed March 11, 2016).

Cochran, B. N., Peavy, K. M., & Cauce, A. M. (2007). Substance abuse treatment providers' explicit and implicit attitudes regarding sexual minorities. *Journal of Homosexuality, 53*(3), 181–207.

Cochran, B. N., Peavy, K. M., & Robohm, J. S. (2007). Do specialized services exist for LGBT individuals seeking treatment for substance misuse? A study of available treatment programs. *Substance Use and Misuse, 42*(1), 161–176.

Comfort, M., Sockloff, A., Loverro, J., & Kaltenbach, K. (2003). Multiple predictors of substance-abusing women's treatment and life outcomes: A prospective longitudinal study. *Addictive Behaviors, 28*(2), 199–224.

Compton, W. M., Thomas, Y. F., Stinson, F. S., & Grant, B. F. (2007). Prevalence, correlates, disability, and comorbidity of DSM-IV drug abuse and dependence in the United States: Results from the National Epidemiologic Survey on Alcohol and Related Conditions. *Archives of General Psychiatry, 64*(5), 566–576.

Condit, M., Kitaji, K., Drabble, L., & Trocki, K. (2011). Sexual-minority women and alcohol: intersections between drinking, relational contexts, stress, and coping. *Journal of Gay and Lesbian Social Services, 23*(3), 351–375.

Conger, J. J. (1956). Reinforcement theory and the dynamics of alcoholism. *Quarterly Journal of Studies on Alcohol, 17*, 296–305.

Conner, K. R., Pinquart, M., & Gamble, S. A. (2009). Meta-analysis of depression and substance use among individuals with alcohol use disorders. *Journal of Substance Abuse Treatment, 37*(2), 127–137.

Delucchi, K. L., & Kaskutas, L. A. (2010). Following problem drinkers over eleven years: Understanding changes in alcohol consumption. *Journal of Studies on Alcohol and Drugs, 71*(6), 831–836.

de Paula Gebara, C. F., de Castro Bhona, F. M., Ronzani, T. M., Lourenço, L. M., & Noto, A. R. (2013). Brief intervention and decrease of alcohol consumption among women: A systematic review. *Substance Abuse Treatment, Prevention, and Policy, 8*(1), 1–8.

DeVito, E. E., Babuscio, T. A., Nich, C., Ball, S. A., & Carroll, K. M. (2014). Gender differences in clinical outcomes for cocaine dependence: Randomized clinical trials of behavioral therapy and disulfiram. *Drug and Alcohol Dependence, 145*, 156–167.

Douglas, K. R., Chan, G., Gelernter, J., Arias, A. J., Anton, R. F., Weiss, R. D., . . . & Kranzler, H. R. (2010). Adverse childhood events as risk factors for substance dependence: Partial mediation by mood and anxiety disorders. *Addictive Behaviors, 35*(1), 7–13.

Drapalski, A. L., Youman, K., Stuewig, J., & Tangney, J. (2009). Gender differences in jail inmates' symptoms of mental illness, treatment history and treatment seeking. *Criminal Behaviour and Mental Health, 19*(3), 193–206.

Eliason, M. J., & Schope, R. (2001). Original research: Does "don't ask don't tell," apply to health care? Lesbian, gay, and bisexual people's disclosure to health care providers. *Journal of the Gay and Lesbian Medical Association, 5*(4), 125–134.

Emanuele, M. A., Wezeman, F., & Emanuele, N. V. (2002). Alcohol's effects on female reproductive function. *Alcohol Research and Health, 26*(4), 274–281.

Emmelkamp, P. M., & Vedel, E. (2012). *Evidence-based treatments for alcohol and drug abuse: A practitioner's guide to theory, methods, and practice.* New York: Routledge.

Epstein, E. E., Fischer-Elber, K., & Al-Otaiba, Z. (2007). Women, aging, and alcohol use disorders. *Journal of Women and Aging, 19*(1–2), 31–48.

Executive Office of the President of the United States. (2014). *National drug control strategy: Data supplement.* Retrieved November 16, 2016, from https://www.whitehouse.gov/sites/default/files/ondcp/policy-and-research/ndcs_data_supplement_2014.pdf.

Fischer, G., Etzersdorfer, P., Eder, H., Jagsch, R., Langer, M., & Weninger, M. (1998). Buprenorphine maintenance in pregnant opiate addicts. *European Addiction Research, 4*(Suppl. 1), 32–36.

Fox, H. C., & Sinha, R. (2009). Sex differences in drug-related stress-system changes: Implications for treatment in substance-abusing women. *Harvard Review of Psychiatry, 17*(2), 103–119.

Friedman, M. S., Marshal, M. P., Guadamuz, T. E., Wei, C., Wong, C. F., Saewyc, E. M., & Stall, R. (2011). A meta-analysis of disparities in childhood sexual abuse, parental physical abuse, and peer victimization among sexual minority and sexual nonminority individuals. *American Journal of Public Health, 101*(8), 1481–1494.

Gilmore, A. K., Koo, K. H., Nguyen, H. V., Granato, H. F., Hughes, T. L., & Kaysen, D. (2014). Sexual assault, drinking norms, and drinking behavior among a national sample of lesbian and bisexual women. *Addictive Behaviors, 39*(3), 630–636.

Gjersing, L., & Bretteville-Jensen, A. L. (2014). Gender differences in mortality and risk factors in a 13-year cohort study of street-recruited injecting drug users. *BMC Public Health, 14*(1), 1–11.

Godley, S. H., Hedges, K., & Hunter, B. (2011). Gender and racial differences in treatment process and outcome among participants in the adolescent community reinforcement approach. *Psychology of Addictive Behaviors, 25*(1), 143–154.

Grant, B. F., Dawson, D. A., Stinson, F. S., Chou, S. P., Dufour, M. C., & Pickering, R. P. (2004). The 12-month prevalence and trends in DSM-IV alcohol abuse and dependence: United States, 1991–1992 and 2001–2002. *Drug and Alcohol Dependence, 74*(3), 223–234.

Graziani, M., Nencini, P., & Nisticò, R. (2014). Genders and the concurrent use of cocaine and alcohol: Pharmacological aspects. *Pharmacological Research, 87*, 60–70.

Green, K. E., & Feinstein, B. A. (2012). Substance use in lesbian, gay, and bisexual populations: An update on empirical research and implications for treatment. *Psychology of Addictive Behaviors, 26*(2), 265–278.

Greenfield, S. F., Back, S. E., Lawson, K., & Brady, K. T. (2010). Substance abuse in women. *Psychiatric Clinics of North America, 33*(2), 339–355.

Greenfield, S. F., Brooks, A. J., Gordon, S. M., Green, C. A., Kropp, F., McHugh, R. K., . . . & Miele, G. M. (2007). Substance abuse treatment entry, retention, and outcome in women: A review of the literature. *Drug and Alcohol Dependence, 86*(1), 1–21.

Grella, C. E. (2008). From generic to gender-responsive treatment: Changes in social policies, treatment services, and outcomes of women in substance abuse treatment. *Journal of Psychoactive Drugs, 40*(suppl. 5), 327–343.

Grella, C. E., & Joshi, V. (1999). Gender differences in drug treatment careers among clients in the National Drug Abuse Treatment Outcome study. *American Journal of Drug and Alcohol Abuse, 25*(3), 385–406.

Grucza, R. A., Norberg, K., Bucholz, K. K., & Bierut, L. J. (2008). Correspondence between secular changes in alcohol dependence and age of drinking onset among women in the United States. *Alcoholism: Clinical and Experimental Research, 32*(8), 1493–1501.

Guerino, P., Harrison, P. M., & Sabol, W. J. (2011). *Prisoners in 2010.* Washington, DC: Bureau of Justice Statistics.

Guttmacher Institute. (2016, February). *State policies in brief: Substance abuse during pregnancy.* Retrieved from http://www.guttmacher.org/statecenter/spibs/spib_SADP.pdf (accessed February 17, 2016).

Harvard Medical School. (2010). Addiction in women. *Harvard Mental Health Letter, 26*(7).

Hatzenbuehler, M. (2009). How does sexual minority stigma "get under the skin"? A psychological mediation framework. *Psychological Bulletin, 135*(5), 707–730. http://doi.org/10.1037/a0016441.

Hecksher, D., & Hesse, M. (2009). Women and substance use disorders. *Mens Sana Monographs, 7*(1), 50–62.

Herek, G. M. (2002). Heterosexuals' attitudes toward bisexual men and women in the United States. *Journal of Sex Research, 39*(4), 264–274.

Herek, G. M., Norton, A. T., Allen, T. J., & Sims, C. L. (2010). Demographic, psychological, and social characteristics of self-identified lesbian, gay, and bisexual adults in a US probability sample. *Sexuality Research and Social Policy, 7*(3), 176–200.

Hien, D. A., Wells, E. A., Jiang, H., Suarez-Morales, L., Campbell, A. N., Cohen, L. R., . . . & Zhang, Y. (2009). Multisite randomized trial of behavioral interventions for women with co-occurring PTSD and substance use disorders. *Journal of Consulting and Clinical Psychology, 77*(4), 607–619.

Hines, L. (2012). The treatment views and recommendations of substance abusing women: A meta-synthesis. *Qualitative Social Work*, 1473325011432776.

Hudson, J. I., Hiripi, E., Pope, H. G., & Kessler, R. C. (2007). The prevalence and correlates of eating disorders in the National Comorbidity Survey Replication. *Biological Psychiatry*, 61(3), 348–358.

Hughes, T. L. (2011). Alcohol use and alcohol-related problems among sexual minority women. *Alcoholism Treatment Quarterly*, 29(4), 403–435.

Hughes, T.L., Szalacha, L.A., & McNair, R. (2010). Substance abuse and mental health disparities: Comparisons across sexual identity groups in a national sample of young Australian women. *Social Science and Medicine*, 71(4), 824–831.

Hughes, T. L., Wilsnack, S. C., Szalacha, L. A., Johnson, T., Bostwick, W. B., Seymour, R., . . . & Kinnison, K. E. (2006). Age and racial/ethnic differences in drinking and drinking-related problems in a community sample of lesbians. *Journal of Studies on Alcohol and Drugs*, 67(4), 579–590.

Hyde, Z., Comfort, J., McManus, A., Brown, G., & Howat, P. (2009). Alcohol, tobacco and illicit drug use amongst same-sex attracted women: Results from the Western Australian Lesbian and Bisexual Women's Health and Well-Being Survey. *BMC Public Health*, 9(1), 317.

Institute of Medicine. (2011). *The health of lesbian, gay, bisexual, and transgender people: Building a foundation for better understanding*. Washington, DC: National Academy Press.

Jones, H. E. (2004). Practical considerations for the clinical use of buprenorphine. *Science and Practice Perspectives*, 2(2), 4–20.

Jones, H. E., Kaltenbach, K., Heil, S. H., Stine, S. M., Coyle, M. G., Arria, A. M., . . . & Fischer, G. (2010). Neonatal abstinence syndrome after methadone or buprenorphine exposure. *New England Journal of Medicine*, 363(24), 2320–2331.

Kaskutas, L. A. (1994). What do women get out of self-help? Their reasons for attending Women for Sobriety and Alcoholics Anonymous. *Journal of Substance Abuse Treatment*, 11(3), 185–195.

Kay, A., Taylor, T. E., Barthwell, A. G., Wichelecki, J., & Leopold, V. (2010). Substance use and women's health. *Journal of Addictive Diseases*, 29(2), 139–163.

Kelly, J. F., & Hoeppner, B. B. (2013). Does Alcoholics Anonymous work differently for men and women? A moderated multiple-mediation analysis in a large clinical sample. *Drug and Alcohol Dependence*, 130(1), 186–193.

Kelly, J. F., Hoeppner, B., Stout, R. L., & Pagano, M. (2012). Determining the relative importance of the mechanisms of behavior change within Alcoholics Anonymous: A multiple mediator analysis. *Addiction*, 107(2), 289–299.

Kerr, D., Ding, K., Burke, A., & Ott-Walter, K. (2015). An alcohol, tobacco, and other drug use comparison of lesbian, bisexual, and heterosexual undergraduate women. *Substance Use and Misuse*, 50(3), 340–349. http://doi.org/10.3109/10826084.2014.980954.

Keyes, K. M., Martins, S. S., Blanco, C., & Hasin, D. S. (2010). Telescoping and gender differences in alcohol dependence: New evidence from two national surveys. *American Journal of Psychiatry*, 167(8), 969–976.

Khan, S., Okuda, M., Hasin, D. S., Secades-Villa, R., Keyes, K., Lin, K., . . . & Blanco, C. (2013). Gender differences in lifetime alcohol dependence: Results from the national epidemiologic survey on alcohol and related conditions. *Alcoholism: Clinical and Experimental Research*, 37(10), 1696–1705.

Khantzian, E. J. (1985). The self-medication hypothesis of addictive disorders: Focus on heroin and cocaine dependence. *American Journal of Psychiatry*, 142(11), 1259–1264.

Killeen, T., Brewerton, T. D., Campbell, A., Cohen, L. R., & Hien, D. A. (2015). Exploring the relationship between eating disorder symptoms and substance use severity in women with comorbid PTSD and substance use disorders. *American Journal of Drug and Alcohol Abuse*, 41(6), 547–552.

Kim, H.-J., & Fredriksen-Goldsen, K. I. (2012). Hispanic lesbians and bisexual women at heightened risk or health disparities. *American Journal of Public Health*, 102(1), e9–e15. http://doi.org/10.2105/AJPH.2011.300378.

Kuhn, C. (2015). Emergence of sex differences in the development of substance use and abuse during adolescence. *Pharmacology and Therapeutics*, 153, 55–78.

Lal, R., Deb, K. S., & Kedia, S. (2015). Substance use in women: Current status and future directions. *Indian Journal of Psychiatry*, 57(Suppl 2), S275.

Lazareck, S., Robinson, J. A., Crum, R. M., Mojtabai, R., Sareen, J., & Bolton, J. M. (2012). A longitudinal investigation of the role of self-medication in the development of comorbid mood and drug use disorders: findings from the National Epidemiologic Survey on Alcohol and Related Conditions (NESARC). *Journal of Clinical Psychiatry*, 73(5), 1–478.

Lehavot, K., & Simoni, J. M. (2011). The impact of minority stress on mental health and substance use among sexual minority women. *Journal of Consulting and Clinical Psychology, 79*(2), 159.

Lembke, A. (2012). Time to abandon the self-medication hypothesis in patients with psychiatric disorders. *American Journal of Drug and Alcohol Abuse, 38*(6), 524–529.

Lewis, C. (2006). Treating incarcerated women: gender matters. *Psychiatric Clinics of North America, 29*(3), 773–789.

Lynch, W. J., Roth, M. E., & Carroll, M. E. (2002). Biological basis of sex differences in drug abuse: preclinical and clinical studies. *Psychopharmacology, 164*(2), 121–137.

McCabe, S. E., Bostwick, W. B., Hughes, T. L., West, B. T., & Boyd, C. J. (2010). The relationship between discrimination and substance use disorders among lesbian, gay, and bisexual adults in the United States. *American Journal of Public Health, 100*(10), 1946–1952.

McCabe, S. E., Boyd, C., Hughes, T. L., & d'Arcy, H. (2003). Sexual identity and substance use among undergraduate students. *Substance Abuse, 24*(2), 77–91.

MacCarthy, S., Reisner, S. L., Nunn, A., Perez-Brumer, A., & Operario, D. (2015). The time is now: Attention increases for transgender health in the United States but scientific knowledge gaps remain. *LGBT Health, 2*(4), 287–291.

McCauley, J. L., Killeen, T., Gros, D. F., Brady, K. T., & Back, S. E. (2012). Posttraumatic stress disorder and co-occurring substance use disorders: Advances in assessment and treatment. *Clinical Psychology: Science and Practice, 19*(3), 283–304.

Marlatt, G. A., & Donovan, D. M. (2005). *Relapse prevention: Maintenance strategies in the treatment of addictive behaviors.* New York: Guilford Press.

Martin, F. S., & Aston, S. (2014). A "special population" with "unique treatment needs": dominant representations of "women's substance abuse" and their effects. *Contemporary Drug Problems, 41*(3), 335–360.

Mason, B. J., & Lehert, P. (2012). Acamprosate for alcohol dependence: A sex-specific meta-analysis based on individual patient data. *Alcoholism: Clinical and Experimental Research, 36*(3), 497–508.

Matheson, J. L., & McCollum, E. E. (2008). Using metaphors to explore the experiences of powerlessness among women in 12-step recovery. *Substance Use and Misuse, 43*(8–9), 1027–1044.

Matthews, C. R., Lorah, P., & Fenton, J. (2005). Toward a grounded theory of lesbians' recovery from addiction. *Journal of Lesbian Studies, 9*(3), 57–68.

Meyer, I. H. (2003). Prejudice, social stress, and mental health in lesbian, gay, and bisexual populations: Conceptual issues and research evidence. *Psychological Bulletin, 129*(5), 674.

Morgan-Lopez, A. A., Saavedra, L. M., Hien, D. A., Campbell, A. N., Wu, E., & Ruglass, L. (2013). Synergy between seeking safety and twelve-step affiliation on substance use outcomes for women. *Journal of Substance Abuse Treatment, 45*(2), 179–189.

National Center on Addiction and Substance Abuse at Columbia University (CASA). (2003). *Food for thought: Substance abuse and eating disorders.* Retrieved from http://www.casacolumbia. org/templates/ Publications_Reports.aspx (accessed May 31, 2016).

National Institutes of Health. (1994, March 18). *NIH guidelines on the inclusion of women and minorities as subjects in clinical research.* Retrieved from http://grants.nih.gov/grants/guide/ notice-files/not94-100.html (accessed April 25, 2016).

National Institutes of Health. (2014, October 20). *Office of Research on Women's Health: Methods and techniques for integrating the biological variable sex into preclinical research.* Retrieved from http://orwh.od.nih.gov/sexinscience/researchtrainingresources/pdf/ORWH_Methods_ Workshop_Mtg_Smry_3-3-15.pdf (accessed April 25, 2016).

National Institutes of Health. (2016). *NIH FY 2016-2020 strategic plan to advance research on the health and well-being of sexual and gender minorities.* Retrieved from https://dpcpsi.nih.gov/ sites/default/files/sgmStrategicPlan.pdf (accessed April 25, 2016).

Ondersma, S. J., Beatty, J. R., Svikis, D. S., Strickler, R. C., Tzilos, G. K., Chang, G., . . . & Sokol, R. J. (2015). Computer-delivered screening and brief intervention for alcohol use in pregnancy: A pilot randomized trial. *Alcoholism: Clinical and Experimental Research, 39*(7), 1219–1226.

Orwin, R., Francisco, L., & Bernichon, T. (2001). *Effectiveness of women's substance abuse treatment programs: A meta-analysis.* Fairfax, VA: Center for Substance Abuse Treatment.

Parsons, J. T., Kelly, B. C., & Wells, B. E. (2006). Differences in club drug use between heterosexual and lesbian/bisexual females. *Addictive Behaviors, 31*(12), 2344.

Petry, N. M. (2010). Contingency management treatments: controversies and challenges. *Addiction, 105*(9), 1507–1509.

Pietrzak, R. H., Goldstein, R. B., Southwick, S. M., & Grant, B. F. (2011). Prevalence and Axis I comorbidity of full and partial posttraumatic stress disorder in the United States: Results from

Wave 2 of the National Epidemiologic Survey on Alcohol and Related Conditions. *Journal of Anxiety Disorders, 25*(3), 456–465.

Reisner, S. L., White, J. M., Bradford, J. B., & Mimiaga, M. J. (2014). Transgender health disparities: Comparing full cohort and nested matched-pair study designs in a community health center. *LGBT Health, 1*(3), 177–184.

Rollnick, S., & Miller, W. R. (1995). What is motivational interviewing? *Behavioural and Cognitive Psychotherapy, 23*(4), 325–334.

Rosario, M., Schrimshaw, E. W., & Hunter, J. (2008). Butch/femme differences in substance use and abuse among young lesbian and bisexual women: Examination and potential explanations. *Substance Use and Misuse, 43*(8–9), 1002–1015. http://doi.org/10.1080/10826080801914402.

Rowe, C., Santos, G.-M., McFarland, M., & Wilson, E. C. (2015). Prevalence and correlates of substance use among trans* female youth ages 16–24 years in the San Francisco Bay Area. *Drug and Alcohol Dependence, 147*, 160–166.

Ruglass, L. M., Hien, D. A., Hu, M., & Campbell, A. N. (2014). Associations between posttraumatic stress symptoms, stimulant use, and treatment outcomes: A secondary analysis of NIDA's women and trauma study. *American Journal on Addictions, 23*(1), 90–95.

SAMHSA. (2007). *Results from the 2006 National Survey on Drug Use and Health: National findings.* Office of Applied Studies, NSDUH Series H-32, DHHS Publication No. SMA 07-4293. Rockville, MD: Substance Abuse and Mental Health Services Administration.

SAMHSA. (2009). *Substance abuse treatment: Addressing the specific needs of women.* Treatment Improvement Protocol (TIP), HHS publication no. (SMA) 15-4426. Rockville, MD: Substance Abuse and Mental Health Services Administration.

SAMHSA. (2014a). *National Survey of Substance Abuse Treatment Services (N-SSATS): 2013. Data on substance abuse treatment facilities.* BHSIS series S-73, HHS publication no. (SMA) 14-4890. Rockville, MD: Substance Abuse and Mental Health Services Administration.

SAMHSA. (2014b). *Results from the 2012 National Survey on Drug Use and Health: Summary of national findings.* NSDUH series H-46, HHS publication no. (SMA) 13-4795. Rockville, MD: Substance Abuse and Mental Health Services Administration.

SAMHSA. (2015a). *Results from the 2013 National Survey on Drug Use and Health: Summary of national findings.* NSDUH series H-48, HHS publication no.(SMA) 14-4863. Rockville, MD: Substance Abuse and Mental Health Services Administration.

SAMHSA. (2015b, September 10). *Results from the 2014 National Survey on Drug Use and Health: Detailed tables.* Retrieved from http://www.samhsa.gov/data/sites/default/files/NSDUH-DetTabs2014/NSDUH-DetTabs2014.pdf (accessed November 4, 2016).

Sanders, J. M. (2006). Women and the twelve steps of Alcoholics Anonymous: A gendered narrative. *Alcoholism Treatment Quarterly, 24*(3), 3–29.

Schindler, S. D., Eder, H., Ortner, R., Rohrmeister, K., Langer, M., & Fischer, G. (2003). Neonatal outcome following buprenorphine maintenance during conception and throughout pregnancy. *Addiction, 98*(1), 103–110.

Schliep, K. C., Zarek, S. M., Schisterman, E. F., Wactawski-Wende, J., Trevisan, M., Sjaarda, L. A., ... & Mumford, S. L. (2015). Alcohol intake, reproductive hormones, and menstrual cycle function: A prospective cohort study. *American Journal of Clinical Nutrition, 102*(4), 933–942.

Sered, S., & Norton-Hawk, M. (2011). Whose higher power? Criminalized women confront the "twelve steps." *Feminist Criminology, 6*(4), 308–332.

Smedslund, G., Berg, R. C., Hammerstrom, K. T., Steiro, A., Leiknes, K. A., Dahl, H. M., & Karlsen, K. (2011). Motivational interviewing for substance abuse. *Cochrane Database of Systematic Reviews, 5*(5).

Smith, J., Meyers, R., & Miller, W. (2001). The community reinforcement approach to the treatment of substance use disorders. *American Journal on Addictions, 10*(s1), s51–s59.

Soyka, M. (2013). Buprenorphine use in pregnant opioid users: A critical review. *CNS Drugs, 27*(8), 653–662.

Susukida, R., Crum, R. M., Stuart, E. A., Ebnesajjad, C., & Mojtabai, R. (2016). Assessing sample representativeness in randomized controlled trials: Application to the National Institute of Drug Abuse Clinical Trials Network. *Addiction, 111*, 1226–1234.

Tan, C. H., Denny, C. H., Cheal, N. E., Sniezek, J. E., & Kanny, D. (2015). Alcohol use and binge drinking among women of childbearing age – United States, 2011–2013. *MMWR: Morbidity and Mortality Weekly Report, 64*(37), 1042–1046.

Terner, J. M., & De Wit, H. (2006). Menstrual cycle phase and responses to drugs of abuse in humans. *Drug and Alcohol Dependence, 84*(1), 1–13.

Terplan, M., Longinaker, N., & Appel, L. (2015). Women-centered drug treatment services and need in the United States, 2002–2009. *American Journal of Public Health, 105*(11), e50–e54.

Tripodi, S. J., & Pettus-Davis, C. (2013). Histories of childhood victimization and subsequent mental health problems, substance use, and sexual victimization for a sample of incarcerated women in the US. *International Journal of Law and Psychiatry, 36*(1), 30–40.

Unger, A., Jung, E., Winklbaur, B., & Fischer, G. (2010). Gender issues in the pharmacotherapy of opioid-addicted women: Buprenorphine. *Journal of Addictive Diseases, 29*(2), 217–230.

Unger, A., Metz, V., & Fischer, G. (2012). Opioid dependent and pregnant: What are the best options for mothers and neonates? *Obstetrics and Gynecology International, 2012,* 195954.

van Dam, D., Vedel, E., Ehring, T., & Emmelkamp, P. M. (2012). Psychological treatments for concurrent posttraumatic stress disorder and substance use disorder: A systematic review. *Clinical Psychology Review, 32*(3), 202–214.

Van Der Walde, H., Urgenson, F. T., Weltz, S. H., & Hanna, F. J. (2002). Women and alcoholism: A biopsychosocial perspective and treatment approaches. *Journal of Counseling and Development: JCD, 80*(2), 145.

Voyer, P., Préville, M., Roussel, M.-E., Berbiche, D., & Béland, S.-G. (2009). Factors associated with benzodiazepine dependence among community-dwelling seniors. *Journal of Community Health Nursing, 26*(3), 101–113.

Wang, Y.-P., & Andrade, L. H. (2013). Epidemiology of alcohol and drug use in the elderly. *Current Opinion in Psychiatry, 26*(4), 343–348.

Warren, C. S., Lindsay, A. R., White, E. K., Claudat, K., & Velasquez, S. C. (2013). Weight-related concerns related to drug use for women in substance abuse treatment: Prevalence and relationships with eating pathology. *Journal of Substance Abuse Treatment, 44*(5), 494–501.

Wills, T. A., & Hirky, A. E. (1996). Coping and substance abuse: A theoretical model and review of the evidence. In M. Zeichn & N. S. Eudler (Eds.), *Handbook of coping: Theory, research, and applications* (pp. 279–302). New York: Wiley.

Wills, T. A., & Shiffman, S. (1985). Coping and substance use: A conceptual framework. *Coping and Substance Use,* 3–24.

Wilsnack, S. C., Hughes, T. L., Johnson, T. P., Bostwick, W. B., Szalacha, L. A., Benson, P., . . . & Kinnison, K. E. (2008). Drinking and drinking-related problems among heterosexual and sexual minority women. *Journal of Studies on Alcohol and Drugs, 69*(1), 129.

Witbrodt, J., Ye, Y., Bond, J., Chi, F., Weisner, C., & Mertens, J. (2014). Alcohol and drug treatment involvement, 12-step attendance and abstinence: 9-year cross-lagged analysis of adults in an integrated health plan. *Journal of Substance Abuse Treatment, 46*(4), 412–419.

Wu, L.-T., & Blazer, D. G. (2011). Illicit and nonmedical drug use among older adults: A review. *Journal of Aging and Health, 23*(3), 481–504.

Index

Printed in the United States
by Baker & Taylor Publisher Services